# Handbook of
# Lower Extremity
# Neurology

## Steven Mandel, MD

Clinical Professor of Neurology
Jefferson Medical College of Thomas Jefferson University
Adjunct Clinical Professor
Temple University School of Podiatric Medicine
Philadelphia, Pennsylvania

## Jeanean Willis, DPM

Assistant Clinical Professor
Electrodiagnostic Laboratory
Temple University School of Podiatric Medicine
Philadelphia, Pennsylvania

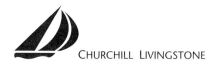

CHURCHILL LIVINGSTONE

A Division of Harcourt Brace & Company
New York, Edinburgh, London, Philadelphia, San Francisco

**CHURCHILL LIVINGSTONE**
*A Division of Harcourt Brace & Company*

The Curtis Center
Independence Square West
Philadelphia, Pennsylvania 19106

**Library of Congress Cataloging-in-Publication Data**

Handbook of lower extremity neurology / [edited by] Steven Mandel,
Jeanean Willis. —1st ed.

p.    cm.

ISBN 0–443–07548–4

1. Nerves, Peripheral—Diseases—Handbooks, manuals, etc. 2. Leg—Diseases—
Handbooks, manuals, etc. 3. Neurologic manifestations of general diseases—
Handbooks, manuals, etc. I. Mandel, Steven. II. Willis, Jeanean. [DNLM:
1. Nervous System Diseases. 2. Leg. WE 850 H236 2000]

RC409.H36  2000  616.8'7—dc21

DNLM/DLC                                                          98-53549

HANDBOOK OF LOWER EXTREMITY NEUROLOGY                    ISBN 0–443–07548–4

Printed in the United States of America.

Last digit is the print number:    9    8    7    6    5    4    3    2    1

*This book is dedicated to my best friend, my wife Heidi,
without whose support and encouragement
this book could never have been written*

*and*

*To my three children, Jesse, Elisabeth, and David,
each special and wonderful in his or her own way.*

**S.M.**

# Contributors

**Todd J. Albert, MD**
Associate Professor of Orthopedic Surgery,
Jefferson Medical College of Thomas Jefferson
University, Philadelphia, Pennsylvania
*Evaluation of Back Pain*

**Robert D. Aiken, MD**
Associate Professor of Neurology, Jefferson Medical
College of Thomas Jefferson University; Attending
Neurologist, Thomas Jefferson University Hospital,
Philadelphia, Pennsylvania
*Paraneoplastic Syndromes*

**Ernest M. Baran, MD, MSBME**
Associate Professor, Department of Rehabilitation
Medicine, Jefferson Medical College of Thomas
Jefferson University, Philadelphia; Medical
Director, Physical Medicine and Rehabilitation,
Nazareth Hospital, Philadelphia; Medical Director,
Lafayette Hill Medical Center, Lafayette Hill,
Pennsylvania
*Rehabilitation: The Lower Extremity and Neurologic
Impairment*

**John M. Barbes, MA, PT, OCS**
Clinical Assistant Professor, Jefferson Medical
College of Thomas Jefferson University,
Philadelphia, Pennsylvania
*Physical Therapy in the Treatment of Lower Extremity
Pain and Impairment*

**Rodney Bell, MD**
Clinical Professor of Neurology, Jefferson Medical
College of Thomas Jefferson University; Chief,
Division of Cerebrovascular Disease, Neurocritical
Care, Thomas Jefferson University Hospital,
Philadelphia, Pennsylvania
*The Lower Extremity in Vascular Disease*

**Richard H. Bennett, MD**
Assistant Clinical Professor of Neurology,
University of Pennsylvania School of Medicine,
Philadelphia, Pennsylvania
*Myopathies*

**Lawrence W. Brown, MD**
Assistant Professor of Neurology and Pediatrics,
University of Pennsylvania School of Medicine,
Philadelphia; Division of Neurology, Children's
Hospital of Philadelphia, Philadelphia,
Pennsylvania
*Pediatric Disorders*

**Richard W. Bunch, PhD, PT**
Clinical Associate Professor, Department of
Cardiopulmonary Science, Louisiana State
University Medical Center, School of Allied Health
Professions, New Orleans, Louisiana
*AMA Guide to Functional Capacity Evaluation*

**Melissa Carran, MD**
Fellow, Jefferson Comprehensive Epilepsy Center,
Thomas Jefferson University Hospital,
Philadelphia, Pennsylvania
*Localization of Neurologic Lesions*

**Edward L. Chairman, DPM**
Active Staff, Graduate Hospital, Philadelphia,
Pennsylvania
*Special Orthopedic Problems*

**Judy Rae Churchill, PhD**
Assistant Professor, Department of Arts and
Sciences Drexel/MCP ◆ Hahnemann School of
Medicine, Philadelphia, Pennsylvania
*Neuroanatomy of the Lower Extremity*

**Mitchell J. M. Cohen, MD**
Clinical Associate Professor, Psychiatry and
Human Behavior, Jefferson Medical College of
Thomas Jefferson University, Philadelphia,
Pennsylvania
*Chronic Pain in the Lower Extremity*

**Timothy Dougherty, MD**
Assistant Professor of Emergency Medicine,
Drexel/MCP ◆ Hahnemann School of Medicine,
Philadelphia, Pennsylvania
*Toxins Producing Clinical Effects Manifested in the
Lower Extremity*

**Michael S. Downey, DPM, FACFAS**
Professor and Immediate Past Chairman,
Department of Surgery, Temple University School
of Podiatric Medicine, Philadelphia; Chief,
Division of Podiatric Surgery and Medicine,
Department of Orthopedics, Presbyterian Medical
Center of the University of Pennsylvania Health
System, Philadelphia, Pennsylvania
*Nerve Injuries in the Lower Extremity*

**Bruce Freundlich, MD**
Clinical Associate Professor, University of
Pennsylvania School of Medicine, Philadelphia;
Medical Director, Mid-Atlantic, Merck & Co., Inc.,
West Point, Pennsylvania
*Neurologic Manifestations of Rheumatologic Diseases*

**Vincenzo Giuliano, MD**
Fellow, Department of Radiology, Thomas Jefferson
University Hospital, Philadelphia, Pennsylvania
*Neurologic Imaging of the Lower Extremity*

**Alan S. Gold, JD**
Attorney, Monaghan & Gold P.C., Elkins Park,
Pennsylvania
*Impact of the Americans with Disabilities Act on
Neurologic Impairments of the Lower Extremities*

**Stephen M. Gollomp, MD**
Clinical Associate Professor of Neurology, Jefferson
Medical College of Thomas Jefferson University,
Philadelphia, Pennsylvania
*Movement Disorders of the Lower Extremities*

**Michael I. Greenberg, MD, MPH**
Professor of Emergency Medicine, Toxicology
Fellowship Program Director, Drexel/MCP ♦
Hahnemann School of Medicine, Philadelphia;
Attending Toxicologist, Mercy Catholic Medical
Center, Philadelphia, Pennsylvania
*Toxins Producing Clinical Effects Manifested in the
Lower Extremity*

**Tucker Greene, MD**
Assistant Professor of Emergency Medicine,
Drexel/MCP ♦ Hahnemann School of Medicine,
Philadelphia, Pennsylvania
*Toxins Producing Clinical Effects Manifested in the
Lower Extremity*

**Steffi Hamarman, MD**
Fellow, Department of Neurology, Thomas Jefferson
University Hospital, Philadelphia, Pennsylvania
*Cutaneous Manifestations of Neurologic Diseases in
the Lower Extremity*

**Terry Heiman-Patterson, MD**
Professor of Neurology and Director, Division of
Neuromuscular Diseases, Drexel/MCP ♦
Hahnemann School of Medicine, Philadelphia,
Pennsylvania
*Acute Neuromuscular Weakness of the Lower
Extremity*

**Mark B. Kahn, MD**
Associate Professor of Surgery, Division of Vascular
Surgery, Jefferson Medical College of Thomas
Jefferson University, Philadelphia, Pennsylvania
*The Lower Extremity in Vascular Disease*

**Brian K. Kelly, MD**
Instructor of Neurology, Jefferson Medical College
of Thomas Jefferson University, Philadelphia,
Pennsylvania
*Clinical Neurogenetics*

**Robert L. Knobler, MD, PhD**
Professor of Neurology, Jefferson Medical College
of Thomas Jefferson University, Philadelphia,
Pennsylvania
*Reflex Sympathetic Dystrophy: Complex Regional
Pain Syndrome, Type 1*

**Peterkin Lee-Kwen, MD**
Clinical Assistant Professor of Neurology, State
University of New York at Buffalo, Buffalo;
Department of Neurology, Buffalo General Hospital,
Buffalo, New York
*Neurologic Examination of the Lower Extremity*

**Lawrence J. Leventhal, MD, FACP, FACR**
Associate Professor of Medicine, Drexel/MCP ♦
Hahnemann School of Medicine, Philadelphia;
Chief of Rheumatology, The Graduate Hospital,
Philadelphia, Pennsylvania
*Neurologic Manifestations of Rheumatologic Diseases*

**R. Mañon-Espaillat, MD**
Clinical Professor of Neurology, Jefferson Medical
College of Thomas Jefferson University,
Philadelphia, Pennsylvania
*Localization of Neurologic Lesions*

**Leo McCluskey, MD**
Assistant Professor of Neurology, University of
Pennsylvania School of Medicine, Philadelphia,
Pennsylvania
*Gait Disorders; Polyneuropathy*

**Jeffrey L. Miller, MD**
Clinical Professor of Endocrinology, Jefferson
Medical College of Thomas Jefferson University,
Philadelphia, Pennsylvania
*Metabolic and Endocrine Disorders*

**Patrick Pullicino, MD, PhD**
Professor of Neurology, State University of New
York at Buffalo; Department of Neurology, Buffalo
General Hospital, Buffalo, New York
*Neurologic Examination of the Lower Extremity*

**Marie Sambor Reilly, JD**
Attorney, Mark J. Hill & Associates, Philadelphia,
Pennsylvania
*Impact of the Americans with Disabilities Act on
Neurologic Impairments of the Lower Extremities*

**Abdolmohamad Rostami, MD, PhD**
Professor of Neurology and Director,
Neuroimmunology Section, University of
Pennsylvania School of Medicine, Philadelphia,
Pennsylvania
*Neuroimmunology*

**Scott A. Rushton, MD**
Clinical Professor of Orthopedic Surgery, Jefferson
Medical College of Thomas Jefferson University,
Philadelphia, Pennsylvania
*Evaluation of Back Pain*

**Richard A. Sater, MD, PhD**
Fellow in Neuroimmunology and Instructor in
Neurology, Department of Neurology, University of
Pennsylvania School of Medicine, Philadelphia,
Pennsylvania
*Neuroimmunology*

**Harold Schoenhaus, DPM**
Professor, Temple School of Podiatric Medicine,
Philadelphia; Chief, Podiatric Surgery, Graduate
Hospital, Philadelphia, Pennsylvania
*Entrapment Neuropathy*

**Mark E. Schweitzer, MD**
Professor of Radiology, Thomas Jefferson
University School of Medicine, Philadelphia,
Pennsylvania
*Neurologic Imaging of the Lower Extremity*

**David J. Secord, DPM**
Active Staff, St. Paul Hospital, Dallas, Texas
*Special Orthopedic Problems*

**Paul Shneidman, MD**
Assistant Professor of Neurology, Jefferson Medical
College of Thomas Jefferson University,
Philadelphia, Pennsylania
*Cutaneous Manifestations of Neurologic Diseases in
the Lower Extremity*

**Leopold J. Streletz, MD**
Professor in Neurology and Director, Clinical
Neurophysiology Residency, Department of
Neurology, Jefferson Medical College of Thomas
Jefferson University, Philadelphia, Pennsylvania;
Wilmington Veterans Administration Hospital,
Wilmington, Delaware
*Somatosensory Evoked Potentials in the Lower
Extremity*

**Russell J. Stumacher, MD, FACP**
Associate Professor of Medicine, Drexel/MCP ◆
Hahnemann School of Medicine, Philadelphia;
Director, Infectious Disease Unit, Graduate
Hospital, Philadelphia, Pennsylvania
*Infections of the Lower Extremity*

**Bruce Vanett, MD**
CoChief of Orthopedic Surgery, Mercy Community
Hospital, Haverford, Pennsylvania
*Soft Tissue Injuries of the Lower Extremity*

**Lubna M. Zuberi, MD**
Fellow, Department of Endocrinology, Thomas
Jefferson University Hospital, Philadelphia,
Pennsylvania
*Metabolic and Endocrine Disorders*

# Preface

Lower extremity complaints may be a presenting sign of a primary neurologic disorder but also can be the first sign of a more systemic disease. As part of the neurologic examination, functional testing, for example, watching someone walk or get on and off an examination table, provides invaluable information often difficult to assess when someone is lying on a bed or sitting on an examination table. Genetic testing allows us to identify the etiology of neuromuscular diseases and aids in looking at the natural history to guide us in medical management. Although there have been advances in the field of diabetes and vascular surgical techniques, neuropathies are prevalent that can produce significant impairments leading to disability, affecting a person's work, leisure, and activities of daily living.

Much has been done in the area of upper extremity disorders; however, not enough attention has been paid to lower extremity disorders other than those associated with back pain syndromes. Fortunately, the medical community is changing its focus. Orthopedic departments in medical schools are setting up specialty clinics in foot and ankle surgery. In the podiatric community, gait laboratories and preventive care programs such as diabetic foot clinics have been developed and expanded. Over the last ten years, my group, which includes Doctors Ramon Mañon-Espaillat and Brian Kelly, has taught the third year neurology curriculum at the Pennsylvania College of Podiatric Medicine. We have also acted as consultants to the Foot and Ankle Institute of the Pennsylvania College of Podiatric Medicine.

Approximately two years ago, Dr. Jeanean Willis suggested the preparation of a guide for the identification, workup, and management of lower extremity problems. Experts throughout the country were contacted and asked to list disorders frequently encountered in their various subspecialties that may often be first recognized by the primary care physician. Dr. Willis and I have identified several major disorders and selected what we believe are of primary interest to the podiatric community and general medical community.

This textbook, therefore, is presented as a reference manual for practicing physicians, students, and other healthcare personnel. Each chapter has been organized in the form of symptoms, physical findings, diagnostic studies, differential diagnosis, and initial course of medical management. We hope that we have accomplished our preliminary goals and that future editions will cover more areas in response to the needs of the medical community in improving patient care through the prompt and efficient diagnosing and treating of lower extremity neurologic disorders.

No major endeavor is undertaken and achieved without significant behind-the-scenes team members. Special thanks go to Lena Rabutino for the many hours of contacting contributing authors, organizing chapters, making sure deadlines were met, and working with Dr. Willis and myself to complete this book. A sincere thank you also goes to my medical transcriptionist, Anne Connors, who has been with me for 11 years and has prepared all of my papers for presentation and publication as well as daily reports.

STEVEN MANDEL

# Contents

# Neuroanatomy of the Lower Extremity

1

*Judy Rae Churchill*

## NEURONS AND THEIR SUPPORTING CELLS

Neurons are the basic functional units of the nervous system and as such are highly diverse in their shape, neurochemistry, and ultimate function. This diversity of neuronal cell form and function underlies the ability of the nervous system as a whole to integrate sensory input and centrally determined goals into coherent and appropriate motor responses. Even though neurons demonstrate the greatest amount of variation in shape of any tissue in the body, most have the same basic pattern of cytoplasmic processes specialized for local or distant signaling, the dendrites and axons, respectively, and a trophic region, the perikaryon, that bears the neuron's nucleus. Neurons communicate with each other and with effector cells, such as glandular and muscle cells, by means of electrical and chemical synapses. A variety of different neurotransmitter substances are released at different synaptic locations, enabling investigators in some cases to characterize pathways and central nervous system (CNS) regions by the neurotransmitter used.

Local and distant electrical signaling along axons involves a transient traveling wave of depolarization and repolarization of the axonal plasma membrane resulting from the movement of $Na^+$ and $K^+$ ions across the membrane. This ion movement is mediated by the activation and inactivation of specialized channel proteins within the axon's plasma membrane. This is the action potential or electrical impulse. It is a stereotyped response with a constant amplitude. Intensity of stimulation is reflected not in a change of action potential amplitude but in the frequency of generation of action potentials. The axon potential is generated at the site of origin of the axon from the cell body in most neurons or adjacent to the receptor ending in sensory axons.

When an action potential reaches the axon terminal at a chemical synapse, the change in electrical potential in the membrane of the presynaptic ending results in an influx of $Ca^{2+}$ ions and the release of neurotransmitter substances from the presynaptic ending. Neurotransmitter chemicals are released into the extracellular space between the pre- and postsynaptic elements. The neurotransmitter substances interact with receptor proteins in the postsynaptic membrane and cause a small change of variable magnitude in the membrane potential in the postsynaptic cell. This change can be stimulatory or inhibitory to the postsynaptic cell, depending on whether it is depolarizing or hyperpolarizing, respectively. The postsynaptic potential is not propagated from its site of origin; instead, the summation of postsynaptic potentials in both time and space determines whether the axon of the postsynaptic cell reaches its threshold and is excited to generate its own action potential.

Because of the special environmental needs of neurons, especially the need for a constant chemical and ionic extracellular environment, neurons have their own supporting tissue, the neuroglia. In the CNS the space between neurons is filled with glial cells and their processes with little room left for extracellular fluid. Astrocytes and ependymal cells function to maintain a constant ionic and chemical extracellular environment, and oligodendrocytes form the myelin sheaths found around certain axons in the CNS. In the peripheral nervous system (PNS), Schwann cells form myelin around certain axons. The myelin covering in both the CNS and the PNS is formed by multiple wrappings of the glial cell's plasma membrane around the axon. This lipid-rich sheath functions to increase the speed of conduction of electrical impulses along the axon. Unmyelinated axons in the CNS lack an oligodendrocyte covering but are invested with astrocytic processes or are exposed to the extracellular fluid. Unmyelinated axons in the PNS are also invested by the plasma membrane of Schwann cells, but the neuroglial cell does not form multiple wrappings in this case. Unmyelinated axons are thinner and conduct more slowly than myelinated axons.

## PERIPHERAL NERVOUS SYSTEM

The PNS connects the CNS to sensory receptors and to effectors such as muscle or gland cells. It is formed by primary sensory and motor neurons, respectively. These are large neurons with axons long enough to reach from the body region that is innervated to the dorsal root ganglia (located in intervertebral foramina) or spinal cord gray matter. For the lower extremity this is an axonal distance of a foot or more.

The primary sensory or first-order neurons of the somatosensory system either terminate as free endings or are involved in more elaborate structures to form encapsulated receptors. The muscle spindle, Golgi's tendon organ, and the corpuscles of Ruffini and Pacini are all encapsulated mechanoreceptors. Cutaneous touch receptors such as the tactile disks associated with specialized cells of the epidermis or the peritrichal endings around hair bulbs are special forms of free endings. The activation of each of these receptors results in a train of action potentials that travel along the sensory axon from the receptor, past the neuron's cell body located in the dorsal root ganglia (spinal ganglia), and along the central limb of the axon to enter into the spinal cord, where synaptic contacts are made with spinal cord neurons. Ganglia for the sensory innervation of the lower extremity are found within the intervertebral foramina associated with vertebral levels L2 through S3. The central limbs of the first-order sensory neurons form the dorsal roots of the cauda equina.

The final common pathway for skeletal muscle innervation is the large alpha motor neuron of the spinal cord ventral gray matter. These neurons give rise to a series of ventral roots (also part of the cauda equina) arising from spinal levels L2 through S3 for the innervation of the lower extremity. Each alpha motor neuron gives rise to a single axon that later branches to innervate several skeletal muscle fibers within the target muscle. This is a motor unit and is the basic unit for the production of motor activity because all muscle fibers of a single motor unit are activated together. Muscles involved in skilled activities have smaller numbers of muscle fibers in each motor unit, and muscles such as the gastrocnemius have large motor units.

Accompanying the axons of the alpha motor neurons within the ventral roots and peripheral nerves are the axons of smaller gamma motor neurons. The gamma motor neurons innervate specialized small skeletal muscle cells located within the connective tissue capsule of muscle spindles. Muscle spindles are complex encapsulated stretch receptors located within the perimysia of the muscle belly. They function as proprioceptors to inform the nervous system about changes in muscle length.

Within the intervertebral foramen just distal to the sensory ganglion, the dorsal root and the ventral root unite to form a mixed spinal nerve. The mixed nerve almost immediately divides into ventral and dorsal primary rami. The ventral primary rami from

**Table 1–1  Major Nerves Providing the Cutaneous Innervation for the Lower Extremity**

| Peripheral Nerve | Area of Cutaneous Distribution |
| --- | --- |
| Femoral | Anterior thigh and medial leg including the medial malleolus |
| Sciatic | Posterior thigh, popliteal fossa, part of posterior leg below the knee |
| Superficial peroneal | Lateral leg, lateral malleolus, and part of dorsum of foot |
| Deep peroneal | First interspace between digits 1 and 2 |
| Tibial | Posterior leg and heel |
| Medial and lateral plantar | Sole of foot |

spinal segments L2 through L4 form the lumbar plexus, and those from L4 through S3 form the sacral plexus. Named peripheral nerves arise from each plexus and are involved in the innervation of the lower extremity. The femoral and obturator nerves arise from the lumbar plexus; the sciatic and its branches, the peroneal and tibial nerves, arise from the sacral plexus. Plexus formation and the segmental origin of sensory and motor innervation result in two patterns of peripheral innervation of the lower extremity: innervation by named peripheral nerve or segmental innervation. The area of skin innervated by a single dorsal root is a dermatome, and the skeletal muscle fibers innervated by a single ventral root form a myotome. Tables 1–1 through 1–5 summarize the peripheral innervation of the lower extremity. The anatomic distinction between peripheral and segmental patterns of innervation is important because it aids in localizing lesions on the basis of clinical findings.

## SPINAL CORD ANATOMY AND DORSAL ROOT ENTRY ZONE

The innervation of the lower extremity is provided by the lumbar and sacral spinal segments of the

**Table 1–2  The Dermatomes of the Lower Extremity**

| Spinal Nerve/ Dermatome | Major Area Innervated |
| --- | --- |
| L2 | Lateral and anterior thigh |
| L3 | Anterior and medial thigh including the knee and medial leg |
| L4 | Anterior and medial knee and leg including the medial malleolus |
| L5 | Lateral leg and dorsal and ventral surface of the foot |
| S1 | Dorsal surface of foot lateral to the first digit and including the lateral malleolus, ventral surface of the foot including the heel, and area over the Achilles tendon |
| S2 | Posterior surface of thigh, knee, and leg, ending at the heel |
| S3 | Posterior surface of the thigh |

There is significant overlap of adjacent dermatomes.

Table 1–3  Major Nerves Providing Motor
Innervation for the Lower Extremity

| Peripheral Nerve | Muscles Innervated |
| --- | --- |
| Femoral | Psoas major, iliacus, pectineus, sartorius, quadriceps femoris |
| Obturator | Obturator externus, adductor magnus, adductor brevis, adductor longus, gracilis |
| Sciatic | Hamstrings, adductor magnus |
| Deep peroneal | Tibialis anterior, extensor hallucis longus, extensor digitorum longus, peroneus tertius |
| Superficial peroneal | Peroneus longus, peroneus brevis |
| Tibial | Gastrocnemius, popliteus, soleus, flexor hallucis longus, flexor digitorum longus, tibialis posterior |
| Medial plantar | Abductor hallucis, flexor digitorum brevis, flexor hallucis brevis, first lumbrical |
| Lateral plantar | Quadratus plantae, abductor digiti minimi, flexor digiti minimi brevis, second, third, and fourth lumbricals, adductor hallucis, all interossei |

Table 1–5  The Major Myotomes of the Lower Extremity

| Spinal Nerve/ Myotome | Muscles Innervated |
| --- | --- |
| L4 | Iliopsoas, quadriceps, tibialis anterior |
| L5 | Tibialis anterior, toe dorsiflexors, hamstrings, tibialis posterior |
| S1 | Gluteus maximus, hamstrings, gastrocnemius, intrinsic muscles of the foot |

spinal cord. Lumbar and sacral spinal segments are numbered corresponding to the vertebrae forming the superior boundary of an intervertebral foramen. Because the spinal cord is shorter than the length of the vertebral column in adults, the five lumbar spinal segments are located at about the position of the spinous processes of vertebrae T11 and T12. The lumbosacral enlargement encompasses spinal segments L4 through S2 and corresponds to the levels of origin of the lumbar and sacral plexuses of the PNS. The remaining three sacral spinal segments are located in the conical tapered end of the cord forming the conus medullaris. This is located opposite the spinous process of the L1 vertebra in an adult.

Externally, the spinal cord of the lumbosacral enlargement and conus medullaris is seen to have several longitudinal markings: a deep anterior (ventral) median furrow, two anterolateral lines marking the exit of the ventral roots, two shallow dorsolateral sulci for entry of the dorsal roots, and a shallow

Table 1–4  Major Nerves Providing Motor
Innervation for the Lower Extremity,
Classified by Major Muscle Actions

| Peripheral Nerve | Major Actions |
| --- | --- |
| Femoral | Hip flexion and knee extension |
| Sciatic | Knee flexion and all ankle and foot motion via its branches |
| Superficial peroneal | Foot eversion and plantar flexion |
| Deep peroneal | Foot inversion and dorsiflexion |
| Tibial | Foot and toe plantar flexion |
| Medial and lateral plantar | Toe plantar flexion, abduction and adduction of the toes |

dorsal (posterior) median sulcus. Four nerve roots arise from each spinal segment. They remain entirely within the spinal (vertebral) canal and are bathed in cerebrospinal fluid. The lumbar and sacral nerve roots are called the cauda equina because of their resemblance to a horse's tail.

The blood supply for the lumbar and sacral spinal cord is provided by one anterior and two posterior spinal arteries. Although the spinal arteries are branches from the vertebral arteries, at lumbar and spinal levels the blood supply is supplemented by several radicular branches arising from lumbar and sacral arteries external to the vertebral column. The largest radicular branch usually enters at the lower thoracic or upper lumbar region of the cord. The posterior spinal arteries provide the blood supply for the posterior columns, with the remainder of the cord being supplied by the anterior spinal artery.

In a cross section of the spinal cord, a central H-shaped area of gray matter is surrounded by a peripheral zone of white matter. The gray matter consists of a feltwork of neuronal cell bodies, dendrites, myelinated and unmyelinated axons, and glial cells. It forms the dorsal and ventral horns and an intermediate zone that surrounds the central canal. The dorsal horns are sensory receptive and processing zones containing interneurons and tract cells, and the ventral horns contain interneurons and the cell bodies of alpha and gamma motor neurons. At upper lumbar levels the intermediate zone extends laterally, forming the caudal limit of the intermediolateral cell column (lateral horn) of preganglionic sympathetic neurons. The lateral horn is a cell column that extends from spinal level T1 through L2.

The peripheral zone of white matter is formed by longitudinally oriented axons from neurons whose cell bodies are in the central gray or in the dorsal root ganglia. It can be considered to be formed of two concentric regions with the area immediately adjacent to the gray matter consisting of short intrasegmental and intersegmental axons forming the propriospinal fasciculus. This zone is formed by the axons of interneurons with a single interneuron having both intrasegmental and intersegmental, ipsilateral and contralateral terminations. This zone thus serves to integrate segmental and intersegmental activity from both sides of the cord. The peripheral area of white matter contains the axons of projection neurons that function to connect spinal segments with suprasegmental levels such as the brain stem, thalamus, cerebellum, and cerebral cortex. The columns of white matter are termed funiculi, and a posterior, a lateral, and an anterior funiculus are found on each side of the cord. The posterior funiculus consists of the fasciculus gracilis caudal to midthoracic levels with a laterally positioned fasciculus cuneatus added at T-6 and extending rostrally to the caudal medulla.

The dorsal root entry zone involves the dorsolateral sulcus and immediately adjacent part of the dorsal funiculus. First-order sensory neurons from the larger dorsal root cells innervate mechanoreceptors such as muscle spindles, Golgi's tendon organs, Ruffini's endings, Merkel's tactile cell endings, and Pacini's corpuscles. They mediate touch, joint position sense, proprioception, and vibratory sensibility. At the dorsal root entry zone these more heavily myelinated proprioceptive and touch axons enter more medially and may end at any of five destinations. The first is to ascend directly, ipsilaterally, within the dorsal column as the beginning of the dorsal column–medial lemniscal pathway conveying tactile discrimination and conscious proprioception. The second is to synapse on projection neurons that ascend either in the dorsal column or in the lateral funiculus in the spinothalamic tract. A third destination is to synapse on the projection neurons of the nucleus dorsalis (Clarke's column) to give rise to the posterior spinocerebellar tract. A fourth destination is to synapse on spinal interneurons or motor neurons for intrasegmental, intersegmental, or myotatic reflexes. The fifth destination also involves spinal interneurons but functions to modulate central transmission of pain by tract cells.

The lightly myelinated and unmyelinated touch, pain, and temperature afferents enter more laterally into the dorsolateral fasciculus or zone of Lissauer. In the dorsolateral fasciculus the incoming axons bifurcate and ascend and descend before synapsing over several spinal segments in the dorsal horn and intermediate gray. This input also has multiple destinations. The first is a synapse on the tract neurons of the spinothalamic and spinoreticular pathways. A second destination is to activate dorsal horn interneurons involved in the modulation of pain transmission. A third destination is to activate somatic and visceral spinal level reflexes.

## LOCAL REFLEXES AND THE GAIT CYCLE

Local reflex arcs are an indicator of intrinsic spinal interconnections and are thought to contribute to a local pattern generator for locomotion. Two important reflex circuits are the myotatic (stretch) reflex and the Golgi tendon organ circuit.

The simplest circuit is found in the myotatic or stretch reflex. This reflex is a monosynaptic, ipsilateral, two-neuron reflex elicited by activation of muscle spindles resulting in a brief muscle contraction. Muscle spindles are complex sensory endings in skeletal muscles. Specialized small muscle cells within the receptor are referred to as intrafusal fibers to distinguish them from the extrafusal fibers of the bulk of the muscle. Muscle spindles have two types of sensory innervation, a primary or annulospiral ending (group Ia afferents) and a secondary or flower-spray ending (group II afferents). The primary endings involve large-diameter, heavily myelinated, rapidly conducting group Ia afferents. Their direct, monosynaptic excitatory synapse on the alpha motor neurons of the muscle of origin (and its synergists) is the basis for the myotatic reflex. Along with the excitatory innervation of the muscle of origin and its synergists, the circuit also involves the reciprocal disynaptic inhibition of antagonists via Ia interneurons. Muscle spindles are positioned in parallel with the extrafusal muscle fibers and both Ia and group II spindle afferents are excited by either stretch on the muscle or contraction of the intrafusal fibers. Gamma motor neurons innervate the intrafusal fibers and provide continued input from the spindle at different muscle lengths. The sudden activation of Ia afferents mediated by stretch of the muscle during the tendon tap with a reflex hammer is the basis for the deep tendon reflex. The circuits activated by muscle spindles also contribute to muscle tone.

Another important receptor in muscle is the Golgi tendon organ. This receptor is found in tendons, where it samples the tension produced by several motor units. The tendon organ is located in series with the extrafusal fibers of the muscle belly and is activated by an increase of tension on the tendon. The increase of tension could result during a passive stretch or during an active muscle contraction. Via Ib interneurons, the tendon organ afferents (Ib afferents) disynaptically inhibit the alpha motor neurons of the muscle of origin and facilitate the motor neurons of its antagonists.

The motor output of gait is supported by two sets of intrinsic spinal neurons: interneurons and propriospinal neurons. Interneurons are interposed between sensory afferents or descending pathways and the lower motor neurons of the lumbar cord. They include the Ia and Ib interneurons and other interneurons. Propriospinal neurons are not interposed between afferent or efferent pathways but mediate intra- and intersegmental connections. Both intrinsic spinal neuron populations are important for locomotion.

The lumbar spinal cord is thought to provide a site for a central (spinal) pattern generator for locomotion. Coordination of the alternating pattern of muscle contractions during the step and stance phases of gait occurs by sequential activation of the motor neurons for the different flexor and extensor muscle groups via a reciprocal linking of agonists (and synergists) to their antagonists. The initiation of a walking pattern is thought to come from a command center in the cerebral cortex via the direct and indirect descending pathways. The spinal pattern generator for locomotion is also modulated by local spinal circuits and by feedback from muscle, joint, and cutaneous receptors.

## LONG SENSORY PATHWAYS
(Fig 1–1)

The direct or lemniscal sensory pathway is involved in tactile discrimination and conscious proprioception. It is also known as the dorsal column–medial lemniscal pathway. The first-order neuron's central axonal branch enters through the medial part of the dorsal root entry zone and ascends directly to the medulla on the ipsilateral side of the cord in the

**Figure 1–1** Schematic diagram illustrating certain aspects of the neuroanatomy of the lower extremity. DRG = dorsal root ganglion cell; MN = motor neuron; LMN = lower motor neuron; DC = dorsal column; ML = medial lemniscus; LCST = lateral corticospinal tract; STT = spinothalamic tract; VPL = ventral posterolateral nucleus of thalamus.

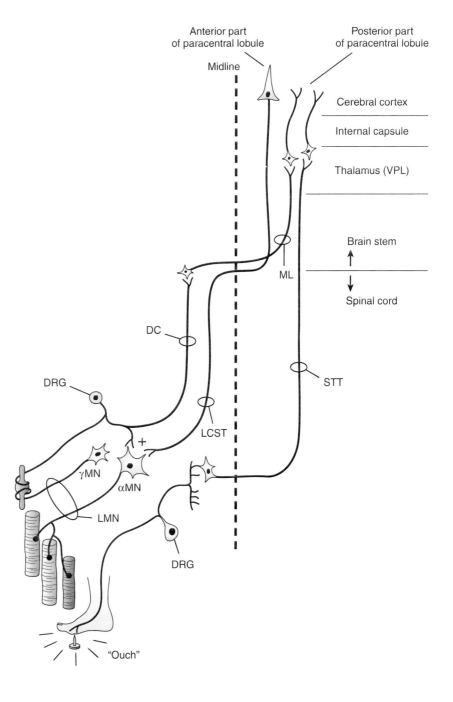

dorsal funiculus. Within the spinal cord in the fasciculus gracilis, the lumbar and sacral levels are medially placed with the most caudal levels positioned most medially. The first-order neurons end in the caudal medulla by synapsing on the nucleus gracilis. Second-order neurons from nucleus gracilis cross the midline to ascend to the thalamus as the medial lemniscus. This crossed pathway begins with a vertical orientation in the medulla with sacral levels positioned most ventrally. As the medial lemniscus passes through the brain stem, it rotates laterally to bring sacral level fibers most lateral in the pons and midbrain. The medial lemniscus terminates in the ventral posterolateral nucleus of the thalamus. In the thalamus, the leg is represented lateral to the hand and head. From the thalamus the third-order neuron ascends through the posterior limb of the internal capsule to the primary somatosensory cortex in the postcentral gyrus. The cortical somatotopic representation of the lower limb is on the medial surface of the hemisphere in the posterior part of the paracentral lobule. This pathway is important for spatiotemporal touch discrimination and fine motor control.

Parallel pathways in the spinal cord convey simple (light) touch in both the dorsal column and spinothalamic pathways, robbing this sensory modality of any utility for the localization of CNS lesions.

In contrast to the lemniscal pathway, the spinothalamic pathway carries information related to pain and temperature sensibility and is found within the anterolateral funiculus of the spinal cord. More is understood about pain than about temperature sensibility. Nociceptive (pain) input has two aspects. One is related to the location and quality of pain; the second is an affective-adversive component. The spinothalamic pathway rapidly conveys information related to the pain and thermal senses and is important for their spatiotemporal localization. The adversive-affective arousal aspects of pain result from a parallel but more indirect and bilateral spinoreticular input to the brain stem reticular formation.

First-order afferents carrying pain and temperature information enter via the lateral portion of the dorsal root entry zone into the dorsolateral fasciculus (zone of Lissauer). Within the dorsolateral fasciculus the axons bifurcate and ascend and descend to provide input over a few spinal segments. The axon of the second-order neuron forms the spinothalamic tract. Its soma is in the dorsal gray, but its axon immediately crosses the midline in the anterior white commissure to ascend in the anterolateral funiculus contralateral to the original input. Sacral level fibers are peripherally located in the tract. The spinothalamic tract ascends through the brain stem in the lateral tegmentum. With the lateral rotation of the medial lemniscus this tract joins the spinothalamic tract in the upper pons. Similarly to the medial lemniscus, the spinothalamic tract terminates in the ventral posterolateral nucleus of the thalamus. Third-order neurons ascend from the thalamus to the somatosensory cortex via the posterior limb of the internal capsule. This pathway is useful clinically for the localization of CNS lesions because it is crossed in the spinal cord and it travels in the lateral medulla near the uncrossed pain projections from the face.

One consequence of bilateral symmetry and of the crossing of the spinothalamic fibers near their level of origin in the spinal cord is that central lesions that expand outward interrupt the crossing fibers from both sides. This results in bilateral loss of pain and temperature sensibility but only over the levels that are interrupted. Such central lesions can occur with a syrinx or cavitation in the region of the central canal (syringomyelia), after trauma, or with growth of a neoplasm.

The dorsal horn is not simply a relay pathway for painful stimuli because CNS systems modulate the transmission of pain within the dorsal horn. This modulation involves both inhibitory input from large-diameter mechanoreceptive afferents and activation of brain stem nuclei that contain receptors for endogenous opioids and that are stimulated by exogenous opioids such as morphine. These brain stem nuclei project to the dorsal horn, where they inhibit pain transmission.

Subconscious (unconscious) proprioception from the lower limb is conveyed to the cerebellum by two pathways for reflex adjustments of posture and to monitor motor performance. Input from muscle spindles, Golgi's tendon organs, joint proprioceptors, and cutaneous mechanoreceptors is sent in parallel to the cerebellum via the uncrossed posterior spinocerebellar tract. Input from the posterior spinocerebellar tract is rapid and arises from a single muscle or a few muscles and from cutaneous areas of the lower extremity. Via cerebellar outflow to subcortical areas and the cerebral cortex, the posterior spinocerebellar tract is thought to mediate a feedback control of movement. The second pathway arises in the spinal gray and immediately crosses midline to ascend to the caudal midbrain, where it recrosses before entry into the cerebellum. This anterior spinocerebellar tract provides the cerebellum with information about the state of excitation of spinal level motor neurons and their associated interneurons. Thus, the cerebellum receives mostly ipsilateral input from the lower extremity.

## LONG MOTOR PATHWAYS AND THEIR EFFECTS ON INTRINSIC SPINAL CIRCUITS

Direct motor pathways descend from the cerebral cortex to spinal level interneurons and motor neurons. Direct projections destined for spinal levels form the pyramidal tracts. Indirect motor pathways include all motor tracts other than the pyramidal tracts. The complete path for some of the nonpyramidal pathways may extend indirectly from the cortex to spinal level motor neurons via synapses in the basal ganglia, cerebellum, and brain stem. Several brain stem nuclei give origin to a number of nonpyramidal indirect motor pathways.

The direct corticospinal pathway is phylogenetically newer and functions in fine, controlled voluntary movements. The corticospinal tract is a direct path from the cerebral cortex to the motor neurons and interneurons of the ventral horn. Its major function is in skilled movements under conscious control. Axons arise from the primary motor cortex, the premotor cortex, and somatosensory cortices to descend through the corona radiata, the posterior limb of the internal capsule, the cerebral peduncle (crus cerebri) of the ventral midbrain, the ventral pons, and the pyramids of the medulla. At the caudal medulla about 90% of axons cross midline to descend in the lateral funiculus as the lateral corticospinal tract. In the course through the ventral brain stem, fibers destined for sacral spinal levels are positioned more laterally. In the lateral corticospinal tracts of the lateral funiculi, sacral level fibers are most superficial. The remaining uncrossed corticospinal fibers descend in the anterior funiculus as the anterior corticospinal tract. The upper motor neurons of the corticospinal tract synapse indirectly on spinal interneurons or directly on spinal lower motor neurons, both alpha and gamma motor neurons.

Pure lesions of the corticospinal tracts in the cortex or the medullary pyramids produce weakness or paralysis of muscles, especially of the distal extremities. Motor impairment is greatest for skilled movements. Muscle tone is depressed, certain superficial reflexes are lost (e.g., superficial abdominal and cremasteric), and an abnormal extensor plantar reflex (the Babinski reflex) occurs on stimulation of the sole of the foot. The normal plantar response is flexion of the toes.

The nonpyramidal motor pathways can be grouped into a medial group and a lateral group. Tracts of the medial group control posture and whole limb movements, act more on proximal than on distal limb musculature, and are facilitory to extensor muscles and inhibitory to flexor muscles. These tracts include the pontine (medial) reticulospinal tract and the lateral vestibulospinal tract. Each descends in the anterior funiculus of the spinal cord. The reticular formation receives input from the basal ganglia via the globus pallidus and the cerebellum's vestibular connections provide indirect influences on spinal motor neurons by these centers. Lateral descending nonpyramidal pathways function in the control of independent flexor movements, especially of the distal extremities. This set of nonpyramidal pathways includes the rubrospinal tract from the midbrain red nucleus and the medullary (lateral) reticulospinal tract. The lateral group descends in the lateral funiculus of the cord.

The clinical effects of damage to the indirect descending pathways are complicated by the lack of well-defined bundles and the change of symptoms with time related to the development of a denervation hypersensitivity by the anterior horn cells. Long-term lesions of these pathways result in loss of postural and voluntary activities but retention of segmental reflexes, such as the deep tendon reflexes, which become hyperactive.

The direct and indirect pathways intermingle in their descent for most of their course, so it is rare for selective damage to involve one and not the other. Unilateral disruption of the descending pathways results in an upper motor neuron lesion resulting in impaired motor activity on one side of the body. In the lower limb, the impairment involves the dorsiflexors of the toes and ankle and the knee and hip flexors. A characteristic circumduction of the lower limb is seen during walking.

## BIBLIOGRAPHY

FitzGerald, MJT: Neuroanatomy, Basic and Applied. Philadelphia, WB Saunders, 1985.
Hollinshead WH: Textbook of Anatomy, 3rd ed. Hagerstown MD, Harper & Row, 1974.
Peele TL: The Neuroanatomic Basis for Clinical Neurology, 3rd ed. New York, McGraw-Hill, 1977.
Westmoreland BF, Benarroch EE, Daube JR, et al: Medical Neurosciences: An Approach to Anatomy, Pathology, and Physiology by Systems and Levels. Boston, Little, Brown, 1995.

# Neurologic Examination of the Lower Extremity

*2*

*Peterkin Lee-Kwen and Patrick Pullicino*

The primary function of the neurologic examination is to detect and localize lesions of the nervous system. This traditionally requires a methodical, complete neurologic examination of the mental state; cranial nerves; and motor, sensory, and cerebellar systems. However, a full neurologic examination may be time consuming and many of the details may be irrelevant for a particular patient. For this reason, it is important to use the history to derive a working hypothesis about localization and diagnosis and to allow the history to guide you to which neural system (e.g., motor or sensory) or part of the body to examine in particular detail.

This chapter first describes the method of examination of the lower extremities with emphasis on signs that indicate the presence of neurologic disease. Second, the distinction between a lower and an upper motor neuron lesion in the lower extremity is discussed. Third, we explain the localization of nervous system lesions presenting with signs in the lower extremity.

## EXAMINATION OF THE LOWER EXTREMITY

The initial objective of the neurologic examination is to localize the lesion. The secondary or subsequent objective is to make a specific neurologic diagnosis. Lesions in specific neural systems can be looked for in the formal part of the neurologic examination by examining the motor, sensory, and cerebellar systems. This formal examination has to be combined with careful observation of the patient's appearance, demeanor, and gait for clues that may help localize a lesion or allow the examiner to jump to a specific neurologic diagnosis. In neurologic disease of the lower extremity, observation of the gait is particularly important and may allow localization of a lesion or even a likely diagnostic hypothesis to be made when the patient is first encountered.

## Gait

The way the patient walks into the consultation room should be carefully observed. If the patient has any difficulty walking or appears unsteady or slow, several things should be noted about the gait. (1) How wide is the walking base? Normally, the medial edge of either shoe should touch an imaginary straight line exactly below the center of the body. If not, the patient has a wide-based gait, which may be a sign of cerebellar disease, posterior column deficit, or a large-fiber peripheral neuropathy. (2) What is the length of the stride? The normal stride length is about 18 inches but varies with age. The stride becomes shorter in older age and in parkinsonism (the festinating gait of parkinsonism is characterized by rapid short steps). (3) The toe should just clear the ground during the stride. Does the toe scuff along the floor (spastic gait in hemiparesis) or is the foot lifted abnormally high (steppage gait of peripheral neuropathy)? (4) Does the heel strike the ground first or is the shoe striking the ground flat or toe first (as in patients with footdrop)? (5) Is there difficulty starting (gait apraxia), stopping (parkinsonism), or turning?

Other gaits that are less easy to characterize include the limping (or antalgic) gait of a patient with back pain or sciatica, the waddling gait of a patient with a myopathy, and the hysterical gait in which the patient leans to impossible angles but does not fall.

Table 2–1 summarizes different types of gait abnormalities seen with lesions of different locations in the nervous system.

## Motor System

### Inspection

It is important to expose the lower extremities fully for examination. Many fundamental errors are made by examining patients with their legs covered. The legs should be examined with the patient lying relaxed and supine.

The first thing to note is the presence of asymmetry of the two legs. Look carefully at thigh girth (easiest from the foot of the bed), calf girth, and prominence of the anterior tibial muscles (the mus-

Table 2–1 Gait Abnormalities Seen with Lesions in Different Nervous System Locations

| Location | Condition | Gait |
|---|---|---|
| Frontal lobes | White matter vascular disease, hydrocephalus | Apraxic |
| Upper motor neuron | Stroke Cerebral palsy | Spastic, hemiparetic |
| Basal ganglia | Parkinsonism | Festinating |
| Cerebellum | Tumors Degenerative disorders | Ataxic or wide based |
| Posterior columns | Sensory ataxia | Steppage |
| Nerve root | Herniated disks | Antalgic |
| Proximal muscles | Myopathy | Waddling |
| Peroneal nerve | Compression neuropathy | High stepping |
| Peripheral nerve | Severe or large-fiber neuropathy | Broad based or steppage |

cle should protrude beyond the anterior edge of the tibia). Suspected asymmetries, which should be confirmed with a tape measure, usually signify wasting of the smaller muscle. Wasting is an important localizing sign and must always be carefully looked for. If wasting is found in one muscle, look carefully for wasting in other muscles, for fasciculations in the leg muscles, and for sensory loss in the dermatomes subserved by the same roots as the involved muscle. Fasciculations are involuntary, random contractions of a group of muscle fibers representing a motor unit. Their presence suggests a lower motor neuron (LMN) lesion such as seen in neuropathy or amyotrophic lateral sclerosis. Fasciculations, particularly in the quadriceps muscle, may be seen in normal individuals and may be brought on by low temperatures, fatigue states, or drowsiness.

Next, compare the degree of dorsiflexion of the feet carefully. A slight asymmetry probably indicates a footdrop on the less dorsiflexed side. If a footdrop is found, look for supporting signs of the different causes of footdrop: (1) pyramidal tract lesion (look for extensor plantar response), (2) L-5 neuropathy (foot inversion is weak), (3) sciatic neuropathy (plantar flexion and dorsiflexion are weak), (4) peroneal neuropathy (inversion spared, sensory loss in lateral leg), (5) peripheral neuropathy (bilateral symmetry), and (6) myopathy (extensor digitorum brevis not atrophied). Also look for any external rotation of a foot compared with the other; this may be the only sign of an upper motor neuron (UMN) lesion on that side.

### Testing for Muscle Tone

This is an important part of the examination and should never be overlooked. Muscle tone is the resistance felt by the examiner when a limb is moved passively by the examiner. Before examining for muscle tone, the patient is instructed to relax

fully. The examiner should always examine from the same side of the couch (usually on the patient's right). Take the foot with the right hand and hold the leg with the left hand just above the knee. Check for tone first with slow movements and then quicker, sudden movements. Check hip rotation, knee flexion and extension, and foot dorsiflexion. In particular, repeated, rapid foot dorsiflexion should be performed with the knee flexed at 90 degrees to look for ankle clonus. Clonus is a repeated reflex plantar flexion in response to passive foot dorsiflexion. If it is elicited, the number of beats should be counted.

Hypertonia or increased tone can be of three types: spasticity, rigidity, and paratonia.

*Spasticity* is a velocity-dependent increase in tone and is felt as a "catch" when a sudden passive joint movement is made. It may also be seen as clonus, particularly at the ankles. If it is severe, it may be difficult to flex the leg at the knee. Spasticity is an important sign of a UMN lesion affecting the pyramidal tract in the brain, brain stem, or spinal cord. If spasticity is found, other UMN signs such as an extensor plantar response must be looked for. A quick test for spasticity in a completely relaxed patient in a supine position is to lift the leg off the couch suddenly from behind the lower thigh. If tone is normal, the heel drags along the couch surface. If spasticity is present, the heel kicks off the couch surface momentarily.

Hypertonia with *rigidity* is the same throughout the entire range of movement. It is also called lead-pipe rigidity because it resembles the resistance to bending of a lead pipe. Rigidity is best appreciated in the lower extremity on testing passive hip rotation. It is a sign of extrapyramidal disease, in particular parkinsonism. If the patient has a tremor, it is superimposed on the hypertonia to give the ratchet-like sensation of "cogwheel" rigidity. Cogwheel rigidity is not specific for extrapyramidal disease and can be seen when there is a combination of tremor and hypertonia of any cause.

*Paratonia* is an increase in tone that varies in severity with the amount of force applied by the examiner. As the examiner tries to move a limb, the patient resists with increasing force or alternatively moves the limb along with the examiner as if to help. The patient appears to not be cooperating with the examiner, but paratonia is involuntary. It is a sign of diffuse cerebral dysfunction, particularly of frontal lobe disease, and is seen in the elderly or those with degenerative diseases such as vascular dementia.

Hypotonia or decreased muscle tone can be seen in any LMN or cerebellar lesion or in muscle disease.

## Muscle Strength Testing

Muscle strength testing is performed to determine the presence of weakness. If weakness is found, its degree should be quantified. The examiner usually looks for muscle weakness by attempting to overcome the strength of different muscle groups. If the examiner cannot overcome the strength of a muscle group, it is usually inferred that the strength of that muscle group is normal. In testing the powerful lower extremity muscles, this conclusion must be qualified by the size and strength of both the examiner and the patient. A considerable degree of weakness of the iliopsoas, quadriceps, or gastrocnemius may not be detectable on routine examination.

The muscle groups should always be tested from the same (usually right) side of the couch, always immediately comparing one side with the other, starting with the proximal flexor muscles. To test the iliopsoas, ask the supine patient to raise one leg to 45 degrees. Try to break the flexed posture by pushing down just above the knee. Considerable force may be necessary. Do the same on the other side and compare, looking for minor degrees of "give." For the knee flexors and extensors, flex the knee 90 degrees. For the quadriceps, hold the leg just above the ankle and ask the patient to extend the knee. For the hamstrings, place your hand behind the heel and ask the patient to flex the knee. The foot dorsiflexors are tested by trying to break the full dorsiflexion of the foot by pushing forward on the distal foot. Inversion and eversion of the foot should be tested in the same way. The gastrocnemius muscles can be tested by asking the patient to push onto your hand, but this detects only severe degrees of weakness. The most sensitive test for the gastrocnemius muscles is to ask patients to walk on their toes. Small foot muscles (abductor hallucis) should be tested by asking the patient to push medially with the great toe.

The hip extensors should always be tested. The best way is to ask the patient to extend the leg 30° from a prone position and attempt to overcome this by pushing down above the knee. A quick screen can be performed in the supine position by putting your hand under the heel, asking the patient to resist you and seeing if you can lift the right hip off the bed.

## Grading Abnormal Strength

Strength is most commonly graded using the Medical Research Council Scale (0 to 5, right-left).

Grade 5    Normal strength (5−, probably normal but doubt exists).

Grade 4    Muscle moves joint against gravity plus added resistance (4 +, definite slight weakness, muscle can just be overcome; 4, weak but easily overcome; 4 −, limb "melts away").

Grade 3    Muscle moves joint against gravity but without added resistance (movement does not have to be full range of motion against gravity).

Grade 2    Muscle moves joint when gravity eliminated.

Grade 1    Flicker of movement seen or felt in the muscle.

Grade 0    No movement or paralysis.

A quicker and more easily reproducible method is the functional scoring method. In this method, muscle strength is tested against the weight of the leg or of the body. The hip flexors are tested by asking the patient to elevate the leg to 60 degrees and maintain the position for 10 seconds. The result can be graded as 0 if there is no movement, 1 if there is loss of position, 2 if the leg hits the couch before 10 seconds, 3 if the leg cannot be lifted off the couch, and 4 if there is no movement at all. The quadriceps can be tested by the ability to climb a step 6 inches high, to stand from a chair 18 inches high without using the hands, or to stand from a squatting position. Foot dorsiflexors and gastrocnemius muscles can be evaluated by the ability to toe or heel walk.

## Palpation and Percussion

Occasionally, palpation or percussion of the muscle belly may be useful in making a diagnosis. Palpation may detect rubbery (glycogen storage disease) or tender (inflammatory myopathy) muscles. In myxedema, percussion of the muscle may produce a pit in the muscle that spreads over the surface like a ripple in a pond, called myoedema.

## Sensory Testing

The sensory examination is probably the most difficult part of the examination of the leg, because it depends on the subjective responses of the patient. As in muscle strength testing, the first decision to be made is whether sensation is normal. In order to obtain meaningful clinical data from sensory testing, it is important (1) to determine from the history the location of any subjective sensory complaint, or likely distribution of any sensory deficit, before examining the patient so that the examination can be focused on this area; (2) to have a thorough knowledge of the cutaneous supply by roots and nerves in order to be able to localize a lesion as well as confirm that the distribution of a sensory deficit fits a known anatomic distribution; and (3) always to keep in mind that many apparently abnormal findings on the sensory examination are not related to underlying pathology.

If the history does not suggest the presence of a sensory deficit, a quick sensory screen may be performed. This should include testing of sensation to pinprick, light touch, vibration, and joint position in the feet. Ideal testing conditions include a relaxed, alert patient and a warm environment. The sensory examination can be divided into (1) pain and temperature (spinothalamic) sensation, (2) light touch, and (3) vibration and joint position (posterior column) sensation.

Pain sensation is tested by using a regular pin or a safety pin, which should be discarded after use. A hypodermic needle is too sharp and should not be used. A broken off Q-Tip stick or tongue blade does not give a reproducible stimulus and should also be avoided.

To test with a pin, begin over the dorsum of the foot and stick the patient gently in the same spot about three times and then in a comparable location on the other foot. If the patient feels the stick, ask the patient to average the sensation and to compare the two sides. If a difference is found, confirm it, making sure the side that feels less is being adequately stimulated. If the sensations on the two sides are the same, repeat the test in the midleg and midthigh. It is not necessary to test temperature routinely.

To test light touch, it is best to use a Q-Tip and draw out the end of the cotton a little way to make a new firm tip. Ask patients to close their eyes and say "yes" each time they feel a touch. Then make randomly placed and timed touches on both left and right leg, foot, and thigh with the cotton tip, noting any areas missed.

To test vibration sensation, use a 128-Hz tuning fork. To screen for abnormal vibration sensation, place the vibrating fork on the medial malleolus and ask the patient to tell you when he or she no longer feels the vibration. If you can still feel the vibration 5 seconds after the patient stops feeling it, the patient's vibration sense is probably reduced.

To test joint position sense, ask the patient to close the eyes. Grasp the lateral sides of the distal phalanx of one great toe with your thumb and index finger. Ask the patient to tell you the direction of the movement and to move the toe randomly up or down. Test larger and then smaller movements. The patient should be able to detect the direction of any movement you make, however small.

If the history suggests a sensory abnormality, you must first try to interpret the history in terms of an anatomic dermatomal or nerve distribution pattern and then specifically test for this distribution, or you may miss the sensory loss. For example, burning in the soles at night suggests tarsal tunnel syndrome and sensory loss must be looked for carefully over the medial sole (medial plantar nerve). To define an area of sensory loss, test with a pin, starting well within the area of sensory loss and working toward normal sensation. Ask the patient to tell you when the pin is felt to be sharp. For example, in a person with diabetes or suspected peripheral neuropathy, start pinprick testing near the toes and work your way proximally.

If the result of any part of the sensory examination is abnormal, more detailed testing of the other sensory modalities is called for.

## Reflexes

The muscle stretch or myotactic reflex requires an intact sensory and motor peripheral pathway for a normal response. The main reflexes in the leg are the patellar jerk (L2-3, femoral nerve) and the ankle jerk (S1-2, tibial nerve). The hamstring reflex may also be elicited (S1, tibial nerve).

To elicit the patellar reflexes, with the patient supine, flex the knees to 90 degrees with the knees resting together by supporting the weight of the legs with your left hand under both popliteal fossae. Make sure the legs are relaxed. Tap the patella tendon with the reflex hammer in the right hand and move from one side to the other, starting with a very gentle tap and then increasing in force. Look for any, even minimal, asymmetry. If no leg jerk is seen, look for a quadriceps contraction. If no contraction is seen, repeat with a reinforcement maneuver.

For the ankle reflexes, with the patient supine and knees flexed, externally rotate the leg to be tested so that it is lying laterally on the couch. With your left hand grasp the end of the foot and dorsiflex the foot firmly, making sure the patient is not helping by contracting the tibialis anterior (this is important, as such contraction often stops the reflex being elicited). Tap the Achilles tendon above the heel and watch for a gastrocnemius contraction. If you cannot elicit the ankle reflex in this way, ask the patient to lie supine with the legs straight and, holding the foot dorsiflexed with your left hand, tap on the ball of the foot (actually on your left hand). Patients find it easier to relax in this position.

Minimal asymmetries should be looked for but quite minor differences are not always indicative of pathology. The abnormal reflex may be either the more or the less brisk one. The presence of spasticity ipsilaterally indicates that a brisk reflex is abnormal.

Reflexes can be graded on a scale as follows, but note that a reflex of any grade apart from grade 0 and possibly grade 4 may be normal:

Grade 0    Absent.

Grade 1    Reflex obtained only with reinforcement. (Jendrassik's maneuver, or asking the patient to pull apart her or his interlocked hands, is a reinforcement maneuver and should be used for any apparently absent reflex.)

Grade 2    Normal.

Grade 3    Physiologically brisk or increased (anxiety states or UMN lesion).

Grade 4    Sustained clonus at ankle or knee (UMN lesion).

### Superficial Reflexes

*Abdominal reflexes* are difficult to elicit in obese patients but are important in localizing spinal cord disease (e.g., epigastric, T6-9; midabdomen, T9-11; hypogastric, T1 to L1).

The *cremasteric reflex* is elicited with the patient in the supine position by gently rubbing the end of the tendon hammer along the inner thigh from the knee upward. This should cause elevation of the ipsilateral testis. This reflex localizes to L1.

The *anal reflex* (S2, S3, S4) can be elicited by gently stimulating the perianal region with a pin. There should be contraction of the anal sphincter (anal wink). Loss of this reflex indicated a lesion in the conus medullaris or cauda equina.

The *Babinski reflex* consists of extension of the great toe with fanning of the other toes. This reflex should be elicited with the minimal stimulus necessary on the lateral, plantar surface of the foot (S1 dermatome). Some patients may withdraw the toes, mimicking the Babinski response, if they have a low tickle threshold. An abnormal response can be seen with any lesion affecting the corticospinal tracts. If a patient withdraws on stimulation of the sole of the foot, extension of the great toe may be elicited by scraping the lateral aspect of the dorsum of the foot below the lateral malleolus (Chaddock's reflex), by rubbing a knuckle gently down the shin (Oppenheim's reflex), by squeezing the gastrocnemius (Gordon's reflex), or by abducting the little toe for 1 to 2 seconds and then releasing (Stransky's reflex).

## Cerebellar Testing

Cerebellar dysfunction may be manifest as nystagmus, staccato or scanning speech, intention tremor, hypotonia, dysmetria, incoordination on finger-to-nose or heel-to-shin test, inability to perform rapid alternating movements, pendular reflexes, or gait ataxia. If there is incoordination in the heel-to-shin or finger-to-nose test, the lesion is usually localized ipsilaterally in the cerebellum or cerebellar outflow tracts. Gait ataxia is localized to the midline cerebellum (vermis).

To perform the heel-to-shin test, ask the supine patient to raise one leg and bring the heel down on the opposite knee. The patient should then run the heel down the shin slowly and accurately. Limb incoordination typically causes the heel to slip off the shin, and as the patient tries to correct this, the heel is pulled back to the shin but slips off the other side. Compare both sides.

To test for gait ataxia, check for a wide-based gait and then ask the patient to walk on a line, the heel of one shoe touching the toe of the other (tandem walking). A patient without ataxia should be able to do this without difficulty.

## Station

The ability to stand still without falling depends mainly on intact joint position sense in the feet and normal cerebellar function. If a patient is feeling vertiginous because of vestibular dysfunction, this also impairs the ability to stand. The visual system can compensate for impaired joint position sense using visual cues. The Romberg test is used to look for posterior column dysfunction. The patient is asked to stand with the heels together without support. If the patient is unable to do this with the eyes open, the posterior columns cannot be implicated as a cause of inability to stand. A patient who is able to stand with the eyes open is then asked to close the eyes. If the patient immediately falls to one side, it is an indication of posterior column dysfunction and joint position sense should be tested in detail. If the patient sways but does not fall, the Romberg test should not be considered positive.

## DISTINGUISHING CLINICAL FEATURES OF AN UPPER OR LOWER MOTOR NEURON WEAKNESS

It is important to distinguish between a UMN lesion and an LMN lesion because this is of great localizing value. The UMN originates from the pyramidal cells

Table 2–2  Characteristics of Upper Motor
Neuron and Lower Motor Neuron Lesions

| Characteristic | Upper Motor Neuron | Lower Motor Neuron |
|---|---|---|
| Location | Corticospinal tract | Anterior horn cell to the neuromuscular junction |
| Bulk | Disuse atrophy | Wasting |
| Strength | Paresis | Paralysis |
| Tone | Increased | Decreased |
| Fasciculation | Absent | Decreased |
| Babinski's sign | Present | Absent |

in the frontal cortex and ends in the motor nuclei of the brain stem of anterior horn cells of the spinal cord. Any destructive lesion such as a stroke, space-occupying lesion (tumor, hemorrhage, or abscess), or demyelinating process (multiple sclerosis) in the brain or spinal cord can cause interruption of the corticospinal pathway.

The clinical features of a UMN lesion include (1) weakness of varying severity, (2) abnormal muscle tone (there may be hypotonia in an acute lesion followed by hypertonia or spasticity), (3) brisk reflexes, (4) Babinski's sign or extensor plantar, and (5) a minor degree of disuse atrophy of muscles after months.

An LMN originates in the anterior horn cell of the spinal cord or bulbar motor nuclei of the brain stem and terminates at the neuromuscular junction. Clinical features of an LMN lesion include (1) paralysis, (2) hypotonia, (3) hyporeflexia, and (4) fasciculations. See Table 2–2.

## USING NEUROLOGIC FINDINGS IN THE LOWER EXTREMITY TO LOCALIZE LESIONS HIGHER IN THE NEURAXIS

Neurologic problems at any level of the neuraxis can present in the lower extremity. The lower limb examination by itself may enable satisfactory localization to a particular level of the neuraxis. In the following, lower extremity examination findings seen with lesions at different levels of the neuraxis are given.

**Cerebral Hemisphere.** Unilateral UMN signs with weakness, spasticity, and a Babinski response are most likely to represent a cerebral lesion. A plantar grasp response (strong, sustained flexion of toes when the ball of foot is stimulated) indicates a frontal lobe location.

**Brain Stem.** Pyramidal signs in one leg and heel-shin incoordination in the other leg suggest a brain stem lesion. There may be associated truncal ataxia.

**Spinal Cord.** Two groups of findings point to the spinal cord. (1) Bilateral leg weakness is usually of the UMN type with extensor plantars, but an early acute lesion may not be associated with increased tone or reflexes. (2) The hemicord syndrome is also typical of a spinal cord lesion. The finding here is of UMN signs in one leg and reduced sensation to pinprick in the other leg. There may be vibration sense loss in the leg with UMN signs.

**Conus Medullaris Syndrome.** The most distal part of the sacral spinal cord is the conus medullaris. Clinical signs are (1) incontinence; (2) loss of sensation of pain in a saddle distribution in the perineum; (3) motor deficits, which are usually symmetric but mild; and (4) loss of ankle, bulbocavernosus, and anal reflexes.

**Cauda Equina Syndrome.** The neuroanatomic location is the lumbosacral roots. The cauda equina lesions may be similar to those of the conus medullaris. Clinical signs are as follows. (1) Sensory loss is asymmetric in a saddle distribution and affects both pain and touch. (2) Motor deficits are asymmetric, moderate to severe, and atrophy may be present. (3) Reflexes may be unaffected. (4) Sphincter dysfunction may be present with loss of the perineal reflexes.

**Radicular Syndrome.** In patients with suspected herniated intervertebral disks, look for (1) sensory loss in the distribution of the affected root, (2) motor weakness and atrophy in the distribution of the affected root, and (3) a diminished or lost ankle reflex in L5 to S1 disk protrusions.

**Peripheral Nerve.** Examination shows a distal symmetric diminution or loss of one or more sensory modalities; typically, vibration loss is an early sign. There may be LMN muscle weakness distally.

**Muscle.** The most frequent pattern of weakness is that of proximal weakness and wasting without loss of the reflexes until advanced stages of the disease. The sensory system is not involved. The peroneal muscles may be involved by themselves. Muscle disease as a cause of distal leg weakness is indicated by sparing of the extensor digitorum brevis muscle, which never happens in peripheral neuropathies. The extensor digitorum brevis can be felt as a round lump on the proximal lateral dorsum of the foot on foot dorsiflexion.

## SUMMARY

Physicians whose practice is centered on the lower extremity often do not have the time to perform a full neurologic examination of every patient. It is important to be able to detect abnormal neurologic signs in the lower extremity even without doing a complete neurologic examination. Diseases of the central nervous system (brain or spinal cord) may present with neurologic signs in the lower extremities. This chapter has reviewed the technique and interpretation of the neurologic examination of the lower extremity with reference to common neurologic conditions.

## BIBLIOGRAPHY

Haerer AF: DeJong's the Neurologic Examination, 5th ed. Philadelphia, JB Lippincott, 1992.

Mayo Clinic and Mayo Foundation: Clinical Examinations in Neurology, 6th ed. St. Louis, Mosby Year Book, 1991.

Murray PM, Duthie EH, Gambert SR, et al: Age related changes in knee muscle strength in normal women. J Gerontol 40:275–280, 1985.

O'Keeffe ST, Smith T, Valacio R, et al: A comparison of two techniques for ankle jerk assessment in elderly subjects. Lancet 344:1619–1620, 1994.

Perret E, Reglis F: Age and the perceptual threshold for vibratory stimuli. Eur Neurol 4:65–76, 1970.

Skinner HB, Barrack RL, Cook SD: Age-related decline in proprioception. Clin Orthop Relat Res 184:208–211, 1984.

Stalberg E, Borges O, Ericsson B, et al: The quadriceps femoris muscle in 20–70 year old subjects: Relationship between knee extension torque, electrophysiologic parameters and muscle fiber characteristics. Muscle Nerve 12:382–389, 1989.

# Localization of Neurologic Lesions 3

*Melissa Carran and R. Mañon-Espaillat*

The neurologic evaluation consists of a history, physical examination, and neurologic examination. With this information, the clinician develops a hypothesis on the basis of the evolution and localization of the lesion. The localization of the lesion is also important in selecting the appropriate test for documenting the lesion. Despite the diversity and sophistication of the techniques of neuroimaging and neurophysiology, all these tests require data obtained from the neurologic evaluation for optimal interpretation. Sometimes lesions are found unexpectedly in neuroimaging or neurophysiology tests. The clinician is called upon to determine whether the lesion found is responsible for the patient's clinical deficit. Knowing the effect that lesions may have in different locations of the central and peripheral nervous systems is of utmost importance in this situation. In this chapter, we provide a general overview of symptoms and signs found in patients with lesions of the central and peripheral nervous systems with emphasis on the lower extremity.

## LESIONS AFFECTING THE UPPER MOTOR NEURON AND CORTICOSPINAL TRACT

The cell body of the upper motor neuron is located in the motor cortex. The axons form the corticospinal tract and descend through the centrum semiovale, internal capsule, cerebral peduncle, basis pontis, and cervicomedullary junction, where they decussate forming the pyramidal decussation. The decussated corticospinal tract continues their course in the lateral and anterior compartments of the spinal cord, and they eventually synapse in lower motor neurons in the anterior horn (Fig. 3–1).

Lesions of the upper motor neuron and corticospinal tract produce predominantly distal weakness, spasticity, increased tone, increased reflexes, and the extensor plantar response (Babinski's sign) (Table 3–1). The Babinski sign is elicited by applying a noxious stimulus starting in the lateral and posterior aspect of the foot, moving it anteriorly toward the small toe, and curving it toward the base of the big toe. The normal response consists of flexion of the toes and foot. The abnormal response consists of extension of the big toe, fanning of the remaining

toes, dorsiflexion of the foot, flexion at the knee and hip, and abduction of the thigh.[1] Because of the anatomic decussation of the corticospinal tract, lesions affecting the upper motor neuron or the corticospinal tracts between the motor cortex and the medulla produce contralateral weakness of the extremities. Lesions affecting the corticospinal tract below the cervicomedullary junction produce ipsilateral weakness.

Lesions in the upper motor neuron and corticospinal tract rarely occur alone, and other associated neurologic signs are of value for further localization of the lesion. With lesions in the left cerebral hemisphere, in addition to weakness of the right lower extremity, there is usually weakness of the right upper extremity and right lower face as well. Because most individuals are left hemisphere dominant for language, patients may also have a language disorder (aphasia). With lesions in the frontal lobe the patient has a nonfluent aphasia, and with lesions in the temporal parietal region the patient has a receptive aphasia. With lesions affecting the prefrontal lobe the patient may have changes in personality, and with lesions affecting the occipital lobe a contralateral homonymous hemianopia can be found. With lesions in the right cerebral hemisphere, the weakness is in the left lower and upper extremities and in the left lower face. Patients with right hemisphere lesions may neglect the left side of their body and left hemispace. Similarly to lesions in the left hemisphere, right frontal lobe lesions produce changes in personality and behavior in addition to the motor deficit. Right occipital lesions cause a left homonymous hemianopia.[2]

Lesions within the brain stem are associated with cranial nerve abnormalities, which are helpful in localization of the lesion (Fig. 3–2). Cranial nerve innervation is usually ipsilateral. Therefore, an important sign of a brain stem lesion is a cross-deficit in which the cranial nerve deficit and the cortical spinal tract deficit are crossed. A midbrain lesion may produce vertical dysplegia because of an oculomotor or trochlear nerve palsy and a contralateral weakness of the lower face and upper and lower extremities (Fig. 3–3). A pontine lesion produces ipsilateral deficits in the trigeminal, abducent, and facial nerve with contralateral weakness of the

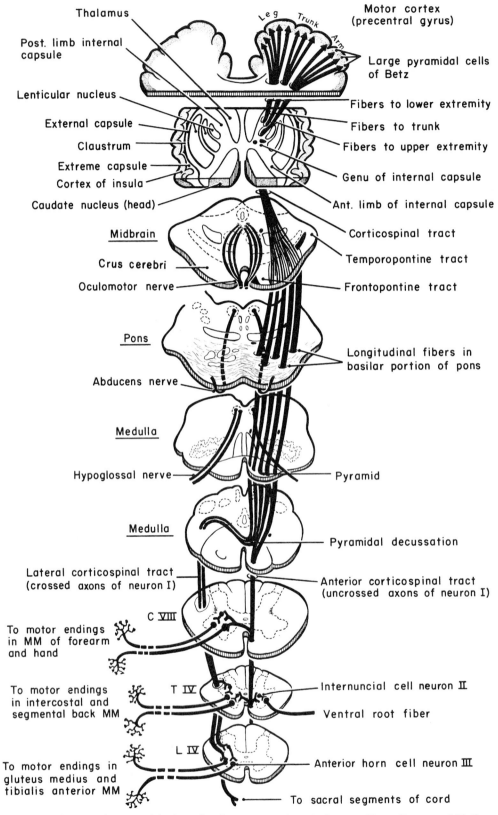

**Figure 3–1** Schematic diagram of the lateral and anterior corticospinal tracts. (From Carpenter MB: Tracts of the spinal cord. *In* Carpenter MB: Core Text of Neuroanatomy, 3rd ed. Baltimore, Williams & Wilkins, 1985, pp 74–101.)

Table 3–1  **Differences Between Upper and Lower Motor Neuron Paralysis**

| Upper Motor Neuron or Supranuclear Paralysis | Lower Motor Neuron or Nuclear-Intranuclear Paralysis |
| --- | --- |
| Muscles affected in groups, never individual muscles | Individual muscles may be affected. |
| Atrophy slight and caused by disuse | Atrophy is pronounced, up to 70–80% of total bulk. |
| Spasticity with hyperactivity of the tendon reflexes and extensor plantar reflex (Babinski's sign) | Flaccidity and hypotonia of affected muscles with loss of tendon reflexes. |
| | Plantar reflex, if present, is of normal flexor type. |
| Fascicular twitches absent | Fascicular twitches may be present. |
| Normal nerve conduction studies: no denervation potentials in electromyogram | Abnormal nerve, conduction studies: denervation potentials (fibrillations, fasciculations, positive sharp waves) in electromyogram. |

Modified from Adams RD, Victor M: Motor paralysis. *In* Adams RD, Victor M: Principles of Neurology, 4th ed. New York, McGraw-Hill, 1989, pp 37–54.

lower and upper extremities. In this case, the facial weakness affects both the upper and lower face and the patient has decreased sensation ipsilaterally in the face. The patient has horizontal diplopia because of weakness of abduction of the affected eye (Fig. 3–4). With lesions in the medulla, there are

deficits in the glossopharyngeal, vagus, and hypoglossal nerves ipsilateral to the lesion with weakness in the upper and lower extremities contralaterally. The patient therefore has difficulty swallowing and the tongue deviates toward the side of the lesion (Fig. 3–5). In addition to these deficits, because the spinothalamic tracts carrying pain and temperature sense and the medial lemniscus tracts carrying proprioception and vibration sense are also in the brain stem and are already decussated, patients have contralateral deficits in pain, temperature, pinprick, vibration, and proprioception sense.

With a spinal cord lesion (Fig. 3–6), the weakness in the lower extremity is ipsilateral to the lesion. Because of damage to the spinothalamic tracts and posterior columns, the patient also has deficits in vibration and proprioception sense, as well as pain, temperature, and pinprick sensation. Characteristically, spinal cord lesions produce a sensory level that corresponds approximately to the location of the lesion. With a hemisection of the spinal cord (Brown-Séquard), there are ipsilateral weakness of the lower extremity; ipsilateral loss of vibration and proprioception sense; and contralateral loss of pinprick, pain, and temperature sensation, the last related to the damage to the already decussated spinothalamic tracts.[3] With lesions in the high cervical cord, in addition to weakness in the lower extremities, there is weakness affecting the upper extremities and possibly the diaphragm.

**Figure 3–2**  Ventral view of the brain stem. (From Brazis PW, Master JC, Biller J: Localization in Clinical Neurology, 2nd ed. Boston, Little, Brown, 1990, p 271.)

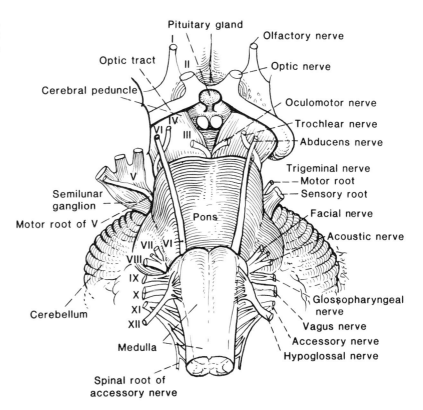

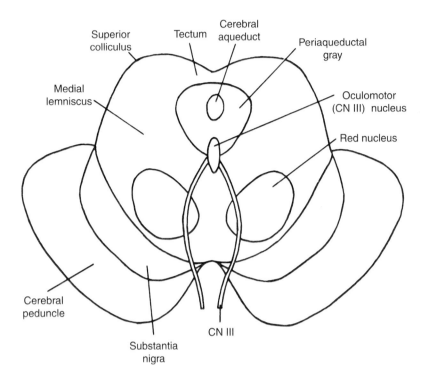

**Figure 3–3** The midbrain. (From Brazis PW, Master JC, Biller J: Localization in Clinical Neurology, 2nd ed. Boston, Little, Brown, 1990, p 281.)

**Figure 3–4** The pons. (From Brazis PW, Master JC, Biller J: Localization in Clinical Neurology, 2nd ed. Boston, Little, Brown, 1990, p 276.)

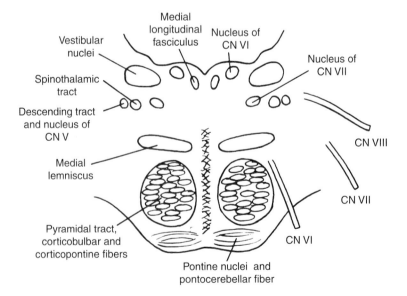

**Figure 3–5** The medulla. (From Brazis PW, Master JC, Biller J: Localization in Clinical Neurology, 2nd ed. Boston, Little, Brown, 1990, p 271.)

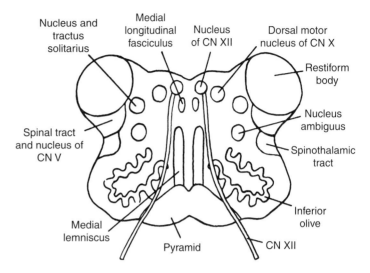

**Figure 3–6** Diagram of ascending and descending pathways of the spinal cord. (From Carpenter MB: Tracts of the spinal cord. *In* Carpenter MB: Core Text of Neuroanatomy, 3rd ed. Baltimore, Williams & Wilkins, 1985, pp 74–101.)

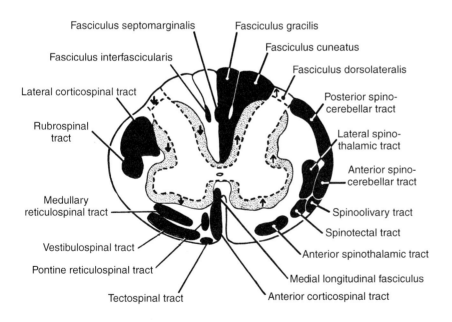

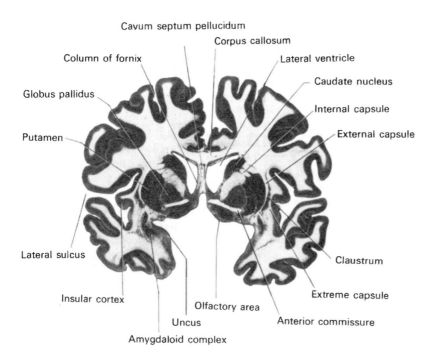

**Figure 3–7** Basal ganglia and related structures. (From Carpenter MB: Corpus striatum and related nuclei. *In* Carpenter MB: Core Text of Neuroanatomy, 3rd ed. Baltimore, Williams & Wilkins, 1985, pp 289–322.)

## LESIONS AFFECTING THE BASAL GANGLIA

For clinical purposes, the basal ganglia structures are considered to be the caudate, putamen, globus pallidus, thalamus, subthalamic nuclei, and substantia nigra (Fig. 3–7). Lesions affecting the basal ganglia characteristically produce movement disorders. There are two major types—hyperkinetic and hypokinetic syndromes.

Hyperkinetic movement disorders include chorea, dystonia, athetosis, myoclonus, and tremor. Chorea refers to random, irregular, rapid involuntary movements. Dystonia refers to torsional and sustained involuntary movements, which can be intermittent or continuous. Athetosis is an intermediate term that is applied to mixed choreiform and dystonic movements affecting the fingers. Tremor is an involuntary, rhythmic oscillation of a body part at a joint. Myoclonus is a rapid "shocklike" muscle contraction. These involuntary movements may be generalized, affect only one side of the body, or be focal or multifocal. They can be continuous or intermittent. When clearly lateralized, the lesion is usually in the contralateral basal ganglia structures. Chorea has been associated with lesions of the caudate nuclei and dystonia with lesions in the putamen; however, more widespread lesions affecting other structures of the basal ganglia can produce similar deficits.[4] Hemiballism, which is characterized by involuntary flail-like writhing, twisting, or rolling movements of the upper and lower extremi-

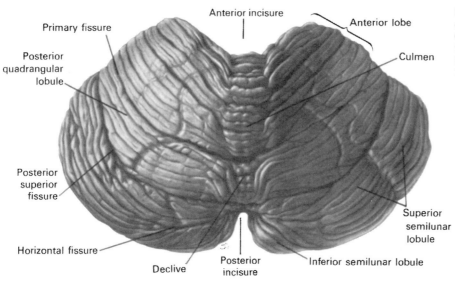

**Figure 3–8** Superior surface of the cerebellum. (From Carpenter MB: Gross anatomy of the brain. *In* Carpenter MB: Core Text of Neuroanatomy, 3rd ed. Baltimore, Williams & Wilkins, 1985, pp 20–51.)

ties, is associated with lesions in the contralateral subthalamic nuclei.[5]

Hypokinetic syndromes are characterized by truncal and appendicular rigidity. Cogwheel rigidity of the extremity is characteristic. The patient may have postural instability, a decrease in automatic movements, disturbances of gait, and slow movements (bradykinesia). The most typical example is that of patients with parkinsonism. This hypokinetic syndrome is indicative of a lesion in the substantia nigra.[4]

Tremor may occur at rest, upon assuming a posture, or upon intention. With lesions in the basal ganglia, tremor occurs at rest and upon assuming a posture. Intention tremor is more typically seen with lesions of the cerebellum.

Myoclonus can be classified broadly as epileptic and nonepileptic. With lesions in the basal ganglia, nonepileptic myoclonus is seen. With seizure disorder, epileptic myoclonus is observed. Epileptic myoclonus is associated with generalized or focal epileptiform discharges in the electroencephalogram indicating cortical neuronal hyperirritability.[6]

## LESIONS AFFECTING THE CEREBELLUM

Lesions in the cerebellum (Fig. 3–8) produce deficits of coordination affecting the movements of the eye, extremities, and trunk. Gaze-evoked nystagmus and ocular dysmetria are found on examination of the eye movements. Truncal instability and ataxia are characterized by a broad-based gait and difficulties with heel-to-toe walking. Intention tremor and dysmetria are found in the upper and lower extremities. Cerebellar lesions produce deficits ipsilateral to the lesion.[4]

## LOWER MOTOR NEURON LESIONS

The lower motor neuron is located in the anterior **horn cell** of the spinal cord. Lesions of the lower motor neuron produce weakness, atrophy, fasciculations, decreased tone, and diminished reflexes (see Table 3–1). The deficit is ipsilateral to the lesion. The lower motor neuron may be affected alone or with the upper motor neuron, as in disorders of motor neurons such as amyotrophic lateral sclerosis. With more diffuse lesions of the spinal cord, deficits are also found in sensations and the corticospinal tract.

## PERIPHERAL NERVE DISORDERS AFFECTING THE LOWER EXTREMITY

### Radiculopathy

Radiculopathies produce pain, sensory, and motor deficits in the distribution of the particular root involved (Table 3–2 and Fig. 3–9). The pain usually radiates from the lower back into the lower extremity. The most common radiculopathies include L5 radiculopathy, which causes weakness of toe extensor and foot dorsiflexion, eversion, and inversion and decreased sensation in the anterolateral aspect of the leg and foot, and S1 radiculopathy, which causes weakness of toe and foot flexion, diminished sensation in the posterior and lateral aspect of the foot, and decreased ankle reflex.

### Lumbosacral Plexopathy

Lesions of the lumbar (L1–4) or sacral (S1–4) plexus (Fig. 3–10) may present with sensory and motor deficits in the distribution of multiple nerves. With lumbar plexus lesions, weakness and sensory loss in the distribution of the femoral and obturator nerve are observed. Lesions of the sacral plexus are

**Table 3–2  Neurologic Features of Lumbar and Sacral Spinal Nerve Root Lesions**

| Nerve Root | Symptoms (Excluding Pain) | Signs |
|---|---|---|
| L-1 | Paresthesias in region of trochanter and upper groin | No motor or reflex changes |
| L-2 | Paresthesias in anterior thigh | Weakness of psoas |
| L-3 | Paresthesias in anterior and medial knee and anterior lower leg ± quadriceps weakness and atrophy | Weakness of psoas and quadriceps; knee jerk depressed |
| L-4 | Paresthesias in medial lower leg and ankle ± quadriceps weakness and atrophy ± footdrop | Weakness of quadriceps, tibialis anterior and posterior; knee jerk depressed |
| L-5 | Paresthesias in anterolateral lower leg and dorsum of foot ± footdrop | Weakness of tibialis anterior, toe extensors, peroneal and gluteal muscles; ankle jerk ± depressed (see text) |
| S-1 | Paresthesias in sole and lateral border of foot and ankle ± weakness of plantar flexion of foot | Weakness of gastrocnemius, toe flexors, peroneal and gluteal muscles; ankle jerk depressed |
| S-2 | Paresthesias in posterior leg ± weakness of plantar flexion of foot | Weakness of gastrocnemius and toe flexors; ankle jerk depressed |
| S-3 | Paresthesias in upper medial thigh and medial buttock | No muscle weakness or reflex changes; bulbocavernosus and anal wink reflexes abnormal |

Modified from Stewart JD: The cauda equina and the lumbar and sacral nerve roots and spinal nerves. *In* Stewart JD: Focal Peripheral Neuropathies, 2nd ed. New York, Raven Press, 1993, pp 261–300

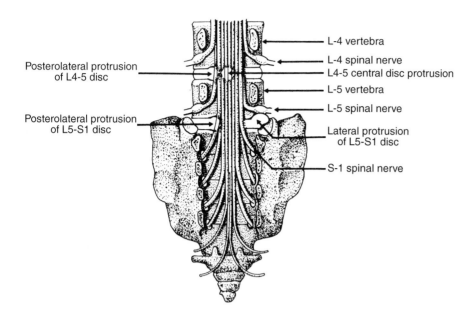

Posterolateral protrusion of L4-5 disc

Posterolateral protrusion of L5-S1 disc

L-4 vertebra

L-4 spinal nerve

L4-5 central disc protrusion

L-5 vertebra

L-5 spinal nerve

Lateral protrusion of L5-S1 disc

S-1 spinal nerve

**Figure 3–9** Dorsal view of the lower lumbar spine and sacrum. (From Stewart JD: The cauda equina and the lumbar and sacral nerve roots and spinal nerves. *In* Stewart JD: Focal Peripheral Neuropathies, 2nd ed. New York, Raven Press, 1993, pp 261–300.)

**Figure 3–10** The lumbosacral plexus. (From Stewart JD: The lumbosacral plexus. *In* Stewart JD: Focal Peripheral Neuropathies, 2nd ed. New York, Raven Press, 1993, pp 301–320.)

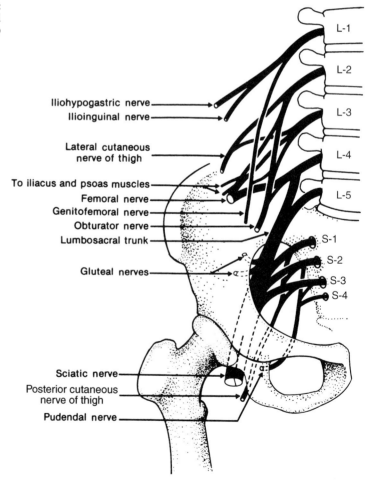

Iliohypogastric nerve

Ilioinguinal nerve

Lateral cutaneous nerve of thigh

To iliacus and psoas muscles

Femoral nerve

Genitofemoral nerve

Obturator nerve

Lumbosacral trunk

Gluteal nerves

Sciatic nerve

Posterior cutaneous nerve of thigh

Pudendal nerve

L-1
L-2
L-3
L-4
L-5
S-1
S-2
S-3
S-4

characterized by weakness and sensory loss in the distribution of gluteal and sciatic nerves. Patients present with back, pelvic, or lower extremity pain followed by sensory symptoms and weakness.

### Iliohypogastric (L1–2), Ilioinguinal (L1–2), and Genitofemoral (L1–2) Nerves

These nerves run across the psoas muscle to supply sensation to the inguinal area, scrotum (labium majus), pubis, external genitalia, and high medial thigh (see Fig. 3–10). Lesions at the plexus, abdominal wall, or inguinal ligament may result in damage to this nerve and resulting pain and sensory loss. Weakness of lower abdominal muscles may occur with lesions of the ilioinguinal nerve. The cremasteric reflex may be lost with lesions of the genitofemoral nerve.

### Femoral Nerve (L2–4)

Femoral nerve lesions result in atrophy of the anterior thigh and weakness of hip flexion and leg extension. The patellar reflex is lost or diminished. Sensory loss or pain occurs on the anterior and medial thigh and medial leg to the ankle. The saphenous branch of the femoral nerve supplies medial leg sensation (Fig. 3–11).

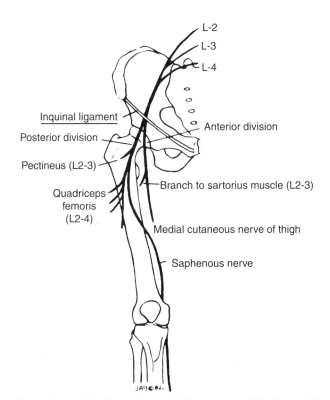

**Figure 3–11** The femoral nerve. (From Brazis PW, Master JC, Biller J: Localization in Clinical Neurology, 2nd ed. Boston, Little, Brown, 1990, p 26.)

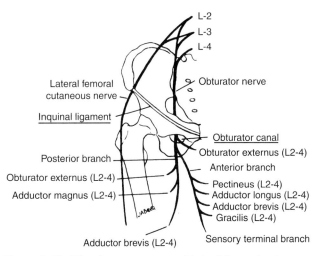

**Figure 3–12** The obturator nerve and lateral femoral cutaneous nerve. (From Brazis PW, Master JC, Biller J: Localization in Clinical Neurology, 2nd ed. Boston, Little, Brown, 1990, p 28.)

### Obturator Nerve (L2–4)

Injury of the nerve produces weakness and wasting of the thigh adductors and sensory deficit of the lower medial thigh (Fig. 3–12).

### Lateral Femoral Cutaneous Nerve (L2–3)

Compression injury of this nerve as it passes beneath the inguinal ligament produces meralgia paresthetica (see Fig. 3–12). This syndrome produces burning pain and sensory loss over the anterolateral thigh.

### Gluteal Nerves (L4 to S1)

These purely motor nerves, which supply the buttocks, may be compressed within the plexus, pelvis, greater sciatic foramen, or buttock (Fig. 3–13). The superior gluteal nerve (L4–5) innervates the gluteus medius, gluteus minimus, and tensor fascia lata. Lesions of this nerve cause weakness of thigh abduction. The inferior gluteal nerve (L5 to S1) innervates the gluteus maximus. Lesions of this nerve result in weak hip extension.

### Posterior Femoral Cutaneous Nerve (S1–2)

Damage to this sensory nerve occurs in the same areas as described for the gluteal nerves. The result is a sensory disturbance in the skin of the posterior thigh and popliteal fossa (see Fig. 3–13).

### Pudendal Nerve (S2–4)

The pudendal nerve supplies the peroneal muscles, the external anal sphincter, and sensation to

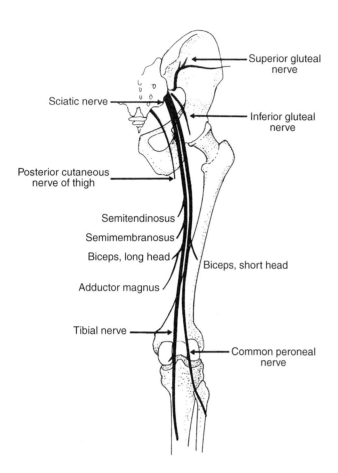

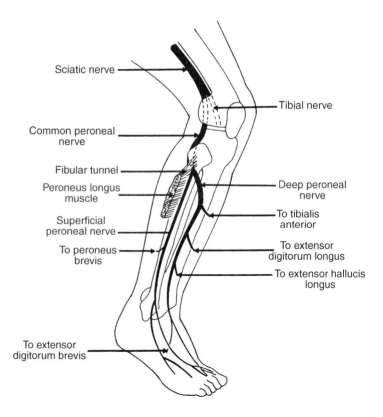

**Figure 3–13**  The sciatic nerve and its branches. (From Stewart JD: The sciatic nerve, the gluteal and pudendal nerve, and the posterior cutaneous nerve of the thigh. *In* Stewart JD: Focal Peripheral Neuropathies, 2nd ed. New York, Raven Press, 1993, pp 321–346.)

**Figure 3–14**  The common peroneal nerve and its branches. (From Stewart JD: The common peroneal nerve. *In* Stewart JD: Focal Peripheral Neuropathies, 2nd ed. New York, Raven Press, 1993, pp 347–366.)

the perineum, pelvis, scrotum (labia majus), and anus. It may be compressed in the greater sciatic notch, producing sensory disturbance or difficulty controlling the bladder and bowel.

### Sciatic (L4 to S2), Peroneal (L4 to S1), and Tibial (L5 to S2) Nerves

The sciatic nerve supplies motor innervation to the posterior thigh, leg, and foot musculature. A high sciatic lesion may result in a flail foot (paralysis of dorsiflexion and plantar flexion) and atrophy and weakness of the hamstrings and all muscles below the knee. The Achilles reflex may be lost or decreased. Sensory deficits are in the outer leg, dorsum, and sole of the foot (see Fig. 3–13).

In the popliteal fossa, the nerve divides into the common peroneal and tibial nerves. The common peroneal is most frequently injured at the fibular neck. Injury produces weakness of foot extension and eversion and weakness of toe extension. Sensory loss is over the lower anterolateral leg and foot dorsum (Fig. 3–14). The tibial nerve innervates the posterior leg muscles for plantar flexion, foot inversion, and toe flexion and abduction. It supplies sensation to the plantar foot (Figs. 3–15 and 3–16). The

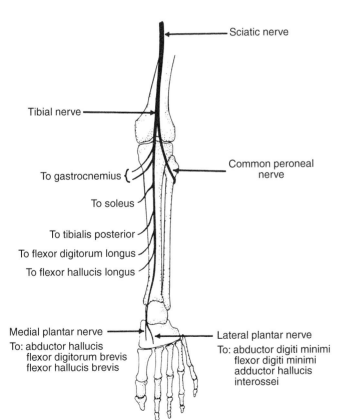

**Figure 3–15** The tibial nerve and its branches. (From Stewart JD: Tibial, plantar, interdigital, and sural nerves. *In* Stewart JD: Focal Peripheral Neuropathies, 2nd ed. New York, Raven Press, 1993, pp 367–386.)

tarsal tunnel syndrome occurs when the tibial nerve is compressed behind the medial malleolus. Here it divides in the distal tunnel into medial and lateral plantar branches. Encroachment by tendons or degenerative bone changes can cause burning pain or sensory deficits in all or part of the plantar foot.

## Sural Neuropathy

The sural nerve is formed from a branch of the common peroneal and tibial nerves. The nerve is predominantly formed from S1 contributions of the tibial nerve. The sural nerve is a pure sensory nerve and lesions cause decreased sensation in the lateral and posterior aspect of the foot, as well as in the distal posterior aspect of the leg (Fig. 3–17).

## Polyneuropathy

In polyneuropathy, the feature is impairment of function of many peripheral nerves simultaneously, resulting in symmetric distal loss of sensory, motor, and autonomic functions. Characteristically, there are distal muscle weakness with or without atrophy, diminished distal sensations, and hyporeflexia or areflexia. In general, the legs are affected earlier and more severely than the arms.

## Disorders of Neuromuscular Junction

The most common disorders of neuromuscular junctions include myasthenia gravis, myasthenic syndrome, and botulinum intoxication. The symptoms and signs of myasthenia gravis are characterized by fluctuating muscle weakness that is exacerbated by physical activity and improved with rest.[7]

Typically, patients with myasthenia gravis have weakness in cranial nerve–innervated muscles, such as extraocular, facial, and pharyngeal muscles. Weakness in the extremities is more proximal than distal. Reflexes are either normal or diminished and there are no sensory deficits. Myasthenia gravis is caused by antibodies against the neuromuscular junction. Myasthenic syndrome typically produces proximal muscle weakness and rarely weakness in the cranial nerve–innervated muscles. Reflexes are usually diminished or absent. Myasthenic syndrome is often a paraneoplastic manifestation. It is caused by antibodies against presynaptic calcium channels.[8]

## Myopathies

Myopathic processes cause predominantly proximal muscle weakness in the upper and lower extremi-

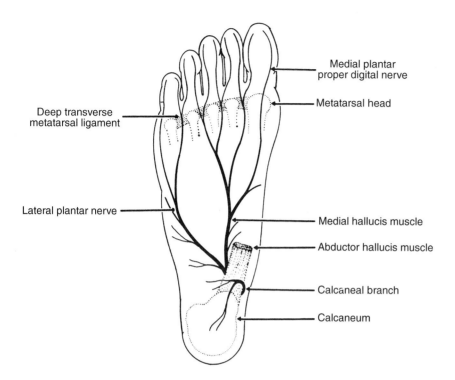

Medial plantar proper digital nerve

Metatarsal head

Deep transverse metatarsal ligament

Lateral plantar nerve

Medial hallucis muscle

Abductor hallucis muscle

Calcaneal branch

Calcaneum

**Figure 3–16**   The lateral and medial plantar nerve. (From Stewart JD: Tibial, plantar, interdigital, and sural nerves. *In* Stewart JD: Focal Peripheral Neuropathies, 2nd ed. New York, Raven Press, 1993, pp 367–386.)

**Figure 3–17**   The sural nerve. (From Stewart JD: The common peroneal nerve. *In* Stewart JD: Focal Peripheral Neuropathies, 2nd ed. New York, Raven Press, 1993, pp 347–366.)

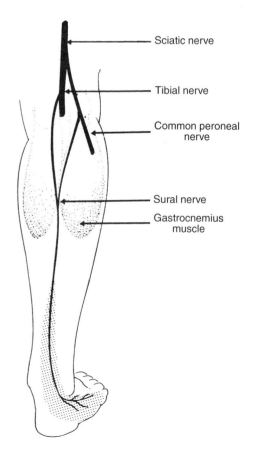

Sciatic nerve

Tibial nerve

Common peroneal nerve

Sural nerve

Gastrocnemius muscle

ties. Weakness may also occur in muscles innervated by cranial nerves, including extraocular, facial, pharyngeal, and neck muscles. Distal weakness
may occur, as in myotonic dystrophy, distal myopathy, facioscapulohumeral dystrophy, scapulopero-
neal dystrophy, and inclusion body polymyositis.
There is associated atrophy of the muscles. There is
no sensory deficit and the reflexes are normal or
diminished.[9]

## SUMMARY

A careful history and physical and neurologic examination constitute the neurologic evaluation. The
neurologic evaluation provides the clinician with
vital data that can be used for localization of the
lesion in the central or peripheral nervous system
and for an assessment of the nature of the lesion.
This leads to appropriate neurologic testing to confirm the diagnosis, which is required for appropriate
management.

## REFERENCES

1. Haerer AF: Corticospinal tract responses. *In* DeJong's the Neurological Examination, 5th ed. Philadelphia, JB Lippincott,
1992, pp 453–464.
2. Masdeu JC: The localization of lesions affecting the cerebral
hemisphere. *In* Brazis PW, Masdeu JC, Biller J: Localization
in Clinical Neurology, 2nd ed. Boston, Little, Brown, 1990,
pp 361–428.
3. Hatter AF: Disorders of the spinal cord. *In* DeJong's the Neurologic Examination, 5th ed. Philadelphia, JB Lippincott, 1992,
pp 578–595.
4. Adams RD, Victor M: Abnormalities of movement and posture
due to disease of the extrapyramidal motor system. *In* Adams
RD, Victor M: Principles of Neurology, 4th ed. New York,
McGraw-Hill, 1989, pp 54–77.
5. Hatter AF: The extrapyramidal level. *In* DeJong's the Neurologic Examination, 5th ed. Philadelphia, JB Lippincott, 1992,
pp 294–305.
6. Adams RD, Victor M: Tremor, myoclonus, spasms and tics. *In*
Adams RD, Victor M: Principles of Neurology, 4th ed. New
York, McGraw-Hill, 1989, pp 78–93.
7. Kimura J: Anatomy and physiology of the neuromuscular
junction. *In* Kimura J: Electrodiagnosis in Diseases of Nerve
and Muscles—Principles and Practice, 2nd ed. Philadelphia,
FA Davis, 1989, pp 169–181.
8. Kimura J: Myasthenia gravis and other disorders of neuromuscular transmission. *In* Kimura J: Electrodiagnosis in Diseases
of Nerve and Muscles—Principles and Practice, 2nd ed. Philadelphia, FA Davis, 1989, pp 519–535.
9. Brooke MH: The symptoms and signs of neuromuscular diseases. *In* Brook MH: A Clinician's View of Neuromuscular
Diseases, 2nd ed. Baltimore, Williams & Wilkins, 1986, pp
1–36.

## BIBLIOGRAPHY

Brazis PW: The localization of lesions affecting the brainstem.
*In* Brazis PW, Master JC, Biller J: Localization in Clinical
Neurology, 2nd ed. Boston, Little, Brown, 1990, pp 269–287.
Brazis PW: The localization of lesions affecting the peripheral
nerves. *In* Brazis PW, Master JC, Biller J: Localization in
Clinical Neurology, 2nd ed. Boston, Little, Brown, 1990,
pp 1–42.
Carpenter MB: Corpus striatum and related nuclei. *In* Carpenter
MB: Core Text of Neuroanatomy, 3rd ed. Baltimore, Wil-
liams & Wilkins, 1985, pp 289–322.
Carpenter MB: Gross anatomy of the brain. *In* Carpenter MB:
Core Text of Neuroanatomy, 3rd ed. Baltimore, Williams &
Wilkins, 1985, pp 20–51.
Stewart JD: The cauda equina and the lumbar and sacral nerve
roots and spinal nerves. *In* Stewart JD: Focal Peripheral
Neuropathies, 2nd ed. New York, Raven Press, 1993, pp
261–300.
Stewart JD: The common peroneal nerve. *In* Stewart JD: Focal
Peripheral Neuropathies, 2nd ed. New York, Raven Press,
1993, pp 347–366.
Stewart JD: The lumbosacral plexus. *In* Stewart JD: Focal Periph-
eral Neuropathies, 2nd ed. New York, Raven Press, 1993,
pp 301–320.
Stewart JD: The sciatic nerve, the gluteal and pudendal nerve,
and the posterior cutaneous nerve of the thigh. *In* Stewart
JD: Focal Peripheral Neuropathies, 2nd ed. New York, Raven
Press, 1993, pp 321–346.
Stewart JD: Tibial, plantar, interdigital, and sural nerves. *In* Stew-
art JD: Focal Peripheral Neuropathies, 2nd ed. New York,
Raven Press, 1993, pp 367–386.

# Neurologic Imaging of the Lower Extremity

# 4

*Vincenzo Giuliano and Mark E. Schweitzer*

## TECHNICAL CONSIDERATIONS

Magnetic resonance (MR) imaging provides a useful noninvasive modality in the evaluation of lower extremity disorders. Detailed evaluation has been augmented by technologic advances in MR scanning technology. One of these is the use of smaller surface coils placed around the anatomic area of interest. This has resulted in significantly improved spatial and contrast resolution for precise delineation of anatomy and morphology while retaining multiplanar capabilities. The second advance is the use of faster and more efficient imaging protocols. Time and expense are still considered limiting factors of MR imaging. However, with further refinements in MR scanning technology, scanners will undoubtedly be more efficient, less costly, and more compact. In particular, limiting pulse sequences and dedicated extremity scanners hold promise for cost-effective MR imaging.

MR has direct application in imaging of the spine and lower extremities. For the spine, the use the T2-weighted fast spin echo (FSE) sequences provides a myelographic effect, in addition to direct visualization of the spinal cord, intervertebral disks, spinal canal, nerve roots, foramina, facet joints, and soft tissues. This technique is faster than that of conventional T2-weighted spin echo sequences. However, fat suppression is required to null the added fat signal and flow compensation to reduce the cerebrospinal fluid pulsation artifact. This technology is available on most current upgraded software packages. In the musculoskeletal system, fat-suppressed T2-weighted fast spin echo and high-resolution intermediate weighted images provide excellent delineation of ligaments, tendons, menisci, cartilage, marrow, and a variety of joint pathologies.

Proper screening procedures should be followed before imaging. These basic measures ensure the safety of patients and image quality. First, because of the strong magnetic fields inherent in most high-field-strength 1.0- to 1.5-T units, the following are considered contraindications to MR imaging: cardiac pacemakers, intraocular metallic foreign bodies, intraspinal electrodes, and first-trimester pregnancy. Although most orthopedic hardware is MR compatible, a metallic artifact in the region of interest greatly distorts image quality and may require protocol modifications that are less sensitive to magnetic susceptibility artifacts. One of these is to use FSE sequences without fat suppression. Also, scans can be performed using a higher bandwidth frequency. A quality control survey should also include removal of articles of clothing or accessories containing metal that would adversely affect image quality. Finally, not infrequently there are questions about whether a metallic implant is MR compatible. A number of excellent references are available concerning the metallic properties of most medically approved metallic devices.[1]

## REFERRED PAIN AND RADICULOPATHY

Radicular pain referred to the lower extremities is invariably the result of some form of lumbar stenosis. The mechanism of radiculopathy involves extradural compression of nerve roots, which can be acquired or developmental. The congenital form of spinal stensosis is caused by short pedicles that narrow the diameter of the spinal canal. This condition is typically asymptomatic until secondary degenerative changes develop, or when accompanied by ligamentum flavum and facet hypertrophy or disk pathology.[2]

Spondylolisthesis is a subtype of acquired spinal stenosis in which vertebral offset narrows the foramina. Spondylolisthesis refers to the offset of one vertebral body over another, which can be forward (anterolisthesis) or backward (retrolisthesis). Spondylolisthesis can be either traumatic or degenerative in nature. The traumatic form involves bilateral laminar fractures of the pars interarticularis (spondylolysis), with 95% occurring at L5. Although the fracture is best demonstrated on plain lumbar radiographs, MR demonstrates the severity of spinal canal compromise and foraminal narrowing (Fig. 4–1). Degenerative spondylolisthesis

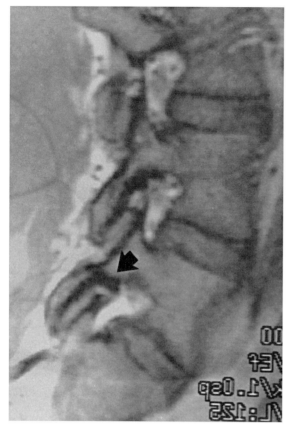

**Figure 4–1** Spondylolysis of L5 (*arrow*) on T1-weighted parasagittal image of the lumbar spine.

The terminology of disk pathology can be confusing. We suggest the following common convention accepted by most radiologists, which characterizes disk pathology on the basis of morphology.[5] A disk protrusion or bulge refers to a broad expansion of the anulus fibrosus. A disk herniation is a frank rupture of the anulus with focal extension of the nucleus pulposus through the defect. If the nucleus pulposus extends completely through the anulus, it becomes an extruded disk. If disk material is separate from the parent disk, it is termed a free fragment or sequestered disk. Disk bulges and herniations can occur in asymptomatic individuals.

Patients with lumbar disk disease present with radicular pain in the thighs, calves, and feet, which can be associated with paresthesias, weakness, and reflex change. Pain is exacerbated by sitting and leg straightening or elevation. More than 90% of disk herniations occur at L4-5 and L-5 to S-1. Lumbar MR evaluation is performed in both the sagittal and axial planes. The sagittal view best demonstrates the herniated disk (Fig. 4–2). The parasagittal view can demonstrate the obliteration of normal neural foraminal fat by lateral extension of the herniated disk. Lateral disk herniations are "blind" to myelography and should be carefully assessed on MR images. The axial view demonstates asymmetry of the

occurs in the older population and results from severe bilateral facet degeneration with resultant joint offset, most commonly at the L4-5 level. Facet and ligamentum flavum hypertrophy often accompanies the degenerative changes.[2] In contradistinction to myelography, MR imaging is performed with the patient in the supine position, which alters the mechanical effects of vertebral body offset on nerve roots.

Disk pathology is another major cause of acquired lumbar stenosis resulting in radiculopathy. The normal intervertebral disk is composed of a gelatinous material called the nucleus pulposus, which is about 85% water. The nucleus pulposus is surrounded by a collagenous capsule, the anulus fibrosus. The aqueous property of the disk accounts for its ability to cushion axial forces on the spine.[3] The basic pathophysiology of disk degeneration includes loss of water content with disk aging, which can occur as result of radial or annular tears. In addition, the anulus can become thin, providing an anatomic site for disk protrusion or frank herniation. Disk degeneration is characterized by a decreased T2 signal and decreased disk height, often accompanied by reactive endplate marrow changes, and osteophytes. Facet arthritis can also accompany disk degeneration.[4]

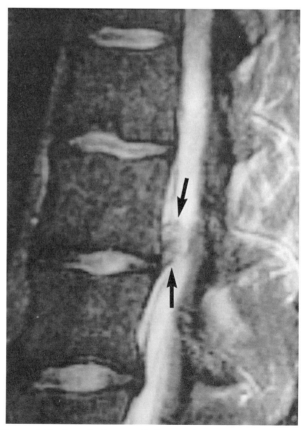

**Figure 4–2** Superiorly extruded L3-4 disc (*arrows*) on sagittal T2-weighted image of the lumbar spine.

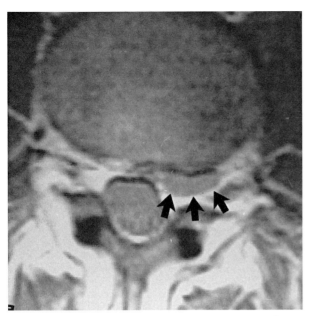

**Figure 4–3** Left foramenal disc herniation (*arrows*) with nerve root compromise on axial T1-weighted image of the lumber spine.

posterior disk margin and displacement of adjacent intraspinal structures (Fig. 4–3). The posterior longitudinal ligament is thick in the middle and therefore acts as a normal anatomic point of resistance. As a result, most disk herniations occur lateral to the posterior longitudinal ligament, in a posterolateral orientation, most often coursing inferiorly toward the foramen at the next lower level to impinge on the lower traversing nerve root. The upper nerve root is compromised only when there is a superolaterally sequestered free fragment in the neural foramen.[6] In addition, the facet joints should be assessed for visible fluid, which is hyperintense on fat-suppressed T2-weighted images. This is considered abnormal and may represent a biomechanical response or arthritic disease.

## REFLEX SYMPATHETIC DYSTROPHY

Reflex sympathetic dystrophy (RSD) is a common vasomotor disturbance that can occur in the lower extremities and is manifested by painful hyperesthesia and trophic skin changes. Although trauma appears to be the most common precipitating cause, the prevalence of the disorder is highest after peripheral nerve injury. Associated injuries include fractures, dislocations, sprains, posttraumatic brain injury or tumors, and myocardial infarction. Failure to diagnose and treat RSD can result in permanent functional impairment and disability. Current treatment involves sympathetic denervation or neural blockade.[7]

MR is the best noninvasive test of RSD, with a sensitivity of 87% and a specificity of 100%. Bone scintigraphy also provides a noninvasive means of diagnosis but has a lower sensitivity of about 60%, especially in the detection of early manifestations of the disease.[8] In contradistinction to earlier reports and to related disorders of transient osteoporosis and regional migratory osteoporosis, marrow edema is not associated with RSD. This can be an important differential feature on MR imaging. Contrast enhancement with gadolinium chelates is utilized in MR imaging protocols. In early or stage I RSD (the warm, vasodilated stage), MR imaging demonstrates periarticular or subcutaneous enhancement, skin thickening, and occasional muscle and fascial edema (Fig. 4–4). In advanced or stage II and III RSD (the vasoconstrictive stage), there is no significant enhancement. Stage III disease is characterized by muscle atrophy. Treatment success generally correlates with the severity of the disease. Therefore, it is most desirable to diagnose this disorder in early-stage disease and expedite treatment to improve function. The ability to characterize stage III disease is also important because treatment is usually ineffective.[8]

## TENDONS

The major tendons of the foot and ankle include the Achilles tendon posteriorly, the posterior tibial tendon (PTT) medially, and the lateral peroneal tendons. The Achilles tendon originates from the gastrocnemius and soleus tendons and inserts on the superior aspect of the posterior calcaneus. The Achilles tendon is unique in that it lacks a synovial sheath and instead is surrounded by a paratenon. Achilles tendon injury occurs with sports that involve running or jumping. Clinically, there is weak or absent plantar flexion. Acute tendinitis is associated with edema in the pre-Achilles fat pad, variable increased internal signal within the tendon, and normal tendon morphology. The internal signal is either normal or characterized as multiple dots, which can also be seen in interstitial tendon degeneration. With more chronic tendinitis, the tendon morphology is altered and the tendon appears to enlarge focally at its insertion (Figs. 4–5 and 4–6). On axial images, the tendon loses its normal lenticular shape and becomes round or ovoid. A vertically oriented linear increased signal is characteristic of either interstitial degeneration, which appears as a dot-dash pattern, or an interstitial tear, which is more continuous. Partial tears have a horizontal orientation.[9]

Tendon rupture occurs in the most avascular zone, approximately 2 to 6 cm from the insertion on

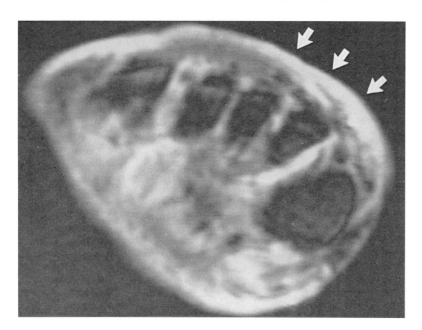

**Figure 4–4** Stage I reflex sympathetic dystrophy with dorsal subcutaneous and skin enhancement and thickening (*arrows*) on fat-suppressed, contrast-enhanced axial T1-weighted image of the foot.

the posterior calcaneus. A positive Thompson test, absence of normal plantar flexion with squeezing of the gastrocnemius-soleus muscle bellies, is consistent with Achilles tendon rupture.[9] The presence of soleus or gastrocnemius atrophy precludes direct tendon repair and tendon reconstruction is considered. Atrophy is characterized by an increased internal signal within the muscle on T1-weighted images, compatible with fatty replacement.[10]

PTT dysfunction is associated with medial ankle instability resulting in collapse of the longitu-

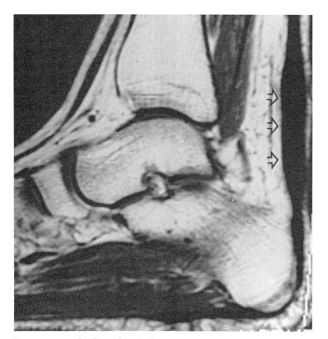

**Figure 4–5** Thickened Achilles tendon (*arrows*) consistent with chronic Achilles tendonitis on sagittal T1-weighted image of the ankle.

dinal arch of the foot. Medial arch pain and painful flatfoot deformity are consistent with this type of injury. The most frequent site of tendon rupture is the avascular zone between the medial malleolus and point of insertion on the navicular.[11] Complete PTT tears with gaps, although commonly seen in the rotator cuff, are unusual in the PTT. More typical is either enlargement or atrophy of the tendon, with variable increased internal signal or edema around the tendon. Using the flexor digitorum tendon as a reference point for morphology, the size of the PTT should be twice that of the adjacent flexor digitorum tendon. Secondary signs of PTT dysfunction include medial subluxation of the navicular in relation to the talus and plantar flexion of the talus with respect to the navicular. Another secondary sign is the presence of an accessory navicular, which is associated with an increased incidence of PTT tears. A cornuate navicular occurs when there is hypertrophy of the medial tubercle leading to an asymmetric navicular that acts biomechanically like a fused accessory navicular. A cornuate navicular is also associated with an increased incidence of PTT tears.[12]

The peroneal tendons are strong evertors and weak plantar flexors of the foot, as well as being the lateral stabilizers of the ankle joint. The peroneal tendons pass around the lateral aspect of the ankle in the retromalleolar sulcus via a fibro-osseous tunnel formed by the fibula, tendon sheaths, and calcaneofibular and posterior talofibular ligaments. The superior peroneal retinaculum maintains the peroneal tendons within the retromalleolar sulcus and is often torn with PTT injury. Injury of the peroneal tendons occurs after simultaneous dorsiflexion of the foot with violent reflex contraction of the pero-

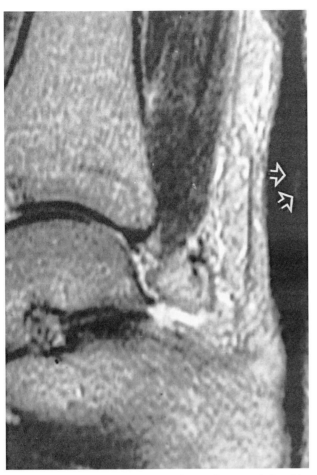

**Figure 4–6** Thickened Achilles tendon with internal signal hyperintensity (*arrows*) consistent with a superimposed tear on fat-suppressed sagittal T2-weighted image of the ankle.

neal musculature. Tenderness and swelling along the posterolateral aspect of the ankle are typical, with inability to evert the foot. A provocative test that distinguishes PTT injury from a lateral ankle sprain is eversion of the foot against resistance, resulting in pain.[13] Like PTT tears, complete peroneal tendon tears are unusual. In addition, tendinitis, which is a frequent precursor for most tendons, is uncommon with the peroneal tendons. More frequently, patients develop specific types of peroneal syndromes. One syndrome is characterized by either lateral subluxation of the tendons from the retromalleolar sulcus, and another by stenosing tenosynovitis secondary to synovial hypertrophy and fibrosis analogous to adhesive capsulitis of the shoulder. The former is related to calcaneal fractures that avulse the calcaneal insertion of the peroneal retinaculum and result in peroneal tendon subluxation. Chronic subluxation can lead to peroneal split syndrome, with longitudinal dissection of the peroneus brevis (Fig. 4–7). MR image evaluation should begin distal to the end of the fibula because false-positive peroneal splits and dislocation or subluxations occur at more cranial levels.[14]

## COMPRESSIVE NEUROPATHIES

The most frequent compressive neuropathies of the ankle and foot are tarsal tunnel syndrome and Morton's neuroma. Tarsal tunnel syndrome is caused by entrapment of the posterior tibial nerve within the tarsal tunnel, occasionally caused by a space-occupying lesion. Causes include ganglion cysts, neurogenic tumors, varicosities, lipomas, synovial or muscle hypertrophy, or scar tissue. Pain and paresthesia are localized in the plantar aspect of the foot. The primary role of MR in this setting is to determine the presence of a tarsal tunnel mass for preoperative evaluation. Although rare, masses are not infrequent causes of tarsal tunnel syndrome. A mass effect can result in edema superficial to the flexor retinaculum and between flexor tendon sheaths.[15]

Morton's neuroma is the result of thickening and degeneration of the plantar digital nerve between the third and fourth metatarsal heads. The MR imaging features are those of a hypointense mass on both T1- and T2-weighted images, with variable enhancement

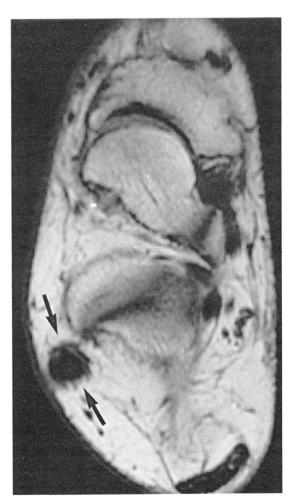

**Figure 4–7** Split peroneus brevis tendon (*arrows*) consistent with peroneal split syndrome on axial intermediate-weighted image of the ankle.

on fat-suppressed T1-weighted images. The signal characteristics are compatible with the fibrous composition of the lesion.[15]

Sinus tarsi syndrome is a clinical entity associated with pain in the sinus. The pathophysiology is nonspecific but can be associated with lateral ligament tears. MR imaging findings include edema or fibrous replacement of the normal fat in the sinus. However, false-positive MR examinations, particularly for edema, are frequent.[14]

## REFERENCES

1. Shellock FG, Kanal E: Bioeffects and safety of MR procedures. *In* Edelman RR, Hesselink JR, Zlatkin MB (eds.): Clinical Magnetic Resonance Imaging, 2nd ed. Philadelphia, WB Saunders, 1996, pp 391–434.
2. Coventry MB: Anatomy of the intervertebral disc. Clin Orthop 67:9–15, 1969.
3. Sether LA, Yu S, Haughton VM, Fischer ME: Intervertebral disc: Normal age-related changes in MR signal intensity. Radiology 177:385–388, 1990.
4. Natarajan RN, Ke KH, Andersson GB: A model to study the disc degeneration process. Spine 19:259–265, 1994.
5. Thornbury JR, Fryback DG, Turski PA, et al: Disc-caused nerve compression in patients with acute low-back pain: Diagnosis with MR, CT, myelography, and plain CT. Radiology 186:731–738, 1993.
6. Jinkins JR, Matthes JC, Sener RN, et al: Spondylosis, spondylolisthesis, and associated nerve root entrapment in the lumbosacral spine: MR evaluation. AJR 159:799–803, 1992.
7. Schwartzman RJ, McLellan TL: Reflex sympathetic dystrophy: A review. Arch Neurol 44:555–561, 1987.
8. Schweitzer ME, Mandel S, Schwartzman RJ, et al: Reflex sympathetic dystrophy revisited: MR imaging findings before and after infusion of contrast material. Radiology 195:211–214, 1995.
9. Frey CC, Shereff MJ: Tendon injuries of the ankle in athletes. Clin Sports Med 7:103–118, 1988.
10. Quinn SF, Murray WT, Clark RA, et al: Achilles tendon: MR imaging at 1.5T. Radiology 164:767–776, 1987.
11. Frey CC, Shereff MJ: Vascularity of the posterior tibial tendon. J Bone Joint Surg [Am] 72:884–888, 1990.
12. Schweitzer ME, Caccase R, Karasick D, et al: Posterior tibial tendon tears: Utility of secondary signs for MR diagnosis. Radiology 88:655–659, 1993.
13. Mann RA, Coughlin MJ: Surgery of the Foot and Ankle, 6th ed. St. Louis, CV Mosby, 1993, pp 1167–1179.
14. Schweitzer ME, Karasick D: MR of the ankle and hindfoot. Semin Ultrasound CT MR 15:410–422, 1994.
15. Beltran J: The ankle and foot. *In* Edelman RR, Hesselink JR, Zlatkin MB (eds.): Clinical Magnetic Resonance Imaging, 2nd ed. Philadelphia, WB Saunders, 1996, pp 2018–2020.

# Somatosensory Evoked Potentials

# in the Lower Extremity

# 5

*Leopold J. Streletz*

Cortical and spinal cord potentials have been used to evaluate reliably the functional integrity of the somatosensory pathways in the lower extremities of humans for 20 years. The technical difficulty of recording surface rostral spinal cord potentials has been overcome by recording from more caudal spine locations, permitting differentiation of peripheral from central disorders of afferent conduction. These studies remain limited by the neurophysiologic fact that the somatosensory evoked potential (SEP) reflects ascending sensory pathway function, which is independent of the descending motor pathways with the exception of contiguous lesions. This discussion is focused mainly on the technical aspects and clinical applications of the lower extremity SEP.

## METHODOLOGY OF SOMATOSENSORY EVOKED POTENTIALS

The following methods conform to the published guidelines of the American Clinical Neurophysiology Society.[1]

### Stimulation

Electroencephalographic disk, needle, or electromyographic stimulating electrodes are commonly used. The impedance of the electrode should be reduced below 10 kilohms to reduce discomfort and the stimulator output isolated to ensure subject safety and minimize stimulus artifact. A band or plate ground electrode is placed between the stimulating and distal recording electrodes.

Whether the posterior tibial nerve at the ankle or the common peroneal nerve at the knee is used depends on the clinical circumstances and personal preference. For posterior tibial nerve stimulation at the ankle, the cathode is placed midway between the medial border of the Achilles tendon and the posterior border of the medial malleolus with the anode 3 cm distal. For common peroneal nerve stimulation at the knee, the cathode is placed over the lateral portion of the popliteal fossa, postmedial to the tendon of the biceps femoris muscle and the inferior leg crease, with the anode 3 cm distal. Der-

matomal peripheral nerve stimulation has not proved to be of great diagnostic value in clinical practice.

A square wave pulse of 200 μs. duration at a rate of 4 to 7 per second (not an integral of 60 Hz) is recommended. The stimulus intensity should be sufficient to produce visible vigorous muscle twitches, which are monitored continually during the recording. The right and left nerve trunks are stimulated independently. However, bilateral stimulation may be useful in some situations (e.g., spinal cord monitoring) to enhance the amplitude of the response. Whether constant current is superior to constant voltage in stimulation remains debatable, but where impedances are unstable, a constant-current stimulator is preferred.

### Recording

Because SEP recordings may be affected by myogenic contamination, the patient should be made to relax, usually in the prone or semiprone position. If this is not successful, a mild hypnotic drug such as chloral hydrate may be used.

The bandpass for the SEP recording amplifier is 5 to 30 to 1500 to 3000 Hz ($-3$ dB) with a gain of $10^4$. The ongoing signal averaging is monitored on the oscilloscope or averager display for artifacts, and artifact rejection is utilized. An analysis time between 60 and 100 ms is recommended, and 1000 to 2000 individual trials should be averaged with replication of two or more averages. Standard electroencephalographic disk electrodes are used, and the recommended montage varies according to the nerve stimulated.

SEPs to posterior tibial nerve stimulation (SEP-T) occur within 50 ms after the stimulus in normal adults. Scalp components are labeled P38 and N45 and the nerve trunk potential in the popliteal fossa is termed the PF potential. For recording the PF potential, an electrode is placed in the popliteal fossa 4 to 6 cm above the popliteal crease midway between the hamstring tendons with a reference electrode on the medial surface of the knee. Elec-

37

trode placements over the spine at L3, T12, and C2 are recommended. Two scalp electrodes are placed on $C_z'$ (2 cm posterior to vertex) and $F_z$ or $F_{pz}'$ (2 cm posterior to $F_{pz}$). The following four-channel montage is suggested: channel 1, $C_z'$-$F_{pz}'$; channel 2, T12–4 cm rostral to T12 or reference; channel 3, L3–4 cm rostral to L3 or reference; channel 4, PF-reference. Alternatively, the following montage has proved useful in our laboratory: channel 1, $C_z'$-$F_z$; channel 2, SC (C2)–$F_z$; channel 3, CE (L3)–IC (iliac crest reference contralateral to stimulus); and optionally channel 4, PF-reference (Fig. 5–1).[1]

SEPs to common peroneal nerve stimulation (SEP-P) occur within 40 ms of the stimulus. Scalp potentials are labeled P27 and N35. Components recorded over the spine are designated L3, T12, and T6 (indicating the spinous process level of the recording). To record the scalp potentials, electrodes are located as for SEP-T. The spinal potentials require six electrodes placed over the L3 spinous process 4 cm rostral to L3, the T12 spinous process, 4 cm rostral T12, the T6 spinous process, and 4 cm rostral to T6. An alternative to bipolar recordings over the spine is use of a reference (shoulder, hand, or ear). The following four-channel montage is suggested: channel 1, $C_z'$-$F_{pz}'$; channel 2, T6–4 cm rostral to T6 or reference; channel 3, T12–4 cm rostral T12 or reference; channel 4, L3–4 cm rostral to L3 or reference.

## Data Analysis and Criteria of Abnormality

In analyzing the SEP, attention is directed to the latency and amplitude of individual components,

interwave intervals, and the configuration of the responses. As with pattern-reversal visual evoked potentials and the brain stem auditory evoked potential, latency differences between sides are a sensitive and reliable measurement. It is suggested that limb measurements be taken between stimulating cathode and the L3 spine electrode and between that site and the vertex ($C_z'$). This allows the calculation of conduction velocities for more precise differentiation of peripheral and central disorders. Generally, the inter- and intrasubject variability in amplitude of the SEP components markedly limits the usefulness of absolute amplitude data. Finally, it cannot be overemphasized that the SEP should never be interpreted as abnormal simply on the basis of "eyeballing."[2]

In SEP-T recordings, analysis is suggested for the following: (1) in the PF lead, the presence and onset or peak latency of the PF potential; (2) in the spine leads, the presence and onset or peak latency of the L3 (CE) and C2 (SC₂) potentials; and (3) in the scalp lead, the presence and peak latencies of the P38 and N45 (Table 5–1).

The criteria of abnormality for SEPs are as follows:

1. Absence of both spine and scalp responses in recordings using analysis times of 100 to 200 ms.

2. Conduction times or conduction velocities above or below 2.5 to 3.0 standard deviations of the mean age for an age-matched control population.

3. Absence of spine potentials in the presence of scalp responses of normal latency should not be interpreted as abnormal. Changes in amplitude or waveform may not be reliable criteria of abnormality and should be interpreted with caution.

The preceding recommendations reflect the method generally used in our laboratory. It should be appreciated that other laboratories use somewhat different methods to obtain nonetheless reliable lower extremity SEP recordings. For instance, rather than determining conduction velocities, some laboratories use a latency-height nomogram.[3, 4]

## NONPATHOLOGIC VARIATION OF SOMATOSENSORY EVOKED POTENTIALS

The previous description of technique is expected to control for variation related to stimulus parameters, bandpass, and electrode placement.

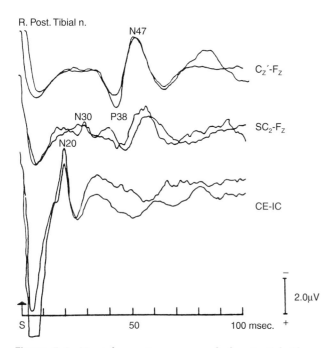

R. Post. Tibial n.

N47

$C_z'$-$F_z$

N30  P38

SC₂-$F_z$

N20

CE-IC

2.0μV

S          50          100 msec.          +

**Figure 5–1** Normal somatosensory evoked potential (three-channel montage).

**Table 5–1    Normal Ranges for Posterior Tibial Nerve Somatosensory Evoked Potentials**

| Parameter | Latency (ms) P38 | Interside Latency Difference (MS) P38 | Latency (ms) N47 | Amplitude (μV) P38-N47 | Latency (ms) P60 |
|---|---|---|---|---|---|
| Mean | 37.6 | 1.0 | 47.3 | 2.7 | 59.5 |
| Standard deviation (SD) | 2.4 | 0.7 | 6.5 | 1.0 | 11.3 |
| Upper limit (mean + 2.5SD) | 43.6 | 2.8 | 63.6 | | 87.8 |

**Age.** Age has been shown to affect spine sensory conduction in children and adults (older than 60).[6] Cracco and colleagues[7] found that conduction velocities in peripheral nerve and spinal cord in the newborn infant were one half of adult values but spinal cord values did not reach adult levels until about 5 years of age.

**Height.** Latency varies directly with limb length, which must be taken into consideration when interpreting the absolute latency of scalp SEP components. The development of a latency-height nomogram is a reliable way to compensate for this variation in adults, as previously discussed.

**Other.** Other factors such as sleep and drugs have not been systematically studied but probably have some effect on scalp SEP components.

## GENERATOR SOURCES

In the SEP recorded from surface electrodes over the lumbar spine (L3), the major negative component (N20) is consistent with potentials arising in the lumbosacral roots of the cauda equina (see Fig. 5–1). The second negative wave following it is thought to arise in postsynaptic ventral roots or volume conducted postsynaptic activity in caudal spinal cord.[7, 8]

Over the rostral spinal cord the small triphasic potential with poorly defined positive phases (N30) has progressively increased in latency from more caudal spine recording locations with decreasing amplitude.[9] It has been suggested that in humans these potentials arise in multiple rapidly conducting afferent pathways, including the dorsal columns and dorsolateral columns, lying primarily ipsilateral to the stimulated nerves.[10–12]

The scalp-recorded SEP using bipolar leads ($C_z'$ - $F_z'$), the P38 and N45 with tibial nerve stimulation and P27 and N35 with peroneal nerve stimulation can be recorded in all normal subjects. Earlier smaller, negative, subcortical components may be resolved in noncephalic reference recordings.[13] The P38 and P27 potentials, however, are more easily recorded in all subjects and may serve as a reliable latency indicator for arrival of the afferent valley in

the somesthetic cortex contralateral to the side of stimulation.[14]

## CLINICAL APPLICATIONS

The main clinical reason for the use of SEPs is to identify and locate a lesion(s) involving the somatosensory pathways. The presence of an abnormality, however, may not provide more information than the clinical neurologic examination. Normal findings never exclude the possibility of organic disease as a cause of symptoms. Furthermore, the presence of a SEP abnormality does not indicate the specific nature of a disease process.

### Peripheral Nerve and Root Lesions

Peripheral nerve and root lesions may produce slowed conduction velocities proximal to segments generally tested by Electroneuromyogography (ENMG). The SEP helps localize the pathology in such a case.[15] Investigation of the usefulness of SEPs in lumbosacral root disease have been limited and indicate that it is no more sensitive than conventional ENMG or late responses.[3, 16] Similarly, plexus lesions and discrete peripheral nerve lesions are best evaluated by conventional nerve conduction studies and needle electromyography. In cases of psychogenic sensory loss, including proprioception, of the leg or foot, normal SEPs may be helpful in confirming the diagnosis.

### Spinal Cord Lesion

A number of studies of spinal cord lesions have used long-latency scalp SEPs to evaluate the extent of lesions and outcome in patients with trauma.[17, 18] Spine and scalp SEPs were investigated in a group of patients with various diseases of the spinal cord.[19] Focal spinal cord compressive lesions generally resulted in prolonged peak latencies of rostral spine and scalp potentials, which slowed the spine-to-scalp conduction velocities. Spine and scalp SEPs may be useful in the evaluation of infants and children with occult spinal dysraphism.[9]

Several studies have compared the upper and lower extremity SEPs in patients with multiple sclerosis and found a higher incidence of abnormalities in lower extremity studies.[20, 21] This higher yield in lower extremity SEP studies probably reflects the greater length of white matter pathways tested and vulnerable to the demyelinating disease.

## Diffuse Neurologic Diseases

Diffuse neurologic diseases may produce slowing of spinal and scalp SEP components. Conduction velocity over peripheral nerve was normal in patients with metabolic degenerative disease (primarily gray matter).[22] Conduction velocities of SEPs over the spinal cord were slowed in these patients. Spinal and peripheral nerve conduction velocities were slowed in some clinically asymptomatic patients with juvenile diabetes.[6] Rossini and colleagues[23] found slowing of conduction in central somatosensory pathways in patients with chronic renal failure and spinocerebellar disorders.

## SUMMARY

The upper and lower extremity SEPs, like other evoked potentials, are extensions of the clinical neurologic examination. They provide accurate, objective, and reproducible data from the somatosensory system in humans and may, under certain circumstances, be more sensitive than the clinical evaluation. Proper performance and technique are prerequisites to clinical interpretation and correlation. With attention to the normal test variability and the neuroanatomic constraints of the pathways, the SEP is a versatile and sensitive diagnostic tool for the evaluation of neurologic disease.

## REFERENCES

1. Gilmore RL: American EEG society guideline for clinical evoked potential studies. J. Clin Neurophysiol 11:11–147, 1994.
2. Andrew E, Roger QC: Overuse of evoked potentials: Caution. Clin Neurology 33:618–621, 1983
3. Chiappa K: Evoked Potentials in Clinical Medicine, 2nd ed. New York, Raven Press, 1990, pp 204–213.
4. Lastimosa AC, Bass NY, Stanback K, Norvell EE: Lumbar spinal cord and early cortical potentials after tibial nerve stimulation: Effects of normative data. Electroencephalogr Clin Neurophysiol 54:499–507, 1982.
5. Dorfman LJ, Bosley TM: Age-related changes in peripheral and central conduction in man. Neurology 29:38–44, 1979.
6. Cracco JB, Cracco RQ, Graziani LJ: The spinal evoked response in infants and children. Neurology 25:31–36, 1975.
7. Dimitrijevis MR, Larsson LE, Lehmkuhl D, Sherwood AM: Evoked spinal cord and nerve root potentials in humans using a noninvasive recording technique. Electroencephalogr Clin Neurophysiol 45:331–340, 1978.
8. Phillips LH, Daube JR: Lumbosacral spinal evoked potentials in humans. Neurology 30:1175–1183, 1980.
9. Cracco JB, Cracco RQ: Spinal somatosensory evoked potentials: Maturational and clinical studies. Ann N Y Acad Sci 388:526–537, 1982.
10. Cracco RQ, Evans B: Spinal evoked potentials in the cat: Effects of asphyxia, strychnine, cord section and compression. Electroenceph Clin Neurophysiol 44:187–201, 1978.
11. Feldman MH, Cracco RQ, Farmer P, Mount F: Spinal evoked potentials in the monkey. Ann Neurol 7:238–244, 1980.
12. Sarnowski RJ, Cracco RQ, Vogel HB, Mount F: Spinal evoked potentials in the monkey. Ann Neurol 43:329–336, 1975.
13. Leuders H, Andrish J, Gurd A, et al: Origin of far field subcortical potentials evoked by stimulation of the posterior tibial nerve. Electroencephalogr Clin Neurophysiol 52:336–344, 1981.
14. Vas GA, Cracco JB and Cracco RQ: Scalp-recorded short latency cortical and subcortical somatosensory evoked potentials to peroneal nerve stimulation. Electroenceph Clin Neurophysiol 52:1–8, 1981.
15. Desmedt JE, Noel P: Average cerebral evoked potentials in the evaluation of lesions of the sensory nerves and of the central somatosensory pathway. In Desmedt JE (ed): New Developments in Electromyography and Clinical Neurophysiology, Vol 2. New York, S, Karger, 1973, pp 352–371.
16. Elleker G, Eisen A: Segmental sensory stimulation and SEPs: Normative data and clinical application. Neurology 30:372–373, 1980.
17. Dorfman LJ, Perkash I, Bosley TM, Cummins KL: Use of cerebral evoked potentials to evaluate spinal somatosensory function in patients with traumatic and surgical myelopathies. J Neurosurg 52:654–660, 1980.
18. Perot PL, Vera CL: Scalp-recorded somatosensory evoked potentials to stimulation of nerves in the lower extremities and evaluation of patients with spinal cord trauma. Ann N Y Acad Sci 388:359–368, 1982.
19. Schiff J, Cracco RQ, Rossini PM, Cracco JB: Spine and scalp somatosensory evoked potentials in normal subjects and patients with spinal cord disease: Evaluation of afferent transmission. Electroencephalogr Clin Neurophysiol 59:374–387, 1984.
20. Eisen A, Odusote K: Central and peripheral conduction times in multiple sclerosis. Electroencephalogr Clin Neurophysiol 48:2553–2265, 1980.
21. Khoshbin S, Hallett M: Multimodality evoked potentials and blink reflex in multiple sclerosis. Neurology 31:138–133, 1981.
22. Cracco JB, Bosch VV, Cracco RQ: Cerebral and spinal somatosensory evoked potentials in children with CNS degenerative disease. Electroencephalogr Clin Neurophysiol 49:437–445, 1980.
23. Rossini PM, Treviso M, DiStefano E, DiPaolo B: Nervous impulse propagation along peripheral and central fibers in patients with chronic renal failure. Electroencephalogr Clin Neurophysiol 56:293–303, 1983.

# Gait Disorders

# 6

*Leo McCluskey*

The examination of gait is an absolutely essential component of a comprehensive neurologic examination. Much can be learned from the observation of this complex yet automatic motor act, which depends on the integrity of the entire neuraxis and involves the interplay of multiple neurologic systems. Unless there is substantial concern about the welfare of the patient, the gait examination should not be eliminated either for the convenience of the examiner or because of concern for an uncomfortable or bedridden patient. In fact, not infrequently an abnormal gait is the only "positive" finding on a complete neurologic examination and thus provides the only clue to a differential diagnosis. It is also common to find that an examination of the gait provides vital additional clues to other neurologic examination findings and thus aids in the formulation of a complete differential diagnosis.

## NORMAL GAIT

The act of walking or running upright in a bipedal fashion depends on the effective performance of stereotyped upper and lower alternating limb movements superimposed on the necessary maintenance of the center of gravity of the body over the narrow lower extremity platform through continuous postural adjustments. The stereotyped limb and postural movements must also be highly adaptable in order to accommodate to the various environmental changes one encounters. It is through the effective integrated performance of the automatic-stereotyped and adaptable components that a normal gait is produced.

Ultimately, it is muscular contraction that provides the force necessary to overcome gravity, maintain an upright posture, and walk. The balance of forces generated by muscular agonists and antagonists acting at each joint can determine static limb position and posture. When walking or when the body is in motion, it is the effective integration of the force output of the same muscular agonists and antagonists that allows not only smooth performance of a motor act but also maintenance of the upright posture.

The motor unit (single anterior horn cell or mo-

tor neuron with its axon innervating a collection of muscle cells) constitutes the final common pathway in this system. Residing completely within the spinal cord and brain stem, local pathways link groups of related motor neurons innervating agonist and antagonist muscles ipsilaterally and bilaterally, thus forming a network that is capable of producing the series of muscular activations required for locomotion. Such a "central pattern generator" is probably of secondary importance in primates and perhaps particularly in humans. Acting on the anterior horn cell and the central pattern generator is a collection of descending pathways emanating from regions within the basal ganglia, red nuclei, pontine nuclei, vestibular nuclei, and other brain stem nuclei responsible for posture and locomotion. The descending corticobulbar pathway most likely acts on these regions to initiate and modulate gait. The cerebral cortex must, of course, provide the capacity to alter voluntarily the stereotyped limb movements generated by the subcortical structures.

The sensory system, consisting of various sensory end organs, sensory axons of the dorsal root ganglion cells, and afferent sensory pathways ascending within the spinal cord and brain stem (dorsal column–medial lemniscus–thalamic, spinothalamic, spinocerebellar, spinoreticular), provides the capacity of feedback or feed forward to the motor system pathways. The labyrinths provide information to the vestibular nuclei via cranial nerve VIII pertaining to head-body position in space as well as linear and angular acceleration. The visual system allows a visuospatial assessment of body position and limb movements during the act of walking or running and in addition provides the ability to anticipate changes necessitated by environmental alterations. The cerebellum provides an analysis of this ascending sensory information (via the spinocerebellar tracts) and thus allows moment-by-moment modulation of the motor output necessary to maintain balance and effective walking.

Mechanically, the normal gait can be divided into the stance phase and the swing phase. Sixty percent of the normal gait is spent in the stance phase. The stance phase is further subdivided into the heel strike, foot flat, midstance, and push-off. The swing phase is further subdivided into acceleration, midswing, and deceleration. The width of the base should be no more than 4 inches from heel to heel.

## HISTORY IN GAIT DISORDERS

The system necessary for maintenance of upright posture and walking spans the entire neuraxis, involving multiple components of both the central nervous system and peripheral nervous system. It follows that neurologic disorders that substantially affect any portion of this system may disrupt gait. Because there is a considerable amount of overlap in the tasks performed by individual components of this large system, partial lesions may not produce noticeable alterations of the gait or station. However, multiple partial lesions affecting different components of the system may summate to produce a gait disorder. Thus, a complete neurologic history and examination are important when patients present with a complaint of gait difficulty.

As with all medical problems, the assessment of gait difficulties begins with the history. The time and mode of onset, relative stability or progression, and exacerbating and relieving factors should be determined. It is important to ascertain the use of assistive devices and when they were employed. A complete neurologic and medical review of systems should be performed. It is particularly important to determine the presence of any medical or neurologic problems known to predispose to gait disorder. Present, recent past, and particularly new medications should be reviewed. A complaint of true weakness suggests a process affecting the motor unit or the central motor pathways. This complaint should be further dissected. It is important to determine what activities the patient has most difficulties with. For example, difficulty climbing stairs or arising from chairs is suggestive of proximal lower extremity weakness, whereas a complaint of frequent tripping related to catching a toe on an uneven pavement is suggestive of distal lower extremity weakness. A sense of heaviness and slowness rather than true weakness in the legs is suggestive of a disorder affecting central motor pathways. Fatigue and in particular a sense of fluctuating fatigue are suggestive of a disorder of neuromuscular transmission.

A sense of imbalance and instability suggests a disorder affecting the sensory pathways or cerebellum. When accompanied by a complaint of lower extremity sensory loss or paresthesias and particularly when the unsteadiness is exacerbated by reduced ambient light or closed eyes, this complaint suggests sensory ataxia related to a disorder of the peripheral sensory (dorsal root ganglia, sensory axons, sensory receptors) or central sensory (spinal cord, brain stem, thalami, sensory cortex) pathways. When unsteadiness or imbalance occurs in isolation, a cerebellar process is suggested. When accompanied by a complaint of true vertigo (an illusion of motion), a disorder of the vestibular system is suggested. When accompanied by cognitive dysfunction and urinary incontinence, a complaint of gait imbalance or unsteadiness suggests hydrocephalus.

## EXAMINATION IN GAIT DISORDERS

The complete neurologic examination, including a specific examination of the gait and station as well as functional testing, should be performed. When deemed appropriate, an examination of the spine, pelvis, hips, knees, ankles, feet, and leg lengths can add important information. It is also important to realize that any bone or joint deformity may affect the patient's ability to perform gait and station testing. Determining supine and standing blood pressures can reveal significant orthostatic hypotension related to dehydration, medication side effect, or an autonomic disorder that can produce a sense of unsteadiness or instability as a single symptom. At times, substantial bilateral anterior and/or posterior cerebrovascular disease can give rise to the same symptom complex without an associated significant loss of standing blood pressure.

Station is evaluated while the patient is both sitting and standing. When the patient is sitting with arms folded across the lap, any sway or corrective movements of the trunk consistent with truncal ataxia are noted. When standing at rest, the position of the feet and width of the stance are noted. A widened stance is consistent with ataxia. If this is present, the patient is asked to narrow the stance. Production of an increase in truncal sway, loss of balance, or falling supports the presence of ataxia related to either sensory system, vestibular system, or cerebellar system dysfunction. If this is measurably increased when the patient's eyes are closed (Romberg's maneuver) an abnormality of the sensory system is strongly suggested. While the patient is standing with feet comfortably apart, reflex righting ability is determined by gently pulling or pushing on the shoulders from behind and asking the patient to stand still. Inability to prevent the taking of one or more steps either forward (anteropulsion) or backward (retropulsion) supports the presence of poor postural reflexes frequently noted in basal ganglia disorders. When the loss of postural reflexes is extreme, spontaneous retropulsion or anteropulsion can occur without any assistance from the examiner.

Patients' gait can, in fact, be observed as they walk into the examination room. This initial evaluation can be augmented by a more specific examination of the gait. Typically, this begins by having the patient walk casually both away from and toward the examiner. The movements of both legs and both arms as well as truncal position are evaluated. The size of steps and the width of the stance are noted. The patient's turning is noted for both the number of steps required and relative stability. Truncal position is noted for stooping or for postural adjustments. When the patient is asked to stop and then restart walking, the size of the initial steps or any difficulty initiating gait is noted. Balance is evaluated by having the patient walk sequentially heel to toe (tandem). Difficulty with this maneuver is consistent with ataxia. Functional testing should include walking on heels (tibialis anterior), walking on toes (gastrocnemius), rising onto the toes repeatedly (gastrocnemius), arising from a low seat (quadriceps and gluteal muscles), and stepping up onto an examining stool (quadriceps and gluteal muscles).

## SPECIFIC ABNORMAL GAIT PATTERNS

During the gait examination it is important to recognize specific patterns of walking that suggest specific neurologic lesion localization. The following is a review of the more classic gait patterns.

### Steppage Gait

Substantial weakness of the ankle dorsiflexor results in footdrop and necessitates a gait in which the leg is lifted higher off of the ground in order to avoid catching the toe on the floor. If the weakness is present bilaterally, this maneuver is performed in each leg sequentially as the patient walks. The patient appears to be stepping over an obstacle on the floor and thus this gait is termed steppage. Although this gait is frequently related to peroneal neuropathy, the differential diagnosis includes sciatic neuropathy, lumbosacral plexopathy, lumbosacral radiculopathy at L5, myelopathy, focal hemispheric lesions, some myopathic disorders, and neuromuscular transmission disorders.

### Myopathic Gait

Weakness of pelvic girdle muscles produces a characteristic waddling gait. In particular, this results from substantial weakness of the gluteus medius and minimus muscles, which contract in the supporting leg to prevent pelvic tilting to the opposite side. Compensation during walking results in a swing of the trunk to the supported side. When bilateral weakness is present, walking produces sequential tilting of the pelvis and trunk from side to side. This is called Trendelenburg's gait. In addition, weakness of other pelvic girdle muscles results in weakness on functional testing such as arising from a squat, arising onto a stool, going up stairs, or arising from a chair. Often, bedside testing of these remarkably strong muscles is normal.

Because myopathic disorders have a predisposition for proximal muscles, this gait is termed the myopathic gait. The differential diagnosis includes inflammatory, dystrophic, and metabolic muscle disease as well as disorders of neuromuscular transmission. However, any disorder that produces symmetric pelvic girdle weakness can result in this gait. The differential diagnosis thus also includes neurogenic disorders such as spinal muscular atrophy, motor neuron disease, lumbosacral radiculopathies, chronic inflammatory demyelinating polyneuropathy, and acute inflammatory demyelinating polyneuropathy (Guillain-Barré syndrome). It should also be cautioned that at times bilateral hip disease may produce a similar gait.

### Hemiparetic Gait

Unilateral upper motor neuron weakness of the arm and leg produces a characteristic gait in which the patient walks with the weakened arm internally rotated and adducted at the shoulder, flexed at the elbow, flexed at the wrist, and the fingers clenched. The weakened leg is extended at the knee and plantar flexed at the ankle, and forward motion of the leg is accomplished by abducting the leg at the hip and circumducting the leg to attempt to clear the plantar flexed toes from the floor. The toes are frequently scuffed along the floor. During walking, the weakened leg noticeably follows behind or is dragged. Typically produced by a contralateral hemispheric lesion, this gait can in fact result from a unilateral upper motor neuron process above the midcervical cord level.

### Paraparetic Gait

When the legs are bilaterally weakened by an upper motor neuron process, the patient walks with each leg extended at the knee and plantar flexed at the ankle. Each leg is circumducted to achieve forward motion. At times there is a prominent increase in adductor tone resulting in a scissoring of the legs both at rest and during walking. Although typically related to spinal cord disorders with resultant bilateral upper motor neuron dysfunction, this gait can also be produced by bifrontal hemispheric processes.

## Ataxic Gait

Patients with this gait pattern stand with a widened base, and even at rest there may be corrective truncal movements (truncal titubation or truncal tremor). When walking, the steps vary so that the leg is placed more forward or backward than on the last movement, resulting in an irregular appearance. The irregularity of the leg movements is accompanied by frequent truncal postural adjustments. Often the individual loses balance and seeks to hold onto furniture or the nearest person in order to avoid falling. The gait is not unlike that of an intoxicated individual, hence the term "drunken" gait. Often, minimal use of a third point of contact (a cane or the hand of the examiner) results in a remarkable improvement in the gait. Narrowing the base and in particular tandem gait testing exacerbate the abnormality.

Classically, this gait results from cerebellar lesions. When it is unaccompanied by cerebellar limb findings (lack of check, dysdiadochokinesia, past pointing, tremor) on bedside testing, a midline cerebellar lesion is most likely. When it is accompanied by limb findings, the cerebellar process most likely affects both the midline and the cerebellar hemisphere ipsilateral to the abnormal limb. Vascular, neoplastic, paraneoplastic, infectious, parainfectious, metabolic, and degenerative cerebellar disorders can produce this type of gait.

A virtually identical gait disorder can be produced by sensory loss resulting from disorders affecting the large sensory afferents, dorsal root ganglia, and posterolateral portions of the spinal cord. Sensory ataxia, however, differs from cerebellar ataxia in that Romberg's maneuver is often grossly abnormal. More often than not, this is accompanied by evidence of large-fiber sensory loss (joint position sense, discriminative touch, vibration sense) in the distal legs and feet.

## Parkinsonian Gait

The stance of the parkinsonian patient is characterized by a stooped posture and relative immobility of the arms at the patient's side. The hands and fingers are held in a characteristic posture (striatal hand) of metacarpophalangeal (MCP) joint flexion and proximal interphalangeal (PIP) joint mild extension while the thumb is adducted and mildly opposed. When the patient is asked to initiate gait, the first steps are small and hesitant. At times, the feet appear to be frozen to the floor. If the patient continues, the speed and size of the steps increase as walking proceeds. When walking, the patient appears to be leaning forward. If the patient is asked to stop and start again, the same pattern is repeated. The arms do not swing. Turning is achieved only by an increased number of small steps. Upon stopping, the patient may spontaneously and uncontrollably take a few steps backward (retropulsion), often exhibiting no corrective limb or truncal movements. At times this results in falling.

Although this gait occurs in its typical form in patients with Parkinson's disease, a similar if not identical gait can be seen in patients with parkinsonism resulting from other disorders of the basal ganglia. A similar gait can be seen in patients with chronic hydrocephalus and frontal lobe lesions.

## Apraxic Gait

At times, the bedside examination of the patient reveals no motor or sensory deficits and the patient can even mimic the movements needed to walk while lying or sitting. Yet, when arising to walk, the patient appears incapable of walking. The feet appear "frozen" and any steps that are taken are small and shuffling. The legs are frequently not lifted from the ground. Such a gait is often referred to as magnetic. Often, the patient requires significant assistance even to maintain an upright posture, demonstrating a tendency to fall backward. Resembling the parkinsonian gait, the gait is frequently termed apractic on the basis of the absence of extrapyramidal features and the presence of cognitive dysfunction, the presence of atavistic reflexes, and the presence of paratonia, which are frequent accompaniments of frontal lobe disorders.

## Antalgic Gait

Painful disorders of the lumbosacral spine, pelvis, hips, knees, ankles, and feet as well as the soft tissues in these regions can produce characteristic gaits that result in splinting of the involved part. Because antalgic gaits can at times mimic various neurologically based gaits, it is important to consider this in the differential diagnosis of gait disorders.

## Hysterical Gait

Related to functional or nonphysiologic causes, the features of hysterical gait often vary from patient to patient and can result in ambulation that can approximate all of the previously discussed organically based gait disorders. The diagnosis is most often based on the detection of various and often multiple neurologic examination inconsistencies, not the least of which is a nonphysiologic and at times bizarre gait pattern. However, at times neuroradiologic as well as neurophysiologic testing may be required to supplement the neurologic examination and history in making the diagnosis.

## LABORATORY EVALUATION OF GAIT DISORDERS

As can be gleaned from the preceeding discussion, gait abnormalities can result from primary or secondary neurologic disorders spanning the entire central and peripheral nervous systems. In addition, gait abnormalities can result from lower extremity mechanical abnormalities affecting the pelvis, hip, knee, ankle, and foot. As a result, a thorough discussion of the laboratory evaluation of patients with gait abnormalities is beyond the scope of this chapter. However, directed by the history and physical examinations, the examiner's goal should be to obtain a differential diagnosis of the possible causes of the gait dysfunction and, using appropriate laboratory studies, to arrive at a definitive diagnosis. This evaluation may include directed blood and urine studies, magnetic resonance and computed tomographic imaging, conventional radiography, myelography, electromyography and nerve conduction studies, electronystagmometry and vestibular testing, and even muscle and nerve biopsy.

## SUMMARY

Gait disorders are a common problem encountered by neurologists and nonneurologists alike. A thorough understanding of the neurologic and mechanical aspects of the gait, coupled with a comprehensive history and physical examination, often leads to a specific diagnosis and thereby appropriate management.

## BIBLIOGRAPHY

Asbury A, McKhann GM, McDonald WI: Diseases of the Nervous System. Philadelphia, WB Saunders, 1986.
DeJong RN: The Neurologic Examination. Philadelphia, JB Lippincott, 1958.
Hoppenfeld S: Physical examination of the Spine and Extremities. Norwalk, CT, Appleton & Lange, 1976.

# 7

# Acute Neuromuscular Weakness of the Lower Extremity

*Terry Heiman-Patterson*

This chapter discusses neuromuscular disorders that can present with acute weakness of the lower extremities. These disorders include diseases that affect any portion of the motor unit including the anterior horn cell peripheral nerve, neuromuscular junction, and muscle. The chapter focuses on disorders that present acutely; diseases that present more slowly are discussed elsewhere (Chapters 15 and 16). In general, although these diseases can affect primarily the lower extremities, they are often more diffuse and also affect the arms and in some cases bulbar regions.

The first step in diagnosing the cause of acute weakness is to localize the process in the motor unit. This is done by performing a thorough history and physical examination, followed by the use of appropriate diagnostic testing. When the process has been localized, a list of possible diseases can be considered and the appropriate additional testing ordered. This chapter first summarizes the localization of diseases within the motor unit and then focuses on the most common diseases that can present acutely, organized by their anatomic localization.

## LOCALIZING DISEASES IN THE MOTOR UNIT

This section provides a brief overview of localization in the motor unit (Table 7–1), but there are additional details in Chapters 3 and 4. It is organized by the pertinent symptoms, signs, and laboratory evaluation.

### Symptoms

The primary symptom of any disorder that affects the motor unit is weakness. The distribution of the weakness can be helpful in localization because myopathic illnesses generally present with proximal weakness, whereas neuropathic disorders are predominantly distal in their location. Often the lower extremities are more involved than the upper extremities. Historically, patients with proximal leg weakness complain of difficulties in getting up from chairs, getting out of cars, or climbing stairs, whereas those with proximal upper extremity weakness complain of difficulty raising their arms above their heads. In patients with distal leg weakness there are problems with ankle sprains, tripping over small ledges, and difficulty on graveled surfaces. Distal arm weakness generally presents with trouble opening jars.

Weakness may be described in several different ways, including heaviness, numbness, or leaden feelings. These descriptions must be carefully explored to rule out sensory involvement. The presence of fatigue with proximal weakness may often signal involvement of the neuromuscular junction. In primary neuropathies with motor involvement there may also be complaints of cramping and twitching (i.e., fasciculations). The presence of paresthesias and numbness often implies accompanying sensory nerve involvement. However, the clinician must be careful to elicit adequate information from the patient in order to determine what is meant by numbness. Patients often describe weakness as numbness, and care must be taken to ascertain whether the patient truly means a sensory disturbance or weakness when the complaint of numbness is elicited. In eliciting a history of the patient's complaint, it is important to determine whether there are additional complaints referable to other areas of the nervous system. This becomes important in generating the differential diagnosis. For instance, the presence of ptosis and diplopia can provide important clues to the diagnosis of myasthenia gravis. Furthermore, a detailed medical and family history can often provide important information leading to a diagnosis.

### Signs

In order to localize the disease process in the motor unit, it is important to perform a thorough neuro-

Table 7-1  **Localization in the Motor Unit**

| Observation | Anterior Horn Cell | Peripheral Nerve | Neuromuscular Junction | Muscle |
|---|---|---|---|---|
| Distribution of weakness | Proximal or distal | Distal | Proximal | Proximal |
| Presence of atrophy | Yes, out of proportion to weakness | Yes, out of proportion to weakness | None | Commensurate with weakness |
| Presence of fasciculations | Yes | Yes | No | No |
| Sensory abnormalities | No | Yes, if there is sensory fiber involvement | No | No |
| Presence of reflexes | Decreased | Decreased | Normal in myasthenia but can be decreased with facilitation in Eaton-Lambert syndrome | Decreased commensurate to weakness |
| Creatine kinase | Normal or only slight elevation | Normal or only slight elevation | Normal | Increased |
| Electro-neuromyography | EMG with large polyphasic units in chronic processes and spontaneous activity (fibrillations, positive sharps) in the case of acute disorders | EMG changes similar to those in anterior horn cell disease  NCV demonstrates either demyelination or axonal changes | EMG generally normal  NCV normal  Repetitive stimulation with a decremental response | EMG with brief small-amplitude polyphasic units  NCV normal |
| Biopsy | Muscle biopsy with type grouping, grouped atrophy, and targets | Muscle biopsy with type grouping, grouped atrophy, and targets  Nerve biopsy can be helpful for vasculitis, amyloid, storage disordes | Muscle biopsy generally normal but occasionally lymphorrhages or scattered angulars | Muscle biopsy with changes of myopathy including regeneration, degeneration, phagocytosis; more specific changes in inflammatory and metabolic diseases |

logic and medical examination. The neurologic examination should include cranial nerve evaluation, muscle strength, sensory examination, reflexes, and gait evaluation.

The cranial nerve examination often provides clues to etiology by virtue of additional involvement, that is, the company a process keeps. For instance, neuromuscular junction disorders are usually accompanied by extraocular motility involvement as well as ptosis. Dysphagia commonly accompanies certain diseases such as oculopharyngeal dystrophy, myasthenia gravis, and the inflammatory myopathies (polymyositis and dermatomyositis).

The motor examination provides information about the distribution of weakness, the presence of atrophy, and the presence of fasciculations. In patients with primary muscle involvement, weakness is proximal in distribution and the legs are often more involved than the arms. Atrophy is commensurate with the amount of weakness and there are no fasciculations. There should be normal sensation. In disorders of the neuromuscular junction, the weakness is usually proximal and can fluctuate with effort. In the case of the postsynaptic disorder myasthenia gravis, strength worsens with use. On the other hand, in patients with Eaton-Lambert syndrome, a presynaptic defect of transmission, strength may improve with repetition. In diseases of the anterior horn cell or lower motor neuron, weakness may be either proximal or distal. There is often striking atrophy, out of proportion to the amount of weakness. Fasciculations are seen in the distribution of the involved root.

If there is sensory fiber involvement, abnormalities are seen on the sensory examination. In this case it is important to determine the topography of the abnormality (distal length dependent, asymmetric mononeuropathy, or radicular) as well as the fiber type affected (i.e., large and/or small). This information can aid in the differential diagnosis (see Chapter 15).

The reflexes are generally commensurate with the weakness in myopathic disorders, whereas they are lost early in neurogenic disorders. They are generally normal in the disorders of neuromuscular transmission, although they can be diminished in Eaton-Lambert syndrome.

## Laboratory Evaluation

The most important tests for localization of motor unit disorders are serum creatine kinase (CK), electrophysiologic studies, and in selected cases muscle or nerve biopsy. Serum CK is elevated in myopathies and generally normal in the other disorders.

Electrophysiologic studies include electromyography (EMG), nerve conduction velocity studies, and repetitive stimulation.

EMG consists of the insertion of a needle electrode into the muscle to record electrical activity on an oscilloscope. Observations are made at rest for spontaneous activity, at minimal effort to evaluate individual units, and at maximal effort to characterize the ability of the muscle to recruit motor units. At rest, the muscle should be electrically silent, although at times there can be potentials related, to motor endplate irritation. The presence of fibrillations and positive sharp waves in resting muscle implicates acute denervation but can be seen in the context of acute myopathies. In these cases the changes imply that the muscle fiber has been damaged in a way that separates it from its innervation (e.g., in segmental necrosis). This activity is especially common in inflammatory or metabolic myopathies. Fasciculations at rest represent the spontaneous discharge of one or more motor units and imply a denervating process. Other spontaneous activity that can be observed at rest includes complex repetitive discharges and myotonic discharges. Complex repetitive discharges are high-frequency spontaneous discharges that vary in frequency and usually stop and start abruptly. They are commonly seen in inflammatory myopathies and metabolic myopathies. Myotonic discharges vary in both amplitude and frequency and are characteristic of the myotonic disorders and periodic paralyses. EMG of individual units at minimal effort demonstrates brief small-amplitude polyphasic units in myopathies and large polyphasic units in chronically denervated muscle that has undergone reinnervation, thereby increasing the size of an individual unit. Large units can also be observed in chronic myopathies with fiber splitting and reinnervation. During full effort, there is early recruitment of many units in myopathies, whereas there is usually less than full recruitment in neurogenic processes.

Nerve conduction velocity studies are performed by applying an electrical stimulus along the course of a peripheral nerve in at least two locations: a proximal and a distal location. Stimulations can be applied to both sensory and motor nerves. In motor conductions, recording electrodes are placed over the muscle that is innervated and the resultant muscle response (the compound muscle action potential or CMAP) is recorded on the oscilloscope. The amplitude of this response can be measured and is directly proportional to the number of axons available for stimulation. A velocity can be calculated by measuring the distance between the proximal and the distal stimulus and determining the difference in time on the oscilloscope between the stimulus and the evoked CMAP of the two stimula-tions. This yields a distance per unit time (meters per second). The velocity is dependent on the integrity of the myelin sheath and the internode distances (i.e., in saltatory conduction). In myelin disorders, saltatory conduction is lost and there is therefore a slowing of the nerve conduction. Finally, as part of the conduction studies, the latency can also be measured. This is the time from the distal stimulus to the muscle belly and is determined not only by the time the response takes to travel down the nerve but also by the time it takes for neuromuscular junction transmission and muscle depolarization.

Nerve conduction studies should be normal in myopathies and disorders of the anterior horn cells. However, if there is peripheral involvement of the nerve, changes are seen. In axonal processes, the major change is a decrease in the amplitude of the evoked response. This is due to the decrease in the number of axons that are available to be stimulated. In demyelinating processes, the predominant change is a decrease in the velocity and prolonged latencies. Similar changes can be seen in sensory nerves by stimulating along the course of the nerve and recording at a distance from the stimulation. It is important in the assessment of peripheral neuropathies to determine the topography (symmetric or asymmetric) as well as the type of involvement (motor, sensory, demyelinating, and axonal) so that a differential diagnosis can be generated (see Chapter 15). Repetitive stimulation is a specialized technique designed to examine neuromuscular junction transmission. In this technique a series of stimuli at specified rates are administered and any changes in CMAP amplitude over a number of stimuli are measured. In presynaptic defects (Eaton-Lambert syndrome and botulism), rapid stimulation produces an increase in amplitude (i.e., an incremental response). In the postsynaptic disorder myasthenia gravis, there is a decrease in response at low rates of stimulation (three to five per second).

Muscle and nerve biopsies are performed in selective cases. In the case of muscle biopsies, there are classic changes that indicate a myopathic or neuropathic process. In myopathies there are regeneration, degeneration, and phagocytosis. In neurogenic processes there are type grouping, grouped atrophy of muscle fibers, and the presence of target fibers with special stains (reduced nicotinamide-adenine dinucleotide [NADH]). Aside from distinguishing myopathic and neurogenic processes, muscle biopsy is essential for the diagnosis of some specific illnesses including the inflammatory myopathies and metabolic myopathies (see later). Nerve biopsies are generally not useful in chronic axonal processes but provide critical information when diseases such as amyloid disease, vasculitis, or the leukodystrophies are under consideration.

When a problem has been localized, the differential diagnosis can be considered and the appropriate work-up pursued. Table 7–2 presents the differential diagnosis of acute weakness organized by anatomic localization in the motor unit. A detailed discussion of the more common disorders follows. In addition, tetanus is discussed, because this disorder results from the retrograde transport of toxin through the motor nerve into the spinal cord.

## DISORDERS OF THE MOTOR UNIT

### Disorders of Muscle

Although inflammatory disorders can present with acute weakness of the lower extremities, they are more commonly progressive over several weeks. An acute presentation of weakness is more common with disorders of energy utilization (i.e., metabolic myopathies), the inherited periodic paralyses, and acute intoxications. In disorders of energy metabolism, there are often exercise-induced symptoms and weakness can be accompanied by rhabdomyolysis with myoglobinuria. In periodic paralysis, weakness can be precipitated by large meals and exercise after a large meal and is often associated with alterations in potassium levels. The periodic paralyses are now known to be ion channel disorders. Detailed descriptions of these more common causes of acute weakness are presented next.

### Inflammatory Myopathies

#### Polymyositis

**Clinical Presentation.** Polymyositis generally presents after age 20 with subacute progressive proximal limb weakness in association with weakness of neck flexors. Although the onset is usually subacute, a fulminant onset can be seen. The lower extremities are usually more involved than the upper extremities. Dysphagia is common and can oc-

---

**Table 7–2   Differential Diagnosis of Acute Neuromuscular Weakness**

| DISORDERS OF MUSCLE | NEUROMUSCULAR JUNCTION |
|---|---|
| Inflammatory myopathies | Presynaptic disorders |
| **Idiopathic**<br>*Polymyositis/dermatomyositis** | *Botulism*<br>*Eaton-Lambert syndrome* |
| **Infectious**<br>Parasitic<br>Bacterial<br>Viral<br>Retroviral | Postsynaptic Disorders<br><br>*Myasthenia gravis* |
| Metabolic myopathies | PERIPHERAL NERVE (see Chapter 15) |
| **Glycolytic**<br>*Phosphorylase deficiency*<br>*Phosphofructokinase deficiency*<br>*PGK deficiency*<br>*PGAM deficiency*<br>*LDH deficiency* | Demyelinating<br><br>*Acute inflammatory demyelinating neuropathy:*<br>*Guillain-Barré*<br>*Diphtheria* |
| **Lipid**<br>*Carnitine deficiency*<br>*CPT deficiency* | Axonal<br><br>Intoxications  Heavy metals |
| Mitochondrial disorders | Axonal Guillain-Barré<br>Porphyria<br>Vasculitis<br>Compressive injuries |
| INHERITED DISORDERS | ANTERIOR HORN CELL |
| *Periodic paralysis* | Polio |
| Medical disorders | SPINAL CORD |
| Endocrinopathies<br>Electrolyte abnormalities | *Tetanus* |
| Toxic | |
| *Medications*<br>*Self-administered toxins* | |

*Italicized topics are discussed in this chapter.
PGK = phosphoglycerate kinase; PGAM = phosphoglycerate mutase; LDH = lactate dehydrogenase; CPT = carnitine palmityltransferase.

cur in 50% to 60% of patients. Only 10% of patients presenting have muscle pain, but over time up to one third develop it. Prominent myalgias should suggest alternative diseases including polymyalgia rheumatica and other connective tissue diseases. Other manifestations include cardiac involvement with arrhythmias, congestive heart failure, and sick sinus syndrome resulting from inflammatory lesions in the heart. Interstitial lung disease, when present, is associated with higher morbidity and mortality as well as Jo-1 antibodies. Finally, there is an increased incidence of malignancy in patients with polymyositis, although it is not as high as in dermatomyositis.

There can be overlap with common connective tissue disorders including systemic lupus erythematosus, Sjögren's syndrome, or rheumatoid arthritis in up to 20% of patients with polymyositis. In contrast, systemic sclerosis and mixed connective tissue diseases are most often associated with dermatomyositis. Polymyositis can also become evident in the context of other autoimmune disorders including Crohn's disease, vasculitis, sarcoidosis, primary biliary cirrhosis, adult celiac disease, chronic graft-versus-host disease, discoid lupus, ankylosing spondylitis, Behçet's disease, myasthenia gravis, acne fulminans, dermatitis herpetiformis, psoriasis, Hashimoto's disease, granulomatous diseases, agammaglobulinemia, monoclonal gammopathy, hypereosinophilic syndrome, Lyme disease, Kawasaki's disease, autoimmune thrombocytopenia, hypergammaglobulinemic purpura, hereditary complement deficiency, immunoglobulin A (IgA) deficiency, and acquired immunodeficiency syndrome.

**Laboratory Evaluation.** Elevated CK levels are an important element of the diagnostic criteria, although they are not always present. Autoantibodies are common, especially in patients with connective tissue disease associated with their inflammatory myopathy and in certain subsets of inflammatory myopathy. For instance, the Jo-1 antibody, found in one third of patients with inflammatory myopathy, is directed toward the nuclear protein histidyl–transfer RNA synthetase. It occurs in the setting of interstitial lung disease, and patients can also have arthritis and Raynaud's disease. Autoantibodies to PM-1 and Ku are more common in the overlap syndrome of polymyositis and systemic sclerosis. SSA antibodies are more common in Sjögren's syndrome but may also be a marker for inflammatory involvement of the myocardium.

The electrogram is abnormal in the majority of patients with myopathic units accompanied by fibrillations and positive sharp waves. This irritative activity is often correlated with disease activity. Muscle biopsy demonstrates scattered inflammation and muscle fiber necrosis. The presence of endomysial inflammatory infiltrates around nonnecrotic fibers is especially helpful. Inflammation can also be seen in the perimysium and perivascular regions. Infiltrates are predominantly macrophages and CD8+ cytotoxic-suppressor cells, indicating a cell-mediated process.

**Treatment and Prognosis.** Treatment for polymyositis relies primarily on immunosuppression. When the diagnosis has been made, the initial treatment strategy is to administer prednisone at 1 mg/kg/day. The patient is advised of the many side effects including fluid retention, gastric irritation, osteoporosis, elevated glucose, cataracts, glaucoma, hypertension, decreased resistance to infection, cushingoid appearance, changes in the skin, and even increased weakness. A rigorous program to monitor side effects should be put into place and patients given calcitriol and elemental calcium supplements. If gastrointestinal symptoms become evident, $H_2$ blockers can be used. The clinical examination and CK evaluation should be performed at 2- to 4-week intervals. When the patient has improved, an alternate-day program of steroids can be adopted. Tapering of steroids should be slow, and if there is any difficulty steroid-sparing agents (azathioprine, methotrexate) can be added. For patients who do not respond or who develop rate-limiting side effects with prednisone, cytotoxic agents can be used including methotrexate, cyclophosphamide (Cytoxan), and azathioprine. Furthermore, studies indicate that there may be a role for intravenous gamma globulin. In any treatment regimen, physical therapy is an important adjunct in maximizing recovery.

The natural history of polymyositis is unknown because patients are almost always treated with steroids, and the mortality rates reported 20 to 30 years ago are outdated. In reviews, mortality rates of 23% to 35% have been reported. Patients with interstitial lung disease have a worse prognosis and may require aggressive treatment with cyclophosphamide. Overall, there are still patients who have not responded to therapy. When treatment is unsuccessful, the patient should be reevaluated, and a repeated biopsy should be considered to make sure that the diagnosis is correct and that inclusion-body myositis, which is resistant to therapy, has not been missed.

## Dermatomyositis

**Clinical Presentation.** Patients with dermatomyositis present with subacute to fulminant proximal weakness in association with a characteristic skin rash. The rash is characterized by erythema and redness over the malar regions and in the periorbital areas of the face, where it has a violaceous hue and is often referred to as a heliotrope rash. The rash extends over the shawl region and onto extensor surfaces. There may also be involvement of the interphalangeal regions along with papular and erythematous changes of the knuckles (Gottron's papules). In severe cases, a necrotizing vasculitis of the skin can be observed. Changes in the capillaries of the nailbed have been described as well. This characteristic rash is accompanied by a progressive proximal weakness of the limbs and neck flexors. Myalgia is present in only 25% of patients. Dysphagia occurs in one third of patients. Respiratory muscle involvement is rare.

There are frequently other manifestations, including joint involvement, contractures, cardiomegaly, arrhythmias, and interstitial lung disease. In patients with prominent dysphagia, aspiration can occur. In some patients, especially children, a necrotizing vasculitis may be present that affects multiple organs including skin, muscle, and the gastrointestinal tract. Finally, patients with dermatomyositis may have as much as a 5 to 11 times greater risk of malignancy, with increasing risk in males and patients older than 50 years. In general, the cancer sites correspond to those at which cancer occurs more frequently at the patient's age. Overall, ovarian cancer is most frequent, followed by intestinal, breast, lung, and liver cancer.

Dermatomyositis usually occurs alone, but it may overlap with systemic sclerosis and mixed connective tissue disease. Fasciitis and skin changes similar to those found in dermatomyositis have occurred in patients with the eosinophilia-myalgia syndrome associated with the ingestion of contaminated L-tryptophan.

**Laboratory Evaluation.** Patients with dermatomyositis demonstrate elevated CK levels in 90% of cases, although the levels do not correlate with severity. The sedimentation rate is generally normal unless there is an associated connective tissue disease. In addition, several autoantibodies may be present, including Jo-1, PM-1, and Mi-2. EMG demonstrates an irritative myopathy, although in late stages there can be large motor units with a decrease in the number of units mimicking chronic neurogenic processes. The larger units are likely to represent sprouting with regeneration of muscle fibers rather than a denervating process.

Muscle biopsy findings are characteristic. Perifascicular atrophy is found in 75% of patients with dermatomyositis and is specific. In fact, the presence of perifascicular atrophy is diagnostic of dermatomyositis, even in the absence of inflammation. This change is due to the microvascular insult, and there is loss of capillaries and portions of the microvasculature in the perifascicular region as well. The changes are often multifocal, and muscle infarcts can be seen in which there are wedge-shaped regions of necrosis. Inflammatory infiltrates are predominantly in the perimysium and perivascular regions and are composed of CD4[+] T helper cells along with macrophages. Finally, there are immune deposits in blood vessels consisting of IgM, less often IgG, and complement components. Similar deposits can be seen in the affected skin. These changes indicate humoral mechanisms directed at the microvasculature and a mechanism different from that of polymyositis.

**Treatment and Prognosis.** The goal of therapy in dermatomyositis is to improve function by improving muscle strength. Although improvement in strength is usually accompanied by a fall in serum CK, decreases in serum CK have to be interpreted with caution because most immunosuppressive therapies result in a decrease in serum muscle enzymes without necessarily improving muscle strength. The treatment strategy is the same as that described for polymyositis with the use of immunosuppressives.

**Differential Diagnosis of Polymyositis and Dermatomyositis.** The differential diagnosis of polymyositis and dermatomyositis is extensive (Table 7–3) and includes all acquired myopathies that involve proximal weakness. Therefore, the diagnosis of polymyositis rests on exclusion of other acquired myopathies including (1) familial neuromuscular diseases, especially muscular dystrophies in which endomysial inflammation can occur; (2) systemic metabolic muscle diseases (endocrinopathies, electrolyte disturbances, mitochondriopathies); (3) any systemic medical illness, including malabsorption syndromes, alcoholism, cancer, vasculitis, systemic infections, sarcoidosis, and granulomatous disease, or treatment with various known myotoxic drugs or a combination of unknown but potentially myotoxic drugs or toxins; (4) neurogenic muscular atrophies or neurogenic conditions; and (5) other inflammatory myopathies. Dermatomyositis can be distinguished by the characteristic rash and muscle biopsy findings. Inclusion body myositis is more slowly progressive with more prominent distal weakness. Connective tissue diseases that can have prominent myopathic involvement include mixed connective tissue disease distinguished by the presence of anti-RNP antibodies, systemic sclerosis, systemic lupus erythematosus, rheumatoid arthritis, Sjögren's syndrome, and polyarteritis nodosa.

## Metabolic Myopathies

The metabolic myopathies include disorders that affect energy utilization in muscle. In order to understand the metabolic disorders, one has to understand some things about how adenosine tri-

**Table 7–3  Differential Diagnosis of Polymyositis and Dermatomyositis**

INHERITED DISEASES OF MUSCLE

Dystrophies: limb girdle dystrophy

METABOLIC DISORDERS OF MUSCLE

Glycogen disorders: deficiencies of acid maltase, debrancher enzyme, brancher enzyme, phosphorylase
Lipid disorders: carnitine deficiency
Mitochondrial

CONNECTIVE TISSUE DISEASES

Systemic lupus erythematosus, periarteritis nodosa, systemic sclerosis, polymyalgia rheumatica, rheumatoid arthritis, Sjögren's syndrome

INFECTIONS

Parasites: trichinosis, schistosomiasis, toxoplasmosis, cysticercosis, Chagas' disease
Viral: coxsackie, influenza, hepatitis B, echovirus
Retroviral: human immunodeficiency virus
Other: *Mycoplasma,* Kawasaki syndrome

MEDICAL DISEASES

Systemic

Neoplastic, sarcoid, amyloid, hypergammaglobulinemia, plasma cell dyscrasias, celiac disease

Endocrine

Hyper- and hypothyroidism, hyperparathyroidism, hyperadrenalism

Metabolic

Starvation, hyperalimentation, hypocalcemia, chronic renal failure, potassium depletion, osteomalacia

Drugs

Penicillamine, clofibrate, steroids, emetine, chloroquine, kaliuretics, aminocaproic acid, zidovudine, rifampin, ipecac, meperidine (Demerol), pentazocine

Toxins

Cocaine, heroin, alcohol, L-tryptophan

phosphate (ATP), that is, energy, is produced in muscle. Muscle utilizes two major substrates, lipids and glycogen, along with breakdown of phosphocreatine and use of the purine nucleotide cycle to generate energy. In the case of lipid and glycogen metabolism, energy production is maximized when the electron transport chain is able to oxidize hydrogen electrons for the production of ATP.

Glycogen is used during the early stages of high-intensity exercise and under anaerobic conditions. Under aerobic conditions, glycogen is metabolized to pyruvate and then converted to acetyl coenzyme A (CoA) by oxidative decarboxylation in the mitochondria. Acetyl CoA can then enter the tricarboxylic acid cycle of the mitochondria to generate NADH and reduced flavin adenine dinucleotide (FADH) for use by the respiratory chain. Under anaerobic conditions, the pyruvate is converted to lac-

tate and generates muscle fatigue. Lipids are used for long-term submaximal exercise and under conditions of starvation. Fatty acids are derived through lipase activity from either stored triglycerides or circulating low-density lipoproteins. In either case, the released fatty acids are activated by acyl CoA synthetase and transported across the mitochondrial membrane through the action of carnitine palmityltransferase (CPT) and linkage to the carrier protein carnitine. Carnitine transports the fatty acids across the inner mitochondrial membrane, where the acetyl CoA is released and oxidized to $CO_2$ and water by beta oxidation, providing additional NADH for processing along the electron transport chain. Thus, both lipid utilization and aerobic glycogen metabolism require mitochondria for maximizing energy production. In either case, molecules of NADH and FADH are generated. These molecules are hydrogen carriers that transfer electrons to the respiratory chain on the inner mitochondrial membrane. The respiratory chain is made up of four multienzyme complexes: I, II, III, and IV. The progressive oxidation of hydrogen electrons through the respiratory chain provides energy to synthesize ATP.

There are two additional ways for muscle to make energy. First, CK catalyzes the reaction of adenosine diphosphate (ADP) with phosphocreatine to form ATP. This pathway is important in very high-intensity exercise but because of limited stores of phosphocreatinine, is generally of brief duration. The second pathway, which is also used for high-intensity, brief exercise, involves conversion of two molecules of ADP to ATP using adenylate kinase. As a result of this reaction, a molecule of adenosine monophosphate (AMP) is formed, which is deaminated to inosine monophosphate by myoadenylate deaminase.

In general, patients with metabolic myopathies present with either exercise intolerance or progressive weakness. In some cases, especially in those with mitochondrial disorders, both symptoms may be present. Exercise intolerance results because the patient cannot fully metabolize substrate for ATP production. Exercise intolerance can be manifest as fatigue with exercise, cramping with exercise, or frank myoglobinuria. Myoglobinuria occurs only when energy production does not keep pace with utilization and there is muscle breakdown. Furthermore, if the disorder presents with exercise intolerance, the type of exercise that precipitates the "energy crisis" is determined by the substrate that is involved. For instance, glycolytic disorders present with cramps, muscle pain, and rhabdomyolysis after relatively brief periods of exercise, and cramping can be provoked by exercise with a tourniquet in place. In lipid disorders, rhabdomyolysis and myalgias occur after prolonged exercise or exercise in a relatively fasted state.

These precipitant types of exercise can provide the basis for provocative testing. For instance, in glycolytic disorders, the patient's forearm can be exercised anaerobically by placing a tourniquet on the forearm. After exercise, the increase in lactate can be measured. In normal patients, there is a four fold elevation above baseline. In patients with glycolytic disorders, the lactate levels may not rise at all or may be less than normal elevations (see later under individual disorders).

The glycolytic disorders that are most likely to present with exercise intolerance and acute symptoms of fatigue, weakness, and muscle pain are deficiencies of phosphorylase (McArdle's disease), phosphorylase b kinase (PBK), phosphofructokinase (PFK), phosphoglycerate kinase (PGK), phosphoglycerate mutase (PGAM), and lactate dehydrogenase (LDH). Among the lipid disorders, CPT deficiency is most apt to present with acute weakness and exercise intolerance. The clinical picture of each of these disorders is briefly reviewed in the following.

### Glycolytic Disorders

#### Phosphorylase Deficiency

**Clinical Presentation.** Phosphorylase deficiency is an autosomal recessive disorder that has been linked to chromosome 11q. There is a male predominance, and patients typically present with exercise intolerance associated with cramping and easy fatigue. Symptoms often occur with brief high-intensity exercise. The onset is frequently during adolescence, when patients complain of decreased endurance compared with their peers. Patients often learn the warning signs of cramping and stop exercising before the onset of rhabdomyolysis and myoglobinuria. Often, patients experience a second-wind phenomenon and can proceed with exercise after a brief rest after the first signs of cramping or myalgia with exercise. Despite the warning cramp, some patients do have frank myoglobinuria and rhabdomyolysis; in fact, 25% of patients experience renal failure. Fixed weakness can occur later in the disease in up to one third of patients.

**Diagnostic Evaluation.** The serum CK is elevated in 90% of patients even between episodes. Provocative testing can be done by exercising a patient with a tourniquet on the forearm (i.e., anaerobically) and evaluating the rise in lactate. Patients with phosphorylase deficiency have a flattened lactate curve because of their inability to produce lactate from glycogen under anaerobic conditions. The ischemic lactate test should be performed with caution because it has resulted in compartment syndromes and rhabdomyolysis. EMG can demonstrate

features of an irritative myopathy with acute fibrillations, positive sharp waves, and myopathic potentials. The exercise-induced cramps are electrically silent contractures, in contrast to typical cramps. Muscle biopsy can appear normal or demonstrate vacuoles that contain periodic acid–Schiff–positive accumulations of glycogen in the subsarcolemmal regions. The histochemical stain for phosphorylase shows an absence of activity. Final verification is made by biochemical assay of phosphorylase activity.

**Treatment and Prognosis.** Acute episodes of weakness and myoglobinuria are an emergency and should be treated with hydration and alkalinization of the urine to prevent renal failure. Patients should be placed in a monitored setting and airway and circulation maintained. Acute tubular necrosis must be prevented by hydration with saline and the urine made alkaline with infusions of sodium bicarbonate. The alkalinization of urine may help to treat hyperkalemia, which can occur with rhabdomyolysis, as well as prevent renal damage by myoglobin and uric acid. Complications of rhabdomyolysis can also include hyperkalemia, hypocalcemia, vascular collapse, and disseminated intravascular coagulation.

In the long term, patients may benefit from a graduated exercise program with emphasis on aerobic activities to promote fatty acid utilization. Attempts to modify diet and raise glucose levels generally have not been helpful, although a high-protein diet has been beneficial in two studies. Most patients learn their limitations and modify their lifestyle accordingly. In one third of patients, permanent weakness can occur.

**Differential Diagnosis.** The differential diagnosis of phosphorylase deficiency includes other metabolic myopathies, especially glycogenosis and disorders of lipid metabolism. On purely clinical grounds, myophosphorylase deficiency is indistinguishable from defects of glycolytic enzymes, such as PFK, PGK, PGAM, and LDH. Laboratory data may offer some clues. Patients with PFK deficiency have hyperbilirubinemia and an increased reticulocyte count because of a hemolytic anemia that results from red blood cell involvement. In the forearm ischemic exercise, patients with defects of terminal glycolysis (PGK, PGAM, and LDH deficiencies) have a blunted but not flat venous lactate response, and patients with LDH, deficiency show a low lactate but an excessive pyruvate response. In PBK deficiency, symptoms are usually milder, myoglobinuria is infrequent, and the result of the forearm ischemic exercise is often normal.

The most common metabolic cause of recurrent myoglobinuria in adults is CPT II deficiency. In patients with myophosphorylase deficiency, rhabdomyolysis and cramps are always preceded by exercise, whereas in patients with CPT deficiency, episodes of myoglobinuria can also occur after prolonged fasting without exertion, or after a combination of exercise and fasting.

Intolerance of exercise also accompanies adenylate deaminase deficiency. Patients with adenylate deaminase deficiency have a normal rise of lactate during ischemic forearm exercise with lack of a rise in ammonia.

Exercise intolerance is a typical syndrome of mitochondrial myopathies, usually related to defects of the respiratory chain. Mitochondrial disorders are characterized by a lactic acidosis at rest with excessive rises after either aerobic or anaerobic exercise. Cramps and myoglobinuria are rare and CK levels are generally normal or only modestly increased. Muscle biopsy can demonstrate mitochondrial proliferation, with "ragged red" fibers shown by the Gomori trichrome stain in some cases.

Exercise-related myoglobinuria can occur in nonmetabolic myopathies as well, including the dystrophinopathies and malignant hyperthermia. Exercise intolerance without myoglobinuria is also a common complaint of malingering and hysterical patients and is the cardinal symptom of the "chronic fatigue" syndrom. However, these diagnoses should be used prudently and only after finding normal serum CK levels and a normal result of the forearm ischemic exercise.

### Phosphorylase b Kinase Deficiency

PBK deficiency in an autosomal recessive disorder that has a heterogeneous clinical picture. Children have presented with hepatomegaly and weakness, whereas adults demonstrated exercise intolerance and myoglobinuria. Some patients have had progressive weakness. CK levels were elevated and the ischemic lactate test has been normal in at least one reported patient. Enzyme levels were reduced in biopsy specimens of muscle.

### Phosphofructokinase Deficiency

**Clinical Presentation.** PFK deficiency is an autosomal recessive disorder with an unexplained male predominance and predisposition in Ashkenazi Jews. The genetic locus is on chromosome 1. Patients experience exercise intolerance with cramps and myoglobinuria similar to that in phosphorylase deficiency. However, there is an associated hemolytic anemia because of the partial PFK deficiency in red blood cells that occurs. Patients have resultant episodes of hemolysis with jaundice. In addition, PFK patients generally have no progressive weakness.

**Laboratory Evaluation.** In addition to an elevated CK, slight anemia and evidence of hemolysis can be seen. The ischemic lactate demonstrates a failure to rise similar to that in phosphorylase defi-

ciency. EMG findings are also similar to those in phosphorylase deficiency. Muscle biopsy demonstrates subsarcolemmal vacuoles with periodic acid–Schiff–positive glycogen and lack of histochemical staining for PFK. The enzyme deficiency can be verified by biochemical assay.

**Treatment and Prognosis.** Acute episodes of weakness and myoglobinuria are an emergency and should be treated with hydration and alkalinization of the urine to prevent renal failure. Patients can improve exercise tolerance by physical conditioning to promote the oxidation of free fatty acids. The anemia is generally mild and therefore no treatment is necessary. Permanent weakness does not occur.

**Differential Diagnosis.** The differential diagnosis of PFK deficiency is similar to and includes that described for phosphorylase deficiency.

## Disorders of Terminal Glycolysis

### Phosphoglycerate kinase Deficiency

PGK deficiency is an X-linked disorder that presents in childhood with seizures and mental retardation. There is usually a severe associated hemolytic anemia. Three cases of PGK deficiency have been reported that involved exercise intolerance, episodes of myoglobinuria, and later progressive weakness. Patients demonstrated laboratory findings of hemolytic anemia, elevated CK levels, and normal interictal electromyograms. The ischemic lactate test shows no rise in venous lactate with anaerobic exercise. Muscle pathology is normal, and the diagnosis is made by biochemical assay. There is no specific treatment. The differential diagnosis of PFK deficiency is similar to and includes that described for phosphorylase deficiency.

### Phosphoglycerate Mutase Deficiency

PGAM deficiency is an autosomal recessive disorder that presents in childhood with exercise intolerance, myoglobinuria, and normal muscle strength. Serum CK is generally elevated and the ischemic lactate test demonstrates a submaximal rise in lactate that is less than the four times baseline in normal patients. Glycogen accumulation is seen on muscle biopsy and enzyme activity is reduced. The differential diagnosis of PGAM deficiency is similar to and includes that described for phosphorylase deficiency.

### Lactate Dehydrogenase Deficiency

LDH deficiency is an autosomal recessive disorder linked to chromosome 11. Only two patients have been reported, and these patients demonstrated exercise intolerance and fatigue with myoglobinuria. Strength was maintained. Interestingly, during episodes of myalgias and weakness after exercise, the CK was elevated while the LDH levels remained normal.

Ischemic exercise testing demonstrates a marked elevation in pyruvate but no elevation in lactate, indicating a block in the conversion of pyruvate to lactate via LDH. LDH is also absent or reduced in red blood cells. Biopsy shows a decrease in LDH activity. The differential diagnosis of LDH deficiency is similar to and includes that described for phosphorylase deficiency.

### Lipid Disorders

*Carnitine Palmityltransferase Deficiency*
**Clinical Manifestations.** CPT deficiency is the most common cause of recurrent myoglobinuria. It is autosomal recessive with a male predominance. Patients present in adolescence with myalgia and stiffness that are triggered by prolonged exercise, fasting, infection, cold, stress, or a high-fat diet. In some cases there may be no apparent precipitant. Episodes occur without a warning cramp and there is no second-wind phenomenon. Examination results are normal between episodes, but weakness can be observed during episodes of rhabdomyolysis.

**Diagnostic Evaluation.** Patients have normal CK between episodes of rhabdomyolysis. Their electromyogram is also normal, as is their ischemic lactate test. Provacative testing with a prolonged fast of up to 72 hours demonstrates elevated CK and a delayed rise in ketones. Although muscle pathology is generally normal, there is a decrease in CPT activity.

**Treatment and Prognosis.** Episodes of rhabdomyolysis should be treated as described earlier for phosphorylase deficiency. The mainstays of treatment are frequent small meals and a low-fat, high-carbohydrate diet. Patients should avoid precipitants such as prolonged exercise, exercise in a poorly fed state, and exercise when infected.

**Differential Diagnosis.** The differential diagnosis is similar to that for phosphorylase deficiency.

### Other Disorders of Muscle Metabolism: Purine Nucleotide Cycle

*Myoadenylate Deaminase Deficiency*
**Clinical Presentation.** Myoadenylate deaminase (MAD) deficiency is an autosomal recessive disorder that can present in some affected patients with exercise intolerance and myoglobinuria. MAD deficiency is present in 1% to 2% of patients undergoing muscle biopsy and its significance is unclear. However, a number of patients have been described with exercise intolerance, fatigue, and rare rhabdomyolysis who demonstrate decreased activity of MAD on biopsy. Symptoms, when present, begin in the second decade. The myalgias affect predominantly the legs and increase with increasing levels of exercise.

**Diagnostic Evaluation.** The CK may be mildly elevated. Electromyograms have been normal. The ischemic lactate test demonstrates a reduced rise in the levels of ammonia. Muscle biopsy demonstrates absence of staining for MAD and reduced enzyme activity.

**Treatment and Prognosis.** There is no specific treatment for MAD deficiency, although exercise tolerance can be improved through training. The disorder is benign.

### Periodic Paralyses and Related Disorders

**Clinical Presentation.** The periodic paralyses are a rare group of autosomal dominant disorders that probably affect no more than 4 to 5 per 100,000 in the population. They involve attacks of flaccid weakness associated with fluctuating potassium levels. Families with decreased serum potassium, increased levels of potassium (adynamia episodica hereditaria), and even normal levels of potassium during attacks have been described. Patients with normal potassium levels clinically resemble hyperkalemic patients. Myotonia* has been observed in patients with hyperkalemic periodic paralysis; furthermore, episodes of flaccid weakness were seen in patients with paramyotonia congenita, leading to early conjecture that these disorders were related. In fact, as pointed out in the following, hyperkalemic periodic paralysis and paramyotonia congenita are allelic disorders linked to chromosome 17 and associated with mutations of the sodium channel. Hypokalemic periodic paralysis has been linked to chromosome 1q in the region of the dihydropyridine receptor.

In all the periodic paralyses, there are attacks of flaccid weakness affecting skeletal muscles associated with loss of reflexes. There are no sensory or other abnormalities. Both hyperkalemic and hypokalemic periodic paralyses can be triggered by rest after intense exercise. Episodes vary in duration, lasting from minutes to hours. During either type of attack, affected muscles are depolarized and electrically inactive. Rarely, potassium levels may be abnormal enough to cause fatal cardiac arrhythmias. Several clinical differences can be found between hyperkalemic and hypokalemic paralyses.

In *hypokalemic periodic paralysis*, onset is at puberty, males are more severely affected, and excessive carbohydrate intake may trigger attacks. Attacks are often severe and can last for up to 24

---

*Myotonia is the inability to relax a contracted muscle. It is accompanied by electrophysiologic discharges on electromyography. These discharges occur spontaneously at rest and vary in both amplitude and frequency. The classic myotonic disorders include myotonic dystrophy, myotonia congenita, paramyotonia congenita, and Schwartz-Jampel syndrome.

hours. Cranial nerves are rarely affected and ocular muscles are never affected. Myotonia, if present, is restricted to the eyelids, and there is no limb myotonia on EMG. The cause of hypokalemic periodic paralysis has not been established, but it is mapped to chromosome 1q. This linked region contains a candidate muscle ion channel, a dihydropteridine-sensitive calcium channel expressed only in skeletal muscle.

Hypokalemia can also be seen in attacks of episodic weakness that are associated with hyperthyroidism in *thyrotoxic periodic paralysis.* Although this disorder can be seen in any race, it has been particularly seen in Asian men. In fact, 10% of Asian men with hyperthyroidism have thyrotoxic periodic paralysis. It is primarily a sporadic disorder, but the tendency to develop periodic paralysis when thyrotoxic may be autosomal dominant. Treatment of the hyperthyroidism decreases the attacks. All patients who present in adulthood with attacks of hypokalemic periodic paralysis warrant an evaluation for possible hyperthyroidism.

*Hyperkalemic paralysis* typically begins in early childhood, affects males and females equally, and episodes can be induced by either immobility or fasting. Carbohydrate ingestion can abort rather than precipitate attacks, and patients can carry candy bars for emergencies. Weakness is generally in the proximal limb muscles, but distal muscles can be affected if they were the site of exercise. CK levels can be elevated during and between attacks. Episodes tend to be shorter and milder than those seen with hypokalemic periodic paralysis. In some patients, potassium levels are normal but potassium can induce weakness. These *normokalemic* patients are thus potassium sensitive, and this is thought to be part of the spectrum of hyperkalemic periodic paralysis. Patients with hyperkalemic periodic paralysis can demonstrate cold-induced myotonia between episodes of weakness. Hyperkalemic periodic paralysis and paramyotonia congenita (see later) are allelic disorders linked to chromosome 17q and are caused by defects in the alpha subunit of a voltage-sensitive skeletal muscle sodium channel.

Myotonia is characteristically seen in two other related disorders, paramyotonia congenita and myotonia congenita. Paramyotonia congenita is an autosomal dominant disorder in which myotonia can be seen in conjunction with episodic weakness with or without hyperkalemia. Patients with paramyotonia congenita exhibit myotonia pardoxica, in which repeated muscle contractions increase the myotonia. In other myotonias, repeated use of a muscle reduces the amount of myotonia. In myotonia congenita, profound myotonia occurs without episodic weakness. There are both dominant (Thomsen's disease) and recessive (Becker's) variants. Patients exhibit a well-muscled appearance often referred to as "juvenile Hercules." The periodic paralyses, myotonia congenita, and paramyotonia congenita are not associated with muscle weakness unless there are repeated frequent episodes of myotonia or weakness. In these cases a slowly progressive, irreversible proximal weakness can occur. By contrast, the other major myotonic disorder, myotonic dystrophy, is characterized by significant distal weakness and mild myotonia with a multisystemic picture. Linkage studies in myotonia congenita have shown that both the dominant and the recessive generalized forms are linked to a locus on chromosome 7 encoding the skeletal muscle–specific, voltage-sensitive chloride channel. The more severe, recessive form of myotonia congenita is believed to result from loss of functional channel protein; the explanation for the dominant mode of inheritance in Thomsen's disease appears to be that the defective protein disrupts multimeric chloride channel subunits.

**Diagnostic Evaluation.** The diagnosis is based on a characteristic history, the presence of a flaccid paralysis during an event, changes in serum potassium levels during attacks, and the presence of clinical or electrical myotonia. In problematic cases, provocative testing to increase or decrease potassium levels or to cool limbs may clarify the diagnosis. Muscle biopsy can show a vacuolar myopathy, but it is not diagnostic. In patients who present during an acute attack, one must consider other causes of acute weakness including hypo- or hypercalcemia, hypophosphatemia, hypermagnesemia, and rhabdomyolysis.

**Treatment and Prognosis.** Management of acute attacks of periodic paralysis is directed at correcting abnormal potassium levels. In hyperkalemic episodes, glucose and insulin are utilized to shift potassium intracellularly. Hypokalemic attacks often respond simply to oral potassium loading over several hours, although severe crises may warrant intravenous potassium loading. It is recommended that such intravenous therapy employ mannitol solutions instead of dextrose in water, as the carbohydrate load in the latter may worsen the weakness.

Chronic therapy of the periodic paralyses is aimed at prevention of episodes of weakness. In both hypokalemic and hyperkalemic paralysis, the carbonic anhydrase inhibitor acetazolamide (typically 250 mg two or three times a day) is effective. In hypokalemic periodic paralysis, attacks may be reduced by reducing dietary carbohydrates and sodium and using medications that promote renal potassium retention (spironolactone or triamterene). In hyperkalemic periodic paralysis, drugs that increase urinary potassium loss (such as thiazides) can be helpful. If myotonia is prominent in periodic paralysis or paramyotonia, then phenytoin (Dilantin), quinidine, procainamide, or mexiletine can be tried.

**Differential Diagnosis.** The characteristic clinical picture of recurrent episodes of weakness with abnormal levels of serum potassium and a positive family history generally establishes the diagnosis of periodic paralysis. When there is no characteristic family history, diseases that can cause secondary potassium changes and thus weakness should be considered (Table 7–4). Furthermore, when serum potassium levels are normal, the diagnosis is more difficult. Several disorders that cause episodic weakness should be considered when potassium is normal, including myasthenia gravis and other disorders of the neuromuscular junction, electrolyte abnormalities, and metabolic myopathies. When myotonia is present, myotonic dystrophy, myotonia congenita and paramyotonia congenita, and rare metabolic disturbances that can produce myotonia (e.g., ingestion of certain cholesterol derivatives) should be considered. In children, a rare disorder that may be present with myotonia is Schwartz-Jampel syndrome.

### Medical Disorders Causing Acute Myopathies

#### Drug- and Toxin-Induced Myopathies

Toxins that are commonly found to cause weakness and acute myopathies include heroin, cocaine, alcohol, and pentazocine. Many clinically indicated medications are also implicated in myopathy and rhabdomyolysis, including corticosteroids, colchicine, clofibrate, zidovudine, cyclosporine, lovastatin, niacin, gemfibrozil, and any agent that lowers potassium. Uncommonly, rifampin, penicillamine, amiodarone, and ipecac can cause a myopathy. Fi-

**Table 7–4 Secondary Causes of Potassium Changes and Episodic Paralysis**

HYPOKALEMIC

Conn's syndrome of hyperaldosteronism
Renal tubular acidosis
Villous adenoma
Bartter's syndrome
Drugs: diuretics, licorice, p-aminosalicylic acid, amphotericin B, corticosteroids, alcohol

HYPERKALEMIA

Potassium-sparing diuretics: spironolactone, triamterene
Addison's disease
Chronic renal failure
Aldosterone deficiency
Rhabdomyolysis
Chronic heparin therapy
Hyporeninemic hypoaldosteronism (diabetes, indomethacin, ibuprofen)

nally, rigidity and rhabdomyolysis are associated with hyperthermia in the neuroleptic-induced neuroleptic malignant syndrome and the anesthetic-induced malignant hyperthermia.

## Neuromuscular Junction Disorders

### Myasthenia Gravis

**Clinical Presentation.** Myasthenia gravis is an autoimmune disorder in which antibody-mediated destruction of the acetylcholine receptor results in a postsynaptic defect of neuromuscular junction transmission. Classically, there are fluctuating symptoms, selective involvement of the cranial muscles along with proximal limb muscles, and worsening of the symptoms during the day. The annual incidence of myasthenia gravis per million population varies from 2 to 5 to a high of 10.4. The ratio of female to male patients is 6:4. The disease presents at any age. The female incidence peaks in the third decade and the male incidence in the sixth or seventh decade of life.

In myasthenia gravis, extraocular involvement is quite characteristic. The extraocular muscles are initially affected in 50% and eventually in 90% of the patients, leading to frequent complaints of diplopia and ptosis. In 20% of patients the disease may remain localized to the eyes (i.e., ocular myasthenia gravis). However, in most patients there is generalization of the symptoms resulting in additional bulbar involvement and extremity weakness. Bulbar involvement can be manifest as dysphagia along with nasal speech and a transverse smile (myasthenic snarl). Extremity weakness is not commonly proximal and more frequently involves the lower extremities. Deep tendon reflexes are preserved. There are no sensory deficits. The weakness commonly worsens over the course of the day or with exercise. Menses, viral infections, exposure to heat, and emotional upsets can worsen symptoms. Myasthenia is associated with other autoimmune disorders including pernicious anemia, systemic lupus, rheumatoid arthritis, vitiligo, and thyroiditis. Furthermore, 10% of myasthenic patients have thyroid dysfunction, most commonly hyperthyroidism. In these cases the cause of the extraocular movement disorder can be confusing but the presence of proptosis implicates Graves' disease.

Transient neonatal myasthenia develops in 12% of infants born to myasthenic mothers. The most frequent findings are weak cry, generalized weakness, and respiratory difficulty. The symptoms present within a few hours after birth, with most presenting by 4 days after delivery. The disorder is transient and has a mean duration of 18 days.

Myasthenia gravis is caused by an autoimmune reaction to the nicotinic acetylcholine receptor in the postsynaptic region of the neuromuscular junction. Both humoral and cellular mechanisms are at work. The passive transfer of disease to mice by myasthenic IgG, immune deposits (IgG and complement components) at the neuromuscular junction, and the presence of antiacetlycholine receptor antibodies in 85% of patients all implicate humoral mechanisms. These autoantibodies cause accelerated destruction of acetylcholine receptors by antigenic modulation; cause antibody-dependent, complement-mediated lysis of the postsynaptic folds; and interfere with the interaction between acetylcholine and acetylcholine receptor. This leads to decreased numbers of acetylcholine receptors available to bind and respond to acetylcholine and compromises the safety margin of neuromuscular transmission.

The thymus gland is also involved in the immunopathogenesis of the disease because lymphofollicular hyperplasia of the thymic medulla occurs in 65% and thymoma in 15%; the thymic microenvironment includes myoid cells expressing acetylcholine receptor near antigen-presenting interdigitating cells and acetylcholine receptor–specific T cells; and thymectomy has a beneficial effect in a high proportion of the cases.

**Diagnostic Evaluation.** The mainstays of diagnosis are the presence of acetylcholine receptor antibodies; a decremental EMG response with stimulation at 2 to 3 Hz (repetitive stimulation test); increased jitter and blocking on single-fiber EMG; and a positive clinical response to edrophonium, a rapidly acting anticholinesterase agent that improves neuromuscular junction transmission in myasthenic patients, reflected as an improvement in strength.

A computed tomographic scan of the mediastinum to screen for thymoma is part of the diagnostic work-up for myasthenia gravis. Antistriational antibodies that bind to various components of the muscle fiber are present in about 84% of cases of thymomatous myasthenia; in those without thymoma, they are found in 5% and 47%, depending on whether the onset was before or after the age of 40.

**Treatment and Prognosis.** Treatment for myasthenia gravis includes symptomatic treatment with an anticholinesterase agent (pyridostigmine or neostigmine bromide), as well as therapies focused on the immune system including alternate-day prednisone therapy, thymectomy, plasmapheresis, and intravenous immunoglobulin (IVIG).

The commonly used anticholinesterase agents include pyridostigmine bromide (Mestinon) and neostigmine bromide. Because these agents are active at both nicotinic and muscarinic junctions, the rate-limiting side effects are often muscarinic, including abdominal cramping, lacrimation, salivation, sweating, bradycardias, increased frequency of urination, and diarrhea. Nicotinic side effects include cramping, fasciculation, and increased weakness. Because Mestinon has fewer muscarinic side effects, it is generally used more frequently. It is initiated at 60 mg every 4 hours with 30-mg increments until therapeutic effects or side effects are observed. If troublesome muscarinic side effects occur, these can be treated with 0.4 to 0.6 mg of atropine orally two or three times daily.

Immune-suppressing drugs play a large role in the treatment of myasthenia gravis. Prednisone can be administered in either a high-dose daily regimen or an alternate-day low-dose regimen. The side effects are greater with the daily high-dose regimen, and there is also an increased risk of worsening during the first 2 weeks of high-dose therapy. However, alternate-day prednisone may not be effective in severe cases and slow increments may be needed. Other immunosuppressives can also be used including azathioprine, cyclosporine, and cyclophosphamide (Cytoxan).

Azathioprine in doses of 2 to 3 mg/kg/day results in improvement in up to 90% of patients after 3 to 6 months. It is commonly used as a steroid-sparing agent. The side effects include hematologic reaction (18%), serious infection (7%), gastrointestinal irritation (8%), and hepatotoxicity (6%). Cyclophosphamide and cyclosporine have also been used in myasthenia gravis, but their therapeutic effects have not been shown to be superior to that of azathioprine.

Thymectomy increases the remission rate and also improves the clinical course of the disease. It is recommended for all generalized myasthenics younger than age 60. There is general agreement that the best response is in young women with a hyperplastic thymus gland and a high antibody titer. Thymoma is an absolute indication for thymectomy.

Progressive weakness can indicate the onset of a cholinergic or myasthenic crisis. Cholinergic crises are usually associated with muscarinic effects along with the weakness, whereas in a myasthenic crises the muscarinic effects are not evident. Patients in crisis who present with progressive respiratory difficulty or difficulty in handling their secretions and do not respond to relatively high doses of anticholinesterases are best treated by tracheal intubation, support with a ventilator, and intravenous feeding. Refractoriness to drug therapy usually disappears in a few days. In these patients a close search for factors that contribute to the crisis should be undertaken. These factors include changes in medication, exposure to drugs that worsen neuromuscular junction transmission (see later), infections, changes in thyroid function, and altered potassium levels. If any of these factors are present, they should be treated. In addition, treatment with either IVIG or plasmapheresis can allow rapid improvement while additional therapeutic interventions that result in slower improvement are undertaken. For patients who are not receiving immunosuppressives, the clinician needs to consider the initiation of an immunosuppressive regimen, traditionally with prednisone. For patients receiving prednisone, an increase in dose needs to be considered. Finally, for patients who have not yet had thymectomy, thymectomy may need to be undertaken.

**Differential Diagnosis.** The differential diagnosis of myasthenia gravis includes neurasthenia, oculopharyngeal muscular dystrophy, mitochondrial myopathies with or without external ophthalmoplegia, compressive and structural lesions of the brain stem and cranial nerves, the Lambert-Eaton syndrome, congenital myasthenic syndromes, and botulism. Patients with neurasthenia complain of abnormal fatigability without objective findings on physical examination or in laboratory tests. In oculopharyngeal muscular dystrophy, the weakness does not fluctuate and diplopia is not a symptom. In the mitochondrial myopathies, dysconjugate gaze is present but diplopia is uncommon, and lactic acidemia, multisystemic features, muscle biopsy, and EMG findings point to the correct diagnosis.

Lambert-Eaton syndrome is associated with antibodies to the voltage-dependent calcium channels and is often associated with malignancy, especially small cell carcinoma of the lung. These patients have improvement of strength with exercise and proximal weakness at rest. Deep tendon reflexes are reduced, and there are frequently autonomic complaints. Among the complaints are dry mouth, a metallic taste, and impotence. EMG reveals a low amplitude of the first evoked compound muscle action potential, and the compound muscle action potential facilitates markedly with fast (20 to 40 Hz) repetitive stimulation.

Patients with congenital myasthenic syndromes have an early onset of symptoms, a positive family history, and absent antiacetylcholine receptor antibodies. EMG demonstrates distinctive findings in the slow-channel syndrome and familial infantile myasthenia gravis. Edrophonium tests can be either positive or negative in the congenital syndromes. Specific diagnosis of congenital myasthenic syndromes relies on specialized in vitro studies.

Botulism presents as a descending, symmetric, flaccid paralysis of all skeletal muscles and many smooth muscles with involvement of the internal as well as the external ocular muscles. The tendon reflexes may decrease. EMG may show an incremental response to high-frequency (40 to 50 Hz) stimulation.

### Lambert-Eaton Syndrome

**Clinical Presentation.** Patients with Lambert-Eaton syndrome present with subacute onset of fluctuating proximal weakness that actually improves with exercise. There is only rare involvement of extraocular muscles. Dysautonomias are common, especially dry mouth, impotence, and hypohidrosis. Occasional complaints of paresthesias can be elicited. Examination demonstrates reduced reflexes that improve with facilitation.

This syndrome is an autoimmune disorder associated with antibodies to the voltage-dependent calcium channel in the presynaptic nerve terminal. It is often associated with neoplasms (50% to 60%), most often small cell lung tumors. These tumors demonstrate reactive calcium channel antigens, and antibodies presumably arise from reaction to the tumor. The damage to the voltage-dependent calcium channel leads to inadequate release of acetylcholine from the presynaptic terminal of both nicotinic and muscarinic junctions, resulting in altered neuromuscular and autonomic junctional transmission.

**Laboratory Evaluation.** The laboratory diagnosis of Lambert-Eaton syndrome rests on the demonstration of an initially low amplitude of the evoked CMAP response and an increment in amplitude of the CMAP with rapid stimulation. Testing for antibodies to calcium channel can be done but the antibodies are not specific. A search for malignancy should be carried out in any patient diagnosed with Lambert-Eaton syndrome.

**Therapy and Prognosis.** Treatment is directed at control of the tumor if present and maximizing release of acetylcholine at the junction. Drugs that can be helpful include aminopyridine and guanidine, but they have significant side effects. Guanidine suppresses the bone marrow and can cause tremors with a cerebellar syndrome. 4-Aminopyridine causes seizures. In addition, because of the immune-mediated mechanisms, plasmapheresis, intravenous gamma globulin, and cytotoxic agents can be of therapeutic value.

**Differential Diagnosis.** The differential diagnosis is similar to that of myasthenia.

### Botulism

**Clinical Presentation.** Botulism presents as a descending, symmetric, flaccid paralysis of all skeletal muscles and many smooth muscles 2 to 6 days after the ingestion of botulinum toxin in tainted food. Weakness progresses over 1 to 3 days and quadriplegia with diminished or absent deep tendon reflexes can follow. Bulbar involvement produces external ophthalmoplegia, dysarthria, dysphagia, ptosis, and facial weakness. Accommodative paresis and sixth-cranial-nerve palsy are frequently early signs. Patients often experience a dry mouth and may develop fixed, dilated pupils. Weakness of respiratory muscles develops and can lead to respiratory failure and intubation. Involvement of smooth muscle in the gastrointestinal tract results in constipation or paralytic ileus, and bladder involvement causes urine retention. Paresthesias and asymmetric limb weakness are occasionally observed. Sensation, mentation, memory, temperature, blood pressure, and heart rate should be normal.

Infantile botulism occurs in infants between 2 weeks and 11 months and results from colonization of the bowel with the toxin-forming organism. The infant may first develop progressively severe constipation that can lead to paralytic ileus. Additional symptoms include poor feeding, decreased movement, and lethargy. Flaccid paralysis then develops along with frequent cranial nerve palsies. Infants can demonstrate ptosis, dilated pupils, diplegia, and an impaired gag reflex along with a weak cry, poor suck, and lethargy. Deep tendon reflexes are decreased or absent. Dry mucous membranes, decreased bowel motility, and urine retention occur because of the involvement of the autonomic nervous system. Weakness of respiratory muscles can progress to respiratory failure. Infants typically recover in the reverse order of the original progression, with their extremity movement improving before their respiratory function.

Patients can also develop botulism when deep wounds are infected with *Clostridium botulinum*. Signs and symptoms are similar to those of patients with food-borne botulism. Although the responsible wound is generally deep, botulism has occurred in the context of much less severe wounds including minimal surgical wounds, superficial skin abscesses, tooth abscess, cellulitis, and maxillary sinusitis after intranasal cocaine abuse.

Botulism is caused by botulinum toxin produced by *C. botulinum*, a spore-forming, strictly anaerobic, gram-positive bacillus commonly found in soil and water. Botulinum toxin is a family of serologically closely related neurotoxins: A, B, C1, D, E, F, and G. Toxin types A, B, E, and F are the main toxins that affect humans. The toxin can be denatured by heating above 80°C but is resistant to stomach acid and digestion by enzymes of the gastrointestinal tract. It is the most potent biologic toxin known. Infection can occur by direct ingestion of tainted food (food-borne), by colonization of the gastrointestinal tract in infants, or by wound inoculation. Whatever the route, the toxin is systemically absorbed and bound to specific presynaptic cholinergic receptors in the peripheral nervous system. Within 30 minutes of binding, the toxin is internalized and interferes with presynaptic cholinergic stimulus-induced and spontaneous quantal acetylcholine release.

**Diagnostic Work-up.** The definitive diagnosis of botulism is made by demonstrating the presence of botulinum toxin in serum, stool, or suspected food. Isolation of *C. botulinum* organisms from stool, food samples, or wound material supports the diagnosis as well. The cerebrospinal fluid and blood are typically normal in both infants and adults. EMG usually shows an increment in M-wave amplitude with rapid (20 to 50 Hz) stimulation. At lower rates of repetitive stimulation there are variable responses. Motor conduction velocities and distal sensory latencies are normal.

**Treatment and Prognosis.** Adult cases of botulism have been drastically reduced through public health measures in food processing. Infantile botulism is now the most common form of human botulism because there is no method for preventing colonization of the gastrointestinal tract. In the United States, about 20 to 30 cases of food-borne botulism and 50 to 80 cases of infantile botulism occur each year. Appropriate débridement and cleaning of the wound and administration of antibiotics, such as penicillin, to kill the *C. botulinum* bacteria prevent wound botulism. Wound botulism is rare, with only one to three cases recognized per year.

When a patient develops botulism, treatment consists of supportive care in a monitored setting. Paralysis can occur rapidly, and intubation should be undertaken if there is evidence of progressive respiratory failure. Many infants experience altered autonomic function that is generally mild and short lived, including sudden unexplained alterations in heart rate, blood pressure, or skin color. A minority of patients develop the syndrome of inappropriate antidiuretic hormone secretion.

Botulinum antitoxin should be given as soon as possible to prevent the progression of weakness in adults. It does not reverse weakness that is already present. Because most cases of human botulism are caused by types A, B, and E, it is possible to give equine anti-A, B, E serum to patients. Infected wounds require débridement and administration of penicillin along with the botulinum antitoxin. In all cases, medications such as the aminoglycoside antibiotics that can cause neuromuscular junction blockade should be avoided.

Death, usually caused by respiratory failure and the resultant complications, occurs in about 20% of patients with food-borne botulism, 15% with wound botulism, and 5% with infantile botulism.

Persistent fatigue may last for 1 to 2 years after recovery in some patients.

**Differential Diagnosis.** The differential diagnosis of food-borne botulism and wound botulism includes Guillain-Barré syndrome, diphtheritic polyneuropathy, tick paralysis, curare poisoning, poliomyelitis, myasthenia gravis, and the Lambert-Eaton syndrome. Infantile botulism can be mimicked by severe dehydration or electrolyte imbalance, neonatal myasthenia gravis, poliomyelitis, hypothyroidism, tick paralysis, Werdnig-Hoffmann spinal muscular atrophy, Leigh's disease (subacute necrotizing encephalomyelopathy), congenital myopathy, and exposures to toxins such as heavy metals and organophosphates.

### Drugs and the Neuromuscular Junction

Several drugs can alter neuromuscular junction transmission and cause acute weakness in patients with myasthenia gravis. These drugs include aminoglycoside antibiotics (e.g., streptomycin, polymyxin, colistin, kanamycin, gentamicin), quinine, quinidine, and procainamide. These agents reduce the safety margin of neuromuscular transmission and should be avoided or used with great caution in patients with known myasthenia gravis. Ampicillin, erythromycin, chlorpromazine, morphine, and β-adrenergic blockers can also worsen defects of neuromuscular transmission and should be used with caution. The contrast agent for magnetic resonance imaging gadolinium diethylenetriaminepentaacetic acid can also worsen myasthenia gravis. Finally D-penicillamine can cause both myasthenia gravis and polymyositis.

## Peripheral Nerve Disorders

### Acute Inflammatory Demyelinating Neuropathy (Guillain-Barré Syndrome)

**Clinical Presentation.** Acute inflammatory demyelinating polyneuropathy (AIDP) presents as an "acute ascending paralysis" with albuminocytologic dissociation in the cerebrospinal fluid. The incidence of AIDP averages from 0.6 to 2.4 cases per 100,000 population per year without any seasonal predisposition. Antecedent events occur within 1 to 3 weeks of onset in two thirds of patients. Upper respiratory events are most common, although up to 20% of patients describe a gastrointestinal event. The preceding event for AIDP is most commonly infectious. However, in 5% to 10% of patients, AIDP may follow a surgical procedure, be associated with malignancies (especially Hodgkin's and other lymphomas), or follow organ transplantation. Other reported preceding events have included vaccinations with rabies vaccine, A/New Jersey influenza vaccine, and tetanus toxoid. Among infectious causes, preceding viral illnesses are most common, with cytomegalovirus the most frequent viral pathogen. After viruses, the most common pathogen is *Campylobacter jejuni*, especially in patients who report a gastrointestinal illness. Other organisms include *Mycoplasma pneumoniae*, gram-negative organisms, *Chlamydia* infection, *Leptospira, Toxoplasma*, and malaria organisms.

The clinical presentation of AIDP usually evolves over several days with an ascending, predominantly motor, polyradiculopathy. Progressive and usually symmetric weakness along with areflexia defines the clinical picture. The weakness is variably severe, tends to be proximal, and generally begins in the lower extremities. Weakness of trunk, intercostal, and diaphragmatic muscles occurs later. There can be associated cranial nerve involvement, and facial diplegia occurs in up to 50% of patients. Ten percent of patients have extraocular involvement. Bulbar dysfunction including difficulties in swallowing and chewing can occur in up to 40% of patients and be the presenting feature in 5%. Respiratory failure correlates with the amount of weakness in shoulder elevation and neck flexion. Sensory loss is variable but occurs in up to 75% of patients. Although most patients have sensory complaints including distal paresthesias, sensory abnormalities on examination are usually mild. Reflexes are often absent at the onset or may decrease in affected areas over the course of progression.

Other manifestations of AIDP include dysautonomias, which can occur in up to 65% of patients. The severity of the dysautonomia parallels the severity of weakness and respiratory involvement and increased mortality. Tachycardia is the most common abnormality and occurs in 50% of patients. Bradycardia, when present, can lead to sinus arrest and asystole requiring a pacemaker. Other dysautonomias include orthostatic hypotension, hypertension, facial flushing, tightness in the chest, sweating abnormalities, ileus, and both diabetes insipidus and inappropriate secretion of antidiuretic hormone. Thirty percent to 55% of patients complain of myalgias and significant pain.

Several important clinical variants of AIDP have been described. The Fisher syndrome consists of ophthalmoplegia, ataxia, and areflexia. Ropper[1] has described the pharyngeal-cervical-brachial variant of AIDP, in which involvement is restricted to these areas and does not extend to the lower extremities. AIDP can remain either a pure motor or pure sensory syndrome. A pandysautonomic syndrome has also been described. Finally, an axonal variant has been described in which the severity is generally worse and recovery poor.

Although the pathogenesis of acute inflammatory demyelinating polyradiculoneuropathy has not been established, evidence suggests that it is a cell-mediated autoimmune disease of the peripheral nerves. Given the high incidence of preceding infections, it is likely that infectious agents play an indirect role through mechanisms such as molecular mimicry between antigens of infectious agents and components of peripheral nerve myelin. For instance, antiganglioside antibodies are detected in 20% to 70% of AIDP patients. Anti-GM$_1$ antibodies are more frequently detected in patients on a background of *C. jejuni*, whose lipopolysaccharide has a GM$_1$ ganglioside–like structure, implicating molecular mimicry.

**Laboratory Evaluation.** The mainstay of the diagnosis is demonstration of an increased spinal fluid protein without mononuclear cells (i.e., albuminocytologic dissociation) in conjunction with evidence of demyelination on electrophysiologic studies. The spinal fluid protein may remain normal for the first week but then increases over 4 to 6 weeks, even when the disease is stabilizing. Concentrations are often higher than 100 mg/dL. The elevated protein is associated with little to no mononuclear cell infiltration. A pleocytosis should raise suspicion of human immunodeficiency virus infection. Electrophysiologic studies may be abnormal even early in the evolution of the disease. The classic findings are those that indicate demyelination and include multifocal conduction block and slowed nerve conduction velocities with prolonged distal and F-wave latencies. Eighty-seven percent of patients meet the clinical criteria for demyelination at some point during the first 5 weeks. The electrophysiologic data can aid in prognosis as well as diagnosis. A mean distal CMAP of 0 to 20% of the lower limit of normal was associated with a poorer prognosis. Variable amounts of axonal damage are reflected by the presence of denervation on needle examination. Features that cast doubt on the diagnosis include marked persistent asymmetry of weakness, persistent bowel or bladder dysfunction, more than 50 mononuclear cells in the cerebrospinal fluid or any polymorphonuclear cells, and finally a sharp sensory level. Other laboratory studies including hematologic and urine studies are generally normal. However, liver enzymes and CK may be elevated, and serum sodium can be decreased if serum inappropriate antidiuretic hormone occurs.

**Treatment and Prognosis.** Patients with suspected AIDP should be placed in a monitored setting where their respiratory function can be watched closely and they can be observed for dysautonomias. Prevention of complications such as respiratory failure and vascular collapse remains the mainstay of management. Ventilatory support and intubation should be carried out if there is a reduced vital capacity of 12 to 15 mL/kg, partial pressure of oxygen (PO$_2$) below 70 mm Hg with inspired room air, or severe oropharyngeal paresis. For patients with significant dysphagia, alternative feeding programs with either nasogastric feeding tubes or surgically placed feeding tubes should be implemented. Other supportive measures include prophylaxis of pulmonary embolism, adequate nutrition, and prevention of decubitus ulcers and tendon shortening. When the patient is stable, a systematic rehabilitation program starting with active resistive strengthening exercise is instituted.

Plasmapheresis and IVIG have shown efficacy in the specific treatment of AIDP. The time spent in the hospital, time receiving ventilation, and time to ambulation are shortened in patients treated with plasmapheresis compared with untreated controls. As a rule, five treatments are given over 7 to 10 days. In cases in which plasmpheresis is unavailable or contraindicated, IVIG may well be of benefit. A favorable response to IVIG was described in a Dutch controlled study in which 52.7% of IVIG-treated patients were improved at 4 weeks compared with 34.2% of patients who had plasmapheresis. Similar responses were found to IVIG and pheresis in a randomized study of 50 AIDP patients treated with IVIG or plasmapheresis.

The course of AIDP follows a regular pattern of progression, plateau, and subsequent resolution. In 50% of cases progression of the syndrome occurs over 2 weeks, in 80% of cases over 3 weeks, and in over 90% the evolution is complete by 4 weeks. There is a subsequent plateau stage that lasts 2 to 4 weeks, followed by recovery. Whereas most patients recover over 4 to 6 months, more severely affected patients have evidence of neurologic residua, although significant neurologic deficit is seen in only 15%. Five percent of patients are permanently disabled. Although AIDP is generally a monophasic illness, it can recur in 3% to 5% of patients and relapse is more likely in patients with a slow evolution (i.e., over 4 weeks).

**Differential Diagnosis.** AIDP must be differentiated from other acute disorders of the motor unit that cause weakness. The characteristic clinical and laboratory findings in AIDP should generally enable the differentiation to be made with minimal difficulty. The main acute myopathic disorder to be considered is periodic paralysis, which also presents with acute flaccid weakness. The history of prior episodes, the shorter duration of the weakness, and the presence of potassium abnormalities in periodic paralysis help to differentiate it from AIDP.

Acute disorders of the neuromuscular junction that can mimic AIDP include myasthenia gravis, tick paralysis, and botulism. Myasthenia gravis is characterized by a history of muscle fatigue with repetitive activity and can be diagnosed by using a bedside edrophonium (Tensilon) test. In botulism there may be a history of tainted food ingestion, hypotension, and fixed and dilated pupils. Spinal fluid is normal.

Causes of acute neuropathies include porphyria, toxins, and polio. Porphyria presents with autonomic involvement including abdominal pain, mental status changes, and neuropathy. The toxins that can mimic AIDP include dapsone, organophosphates, hexacarbons, and solvents. Polio is now rare but can occur in nonimmunized and partially immunized patients. The lack of sensory symptoms, the presence of meningismus, and a cerebrospinal fluid pleocytosis in acute polio help to distinguish it from AIDP.

### Diphtheria

**Clinical Presentation.** Diphtheria is caused by exotoxin produced during *Corynebacterium diphtheriae* infection. The acute illness begins as a local inflammatory infection of the upper airways, but approximately 20% of patients develop cardiomyopathy and neuropathy secondary to the production of the exotoxin. Diphtheria generally begins as a local throat infection. The three major varieties of diphtheria are faucial, laryngeal, and nasal diphtheria. These syndromes occur after an incubation period of 2 to 6 days with general malaise, irritability, anorexia, and aching. These generalized symptoms are accompanied by local symptoms including an exudative membrane adherent to the mucosa of the throat and, in severe cases, cervical adenopathy. If the disease is mild, resolution occurs within the first week. However, in more severe cases, respiratory collapse, cardiac arrhythmias, congestive heart failure, and death can occur.

Two types of neuropathic sequelae can result from the elaboration of an exotoxin. First, there can be a local neuropathy of the cranial nerves that develops between 20 and 30 days from the time of the throat infection with resultant nasal speech, dysphagia, and possibly respiratory compromise. The second type of neuropathy is a generalized neuropathy that develops 8 to 12 weeks after the onset of the infection. The incidence of neuropathy in diphtheria varies between 8% and 66% and is usually about 20%.

Local neuropathy begins with palatal paralysis, nasal speech, and impaired palatal sensation 3 to 4 weeks after the initial infection. The decrease in palatal sensation and poor cough contribute to respiratory compromise and aspiration. As the syndrome progresses, there can be autonomic involvement including poor pupillary accommodation and blurred vision while the pupillary light reflex is spared. Subsequently, between the fifth and seventh weeks after infection, in severe cases, there can be progressive paralysis of the pharynx, larynx, and diaphragm. This leads to dysphagia, hoarseness, aphonia, and respiratory failure. In the most severe cases, there may be weakness of oculomotor muscles, jaw and facial movements, sternocleidomastoid muscles, and tongue.

Generalized neuropathy usually occurs 8 to 12 weeks after the initial infection, although it can occur as early as 3 to 4 weeks after infection. It tends to be a distal sensory and motor neuropathy with both large-fiber and small-fiber involvement. In some patients there is a marked sensory ataxia. The distal weakness can be accompanied by myalgias and progress to involve proximal and trunk muscles. Reflexes are diminished or absent. Rarely, bowel and bladder involvement occurs. Recovery occurs over days to weeks, depending on severity. The neuropathy can be accompanied by severe myalgias. There is usually complete recovery over a period of weeks, with return of reflexes last to occur. Cerebrospinal fluid has been reported to demonstrate albuminocytologic dissociation in some patients and pleocytosis in other cases.[2] Electrophysiologic studies are consistent with a demyelinating neuropathy. The changes may not become evident for 2 to 3 weeks after the onset of weakness.

**Treatment and Prognosis.** Prompt administration of antitoxin in faucial diphtheria within the first 48 hours of onset sharply reduces the incidence of neuropathy. Mortality in both early and late stages appears most often related to cardiac complications, but respiratory failure can occur as well.

## Spinal Cord

### Tetanus

**Clinical Presentation.** Tetanus is more prevalent in developing countries, with approximately 1 million cases (18 per 100,000) occurring annually. Almost half of the cases worldwide are neonatal. The clinical hallmark of tetanus is sustained muscular rigidity and, in severe cases, reflex spasms and dysphagia with respiratory compromise. Tetanus is caused by wound infection with *Clostridium tetani* and resultant toxin production. Although in most cases an initial wound can be identified, there are some patients in whom no wound is found. After entry of bacteria and production of spores, there may be an incubation period varying from a few days to weeks before symptoms are evident. The period of onset between the first symptoms and reflex spasms is variable as well (3 to 14 days); the shorter the interval, the more severe the syndrome.

Tetanus can occur in either a generalized or local form. Disease severity is determined by the temporal progression of symptoms. The earliest signs of generalized tetanus include rigidity of the masseter muscles (trismus, or lockjaw) and facial muscles. There may be straightening of the upper lip with a grimace (risus sardonicus). Localized stiffness near the injury may or may not be present. Subsequently, rigidity progresses to include axial musculatures with involvement of neck, back muscles (opisthotonos), and abdomen. Finally, there is stiffness of limb muscles with relative sparing distally. In severe cases there are repetitive paroxysmal, violent contractions of involved muscles (reflex spasms) when the patient tries to move or in response to even the slightest external or internal stimuli (e.g., fear, hunger). Dysphagia and speech difficulties may be present because of trismus and spasms of the muscles of deglutition. In the most severe cases, laryngospasm can lead to respiratory compromise. Autonomic involvement causes predominantly an increase in sympathetic activity with fluctuating blood pressure and heart rate, hyperhidrosis, and hyperthermia. If severe, the dysautonomias can result in respiratory collapse. The disease progresses for up to 14 days after the initial symptoms and improvement usually begins after 4 weeks.

Localized tetanus occurs when the muscular rigidity is restricted to the wound-bearing extremity and may persist for months. However, more commonly, local tetanus is a forerunner of the generalized form.

Tetanus is caused by the neurotoxin tetanospasmin, produced by spores of the anaerobic gram-positive rod *C. tetani*. The spores are introduced into wounds, and under appropriate anaerobic conditions (especially in necrotic wounds), contaminated spores germinante, proliferate, and produce tetanospasmin. Tetanotoxin can then bind to peripheral nerve terminals (see later) or be spread through the blood stream to neuromuscular junctions. Once bound to the nerve terminus, the toxin travels centrally via retrograde axonal transport along the motor nerves and proceeds transsynaptically into presynaptic inhibitory interneurons, where it inhibits the release of neurotransmitters (mainly γ-aminobutyric acid in brain stem and glycine in spinal cord). This results in increased muscle activity. Similarly, catecholamine levels may be increased, causing sympathetic overactivity.

**Diagnostic Work-up.** Tetanus is usually diagnosed by the characteristic clinical picture. Although a history of wound exposure or the presence of a portal of entry supports the diagnosis, only one third of cultures reveal *C. tetani*. There is no serologic test for toxin in serum or cerebrospinal fluid.

**Treatment and Prognosis.** The mainstays of prevention are proper wound care and vaccination. Booster doses are recommended at 10-year intervals throughout adult life. In cases with an uncertain history of vaccination, a complete series of tetanus vaccinations should be administered; if the wound is tetanus prone (severe tissue necrosis, suppuration, and retained foreign bodies), human tetanus immune globulin, 250 U intramuscularly, is also needed.

The primary treatment strategies when tetanus occurs include elimination of the source of toxin, toxin neutralization, control of muscle rigidity and spasm, and ventilatory support. The first steps in treatment include determining the severity of the clinical symptoms and identifying the portal of entry so that the wound can be properly treated. Before wound manipulation, human tetanus immune globulin should be administered to neutralize toxin. When the wound is identified, it is cleaned and penicillin is begun to eradicate vegetative spores. A primary immunization series is required in addition to human tetanus immune globulin.

Those with tetanus of moderate severity who can still maintain adequate ventilation should have benzodiazepine treatment, preferably with diazepam, by the nasogastric or intravenous route. These patients can tolerate doses of diazepam as high as 100 mg daily without depression of consciousness. Lorazepam, which has a longer duration of action, can be used as an alternative. Intrathecal baclofen (infusion or intermittent injections) may be effectively used as a single therapy in moderately severe cases. In severe cases, with ventilatory failure and violent spasms, neuromuscular blockade with atracurium, vecuronium, or pancuronium is required. Tracheostomy is usually considered early in these severe cases because when the disease reaches its peak, it takes at least 4 weeks for recovery to occur. There is no standard regimen for treatment of autonomic instability. Combined α- and β-adrenergic blocking agents (e.g., esmolol, labetalol) have been tried with some success.

The prognosis depends on progression, severity, presence of autonomic instability, portal of entry, and age. Common complications include pneumonia, fractures, muscle ruptures, rhabdomyolysis, and renal failure.

**Differential Diagnosis.** Diseases that can mimic tetanus include strychnine intoxication, malignant neuroleptic syndrome, dystonias, hypocalcemia, and stiff-man syndrome.

## REFERENCES

1. Ropper AH: Unusual clinical variants and signs in Guillain-Barré syndrome. Arch Neurol 43:1150, 1986.
2. Solders G, Nennesmo I, Perrson A: Diphtheritic neuropathy, an analysis based on muscle and nerve biopsy and repeated electrophysiologic and autonomic function tests. J Neurol Neurosurg Psychiatry 52:876, 1989.

## BIBLIOGRAPHY

Adams JH, Duchen LW (eds): Greenfield's Neuropathology. New York, Oxford University Press, 1992, pp 455–462.

Albers JW, Donfrio PD, McGonagle TK: Sequential electrodiagnostic abnormalities in acute inflammatory demyelinating polyradiculoneuropathy. Muscle Nerve 8:528–539, 1985.

Arnason BGW, Solvien B: Acute inflammatory demyelinating polyradiculoneuropathy. In Dyck PJ, Thomas PK, Griffin JW, et al (eds): Peripheral Neuropathy, 3rd ed. Philadelphia: WB Saunders, 1993, pp 1437–1497.

Arsura E: Experience with intravenous immunoglobulin in myasthenia gravis. Clin Immunol Immunopathol 53:S170–S179, 1989.

Asbury AK, Cornblath DR: Assessment of current diagnostic criteria for Guillain-Barré syndrome. Ann Neurol 27 (Suppl):S21–S24, 1990.

Banker BQ, Engel AG: The polymyositis and dermatomyositis syndrome. In Engel AG, Banker BQ (eds): Myology. New York: McGraw-Hill, 1986, pp 1385–1422.

Cherin P, Herson S, Weschsler B, et al: Intravenous immunoglobulin for polymyositis and dermatomyositis. Lancet 336:116, 1990.

Cole L, Youngman H: Treatment of tetanus. Lancet 1:1017–1020, 1969.

Cornblath DR: Electrophysiology in Guillain-Barré syndrome. Ann Neurol 27(Suppl):S17–S20, 1990.

Dalakas M: Pharmacologic concerns of corticosteroids in the treatment of patients with immune-related neuromuscular diseases. Neurol Clin 8:93–118, 1990.

Dalakas MC: Polymyositis, dermatomyositis, and inclusion-body myositis. N Engl J Med 325:1487–1498, 1991.

Dalakas MC: Inflammatory myopathies: Pathogenesis and treatment. Neuropharmacology 5:327–351, 1992.

Dowell VR Jr: Botulism and tetanus: Selected epidemiologic and microbiologic aspects. Rev Infect Dis 6(Suppl 1):S202–S207, 1984.

Drachman DA, Patterson PY, Berlin BS, Roguska J: Immunosuppression and the Guillain-Barré syndrome. Arch Neurol 23:385–393, 1970.

Engel AG: The periodic paralyses. In Engel AG, Banker BQ (eds): Myology. New York: McGraw-Hill, 1986, pp 1843–1870.

Engel AG: Myasthenic syndromes. In Engel AG, Franzini-Armstrong C (eds): Myology, 2nd ed. New York, McGraw-Hill, 1994, pp 1798–1835.

George AL Jr, Crackower MA, Abdalla JA, et al: Molecular basis of Thomsen's disease (autosomal dominant myotonia congenita). Nat Genet 3:305–310, 1993.

Griggs RC, Mendell JR, Miller RG: Evaluation and treatment of myopathies. In Metabolic Myopathies. Philadelphia, FA Davis, 1995, pp 247–249.

Horwitz MA, Hughes JM, Merson MH: Food-borne botulism in the United States. J Infect Dis 136:153–159, 1977.

Hughes RAC, Newsom-Davis JM, Prkin GD, Pierce JM: Controlled trial of prednisone in acute polyneuropathy. Lancet 2:750–753, 1978.

Kaldor J, Speed BR: Guillain-Barré syndrome and Campylobacter jejuni: A serologic study. BMJ (Clin Res Ed) 288:1867–1870, 1984.

Lanska DJ: Indications for thymectomy in myasthenia gravis. Neurology 40:1828–1829, 1990.

Lehmann-Horn F, Rudel R, Ricker K: Non-dystrophic myotonias and periodic paralyses. Neuromuscul Disord 3:161–169, 1993.

Luisto M, Seppalainen AM: Electroneuromyographic sequela of tetanus, a controlled study of 40 patients. Electromyogr Clin Neurophysiol 29:377–381, 1989.

McArdle B: Myopathy due to a defect in muscle glycogen breakdown. Clin Sci 10:13–33, 1951.

McDonald I, Kocen RS: Diphtheritic neuropathy. In Dyck PJ, Thomas PK, Griffin JW, et al (eds): Peripheral Neuropathy, 3rd ed. Philadelphia, WB Saunders, 1993, pp 1412–1417.

McFadzian AJS, Yeung R: Familial occurrence of thyrotoxic periodic paralysis. BMJ 1:760, 1969.

McKhan GM, Griffin JW, Cornblath DR, et al: Guillain-Barré Syndrome Study Group: Analysis of prognostic factors and the effect of plasmapheresis. Ann Neurol 23:347–353, 1988.

Miller HG, Stanton JB: Neurologic sequelae of prophylactic inoculation. QJM 23:1, 1954.

Plotz PH, Dalakoas M, Leff RL, et al: Current concepts in the idiopathic inflammatory myopathies: Polymyositis, dermatomyositis, and related disorders. Ann Intern Med 111:143–157, 1989.

Ptacek LJ, Johnson KJ, Griggs RC: Genetics and physiology of the myotonic muscle disorders. N Engl J Med 328:482–489, 1993.

Ricker K, Lehmann-Horn F, Moxley RT: Myotonia fluctuans. Arch Neurol 47:268–272, 1990.

Seybold ME, Drachman DB: Gradually increasing doses of prednisone in myasthenia gravis: Reducing the hazards of treatment. N Engl J Med 290:81–84, 1974.

Spaans F: Guillain-Barré syndrome with exclusively motor involvement. Electroencephalogr Clin Neurophysiol 61:15, 1985.

Tonin P, Lewis P, Servidei S, DiMauro S: Metabolic causes of myoglobinuria. Ann Neurol 27:181–185, 1990.

Truax BT: Autonomic disturbances in the Guillain-Barré syndrome. Semin Neurol 4:462–468, 1984.

Weber JT, Goodpasture HC, Alexander H, et al: Wound botulism in a patient with a tooth abscess: Case report and review. Clin Infect Dis 16:635–639, 1993.

Wright GP. The neurotoxins of Clostridium botulinum and Clostridium tetani. Pharmacol Rev 7:413–465, 1955.

# Neurologic Manifestations of

# Rheumatologic Diseases

8

*Lawrence J. Leventhal and Bruce Freundlich*

The most common rheumatologic process that can lead to neuropathy in the lower extremity is due to spinal pathology in the form of foraminal stenosis caused by degenerative joint disease in the vertebral facet joints, degenerative disk disease, or bulging or herniated lumbar disks. This chapter, however, concentrates more on the neurologic consequences of vasculitis and connective tissue disease. Although many of the diseases in these categories are uncommon or rare, failure to recognize and treat these conditions can lead to grave consequences. Both vasculitis and connective tissue disease can cause lower extremity pain and weakness of neuropathic or myopathic origin by affecting the spinal cord, nerve roots, plexus, peripheral nerves, or muscles. Evaluation for these diseases is usually prompted by the presence of *unexplained multisystem disease, arthritis symptoms, other musculoskeletal pain, or unexplained laboratory abnormalities* (Table 8–1). These conditions are frequently complex and multisystemic; therefore, a detailed history and review of systems are critical in establishing a pattern of clinical involvement that leads to the correct diagnosis. With the exception of a positive tissue biopsy in vasculitis, it is unusual for a single clinical finding or laboratory abnormality to be diagnostic of these conditions.

## DISEASE PROCESSES

Vasculitis is an inflammation of blood vessels that can lead to severe, life-threatening illness. There are multiple forms of vasculitis, which are usually categorized by the size of blood vessel, the pattern of organ involvement, or the histopathology.

Not all types of vasculitis affect the nervous system. For example, neurologic involvement is rare in hypersensitivity vasculitis, the most common form of vasculitis that affects the small vessels. Other types of small-vessel vasculitis, however, can affect nerves and may present in the lower extremities with footdrop or less dramatically with distal paresthesias. These conditions can be associated, for example, with hepatitis B and C, cryoglobulinemia, lymphomas, infections, and human immunodeficiency virus (HIV). Vasculitis of medium-sized vessels is frequently associated with neurologic involvement. The two most important forms of medium-sized vessel disease are polyarteritis nodosa and allergic angiitis and granulomatosis (Churg-Strauss syndrome). Wegener's granulomatosis, in which granulomas are found surrounding the blood vessels, is another important type of vasculitis that can damage nerves.

Connective tissue diseases are a group of systemic illnesses that are characteristically associated with autoantibodies and can have overlapping clinical manifestations. These include systemic lupus erythematosus (SLE), rheumatoid arthritis (RA), systemic sclerosis (scleroderma), polymyositis, dermatomyositis, and Sjögren's syndrome. The pathogenic process in these diseases is complex, but infrequently they have a component of vasculitis. Therefore, the damage to nerves seen in the connective tissue diseases may be direct autoimmune-mediated nerve damage or damage related to vasculitis of the vessels feeding particular nerves. All of these conditions are occasionally associated with inflammation of the muscle. This is a sine qua non of polymyositis and dermatomyositis.

## CLINICAL APPROACH TO DIAGNOSIS

When one is dealing with systemic disease in the context of neurologic or myopathic dysfunction of the lower extremity, the patient's history and physical findings are quite important in the diagnosis of vasculitis and connective tissue disease. Rheumatic disease is often suspected because of accompanying musculoskeletal complaints. The initial approach to a patient with suspected rheumatic disease involves determining whether the patient has true arthritis, arthralgias without arthritis, or periarticular and/or nonarticular pain.

When the clinician decides that the patient indeed has arthritis pain, the next determination is

**Table 8–1  Clinical Presentations of Selected Rheumatologic Diseases**

| Rheumatologic Disease | Articular Symptoms and Signs* | Representative Extra-articular Manifestations* | Representative Laboratory Abnormalities* | Common Neurologic Presentations of Lower Extremity* |
|---|---|---|---|---|
| Rheumatoid arthritis (RA) | Erosive, symmetric polyarticular synovitis, predominantly small joints of hands and wrists | Subcutaneous nodules<br>Raynaud's phenomenon<br>Pleuritis, pulmonary fibrosis<br>Pericarditis<br>Vasculitis | +RF (75%); increased ESR<br>Anemia; increased WBC<br>+ANA (low titer)<br>Synovial fluid inflammatory | Entrapment, neuropathy<br>Distal symmetric polyneuropathy<br>Mononeuritis multiplex<br>Myelopathy (rare)<br>Drug-induced neuropathy and myopathy |
| Systemic lupus erythematosus (SLE) | Similar to RA but nonerosive, nondestructive | Raynaud's phenomenon<br>Rash<br>Photosensitivity<br>Oral ulcers<br>History of thrombosis<br>Renal disease<br>Pleuro- or pericarditis<br>Interstitial lung disease<br>Vasculitis | Anemia<br>Decreased WBC; decreased platelets<br>+ANA; +RF (low titer)<br>Decreased complement; increased ESR<br>+VDRL<br>+Anti-dsDNA antibody<br>+Anti-Smith, RNP antibody<br>Urinalysis: active sediment | Entrapment neuropathy<br>Distal symmetric polyneuropathy<br>Transverse myelitis<br>Mononeuritis multiplex<br>Radiculopathy (rare)<br>Ascending paralysis (rare) |
| Polymyositis (PM) or dermatomyositis (DM) | Similar to RA but nonerosive, nondestructive | Dysphagia<br>Pulmonary fibrosis<br>Proximal muscle weakness<br>Also for dermatomyositis<br>Periorbital edema<br>Heliotrope rash<br>Gottron's papules | Anemia<br>Increased CPK<br>Increased aldolase, SGOT, SGPT<br>+ANA; increased ESR<br>EMG: myopathic process<br>Muscle biopsy: inflammatory myositis | Proximal muscle weakness<br>Mononeuritis multiplex (rare)<br>Distal symmetric polyneuropathy (rare) |
| Sjögren's syndrome (SS) | Similar to RA but nonerosive, nondestructive | Dry eyes, dry mouth<br>Dry skin<br>Parotid enlargement<br>Pulmonary interstitial fibrosis<br>Renal tubular dysfunction | +ANA<br>+SSA or SSB antibody<br>+RF<br>Anemia | Entrapment neuropathy<br>Sensory neuronopathy<br>Peripheral sensory and motor polyneuropathy<br>Mononeuritis multiplex |
| Systemic vasculitis | Nonerosive, nondestructive and tends to involve only a few joints | Digital ischemia<br>Rash, especially palpable<br>Purpura and livedo reticularis<br>Hypertension<br>Renal disease<br>Multiorgan involvement depending on type of vasculitis | Increased ESR<br>Increased WBC<br>Anemia<br>Urinalysis: active sediment<br>+ANCA<br>Synovial fluid: mildly inflammatory if available | Mononeuritis multiplex<br>Mononeuritis<br>Ascending paralysis<br>Rarely:<br>Transverse myelitis<br>Distal symmetric polyneuropathy |
| Lyme disease | Stage I: arthralgias<br>Stage II: Chronic arthritis that can be erosive and tends to be mono- or oligoarthritis | Aseptic meningitis or menigoencephalomyelitis<br>Cranial nerve palsy<br>Heart block | +Lyme serology<br>CSF: increased WBC<br>Increased protein<br>Synovial fluid: inflammatory | Radiculoneuritis<br>Rarely<br>Lumbosacral plexopathy<br>Mononeuritis multiplex<br>Guillain-Barré like |
| Osteoarthritis of lumbar spine | Sclerosis and joint space narrowing of facets<br>Associated with degenerated disks and vertebral osteophytes | Usually none | Normal except radiographic changes as indicated | Lumbar radiculopathy<br>Lumbar spinal stenosis<br>Rarely: myelopathy |
| Bursitis, tendonitis, repetitive strain | Usually none | Normal | Normal | Entrapment neuropathy, tarsal tunnel, meralgia paresthetica |

*Not all of these features neccesarily occur in every patient with this particular disease process.

ANA = antinuclear antibody; ANCA = antineutrophilic cytoplasmic antibody; CSF = cerebrospinal fluid; CPK = creatine phosphokinase; dsDNA = double-stranded DNA; EMG = electromyography; ESR = erythrocyte sedimentation rate; RF = rheumatoid factor; SGOT = serum glutamic-oxaloacetic transaminase; SGPT = serum glutamic-pyruvic transaminase; SSA (B) = Sjögren's syndrome antigen A (B); VDRL = Venereal Disease Research Laboratory; WBC = white blood cell count.

whether the arthritis is inflammatory or noninflammatory. This distinction is also made on clinical grounds. If a patient is thought to have an inflammatory arthritis, the next step is to sort out the cause of the inflammatory arthritis. This is usually approached by evaluating the distribution of the joints involved and assessing nonmusculoskeletal complaints. The following are some examples of this concept.

Photosensitive rashes, a prior history of proteinuria, and pleuritic chest pain are helpful in the diagnosis of SLE. Dry eyes and dry mouth suggest Sjögren's syndrome. Raynaud's phenomenon by history is associated with SLE and systemic sclerosis. A history of prior jaundice, blood transfusions, promiscuous sexual contact, or intravenous drug use suggests hepatitis or cryoglobulinemia. Prior asthma suggests Churg-Strauss syndrome, and a history of sinusitis may suggest Wegener's granulomatosis. Difficulty in rising from a chair, climbing steps, or combing the hair is frequently reported by patients with myositis.

The history is also used to probe for other systemic nonrheumatologic conditions that are associated with neuropathy. Examples include a complaint of polyuria and polydipsia as seen in diabetes mellitus, unexplained dyspnea in sarcoidosis, consumption of moonshine and gout with lead poisoning, and the episodic abdominal pain of acute intermittent porphyria.

The physical examination may also provide important diagnostic clues. A malar rash (on the cheeks and bridge of the nose) or petechiae in the distal lower extremities (resulting from thrombocytopenia) suggests SLE. Multiple inflamed joints in a symmetric pattern are compatible with with a diagnosis of RA or SLE, whereas a more transient asymmetric arthritis involving only a few joints may suggest vasculitis. Feet that become purplish in the cold on examination may indicate Raynaud's phenomenon. Palpable purpura or footdrop strongly suggests a vasculitis. Nonhealing ulcerations can be seen in both connective tissue disease and vasculitis.

Proximal muscle weakness should make one suspect myositis. Clinically, it is crucial to distinguish weakness related to a neuropathic process from that related to a myopathic process. Weakness associated with myopathy is usually proximal, whereas that related to neuropathy is predominantly distal. The deep tendon reflexes are preserved in myopathy, whereas in neuropathy they are decreased or absent. The presence of sensory abnormalities and fasciculations favors neurogenic weakness.

## LABORATORY ASSESSMENT

Laboratory findings are the third cornerstone in suggesting a diagnosis of the preceding entities. It must be kept in mind that laboratory tests are merely adjuncts to the clinical diagnosis of rheumatic diseases. With few exceptions, a single test result does not confirm or exclude the diagnosis of any disease. There is an increased prevalence of positive rheumatologic tests in patients with neurologic disease. This does not always indicate that a rheumatic disease is the cause of the neurologic findings. The abnormality may simply be a nonspecific finding secondary to coexistent disease or an age-related outlier. In others, it may be secondary to the autoimmune pathogenesis of the neurologic disease (e.g., in multiple sclerosis).

Antinuclear antibodies (ANAs), rheumatoid factor, the erythrocyte sedimentation rate, and complement levels are useful in screening for connective tissue disease and vasculitis. Although none of these are specific, high ANA titers suggest a connective tissue disease and make vasculitis less likely. A positive test for ANAs or rheumatoid factor, especially in high titer, or low serum levels of complement should alert the clinician to a potential serious systemic illness of rheumatic origin. If an ANA is found, a positive test for antibody to deoxyribonucleic acid (anti-DNA) (double stranded), antiribonucleoprotein (anti-RNP), or anti-Smith antibody is usually confirmatory of SLE. Cryoglobulin, liver function, and antineutrophil cytoplasmic antibody (ANCA) tests should usually be performed if vasculitis is suspected.

If there is a joint effusion, arthrocentesis should be performed to look for inflammatory fluid. This finding is important evidence that the patient has an inflammatory arthropathy as opposed to degenerative arthritis. Synovial biopsy is usually unnecessary.

## ELECTROMYOGRAPHY AND NERVE CONDUCTION VELOCITY STUDIES

Electromyography (EMG) and nerve conduction velocity (NCV) studies are described in detail in other chapters. In brief, the electrodiagnostic studies provide key diagnostic information by distinguishing neuropathic from myopathic processess and axonal from demyelinating neuropathies. The nerve conduction velocity is often decreased in peripheral neuropathy, and the EMG shows fibrillations, positive sharp waves, and a reduced number of motor units. In myopathies, short-duration, small-amplitude, polyphasic motor units are seen. Fibrillation potentials and positive sharp waves are frequently seen in myositis.

Determining the overall pattern of neuropathic involvement can help guide the further evaluation of the patient. For example, extensive serologic testing or nerve biopsy is rarely indicated for a mild distal sensory neuropathy but is extremely important in the evaluation of a distal neuropathy that causes progressive neurologic deficit or in mononeuritis multiplex. Furthermore, the pattern of neurologic involvement may be a clue to the underlying diagnosis. In addition, electrophysiologic studies may aid in the decision about further work-up. For example, when a patient with suspected vasculitic neuropathy undergoes nerve biopsy, the nerve for biopsy can be chosen on the basis of abnormal nerve conduction in order to avert false-negative sampling error.

## BIOPSY

In most instances, for a definitive diagnosis of vasculitis or inflammatory myopathies, tissue must be obtained for histopathologic assessment. If these diseases are suspected, it is most important, when possible, to obtain a biopsy specimen, because treatment of the disease frequently involves potent cytotoxic agents.

Specific patterns of neurologic abnormalities that may affect the lower extremity are delineated and discussed in the following. An algorithmic approach for determining whether a rheumatic disease is the cause of a neurologic abnormality of the lower extremity is outlined in Figure 8–1.

## CENTRAL NERVOUS SYSTEM

Rheumatic diseases are rare causes of myelopathy involving the lower extremities. The spinal cord may be affected by mechanical compression or by infarction secondary to ischemia, such as in vasculitis. The onset is rapid with vasculitis but may be

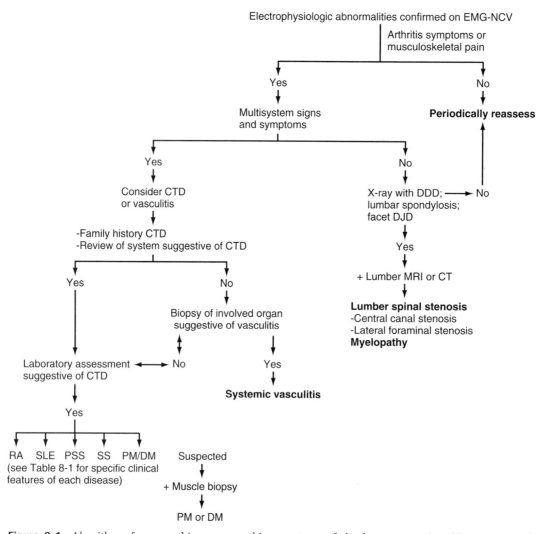

**Figure 8–1** Algorithm of neuropathic or myopathic symptoms of the lower extremity. CT = computed tomography; CTD = connective tissue disease; DDD = degenerative disc disease; DJD = degenerative joint disease; DM = dermatomyositis; EMG = electromyography; MRI = magnetic resonance imaging; NCV = nerve conduction velocity; PM = polymyositis; PSS = progressive systemic sclerosis; RA = rheumatoid arthritis; SLE = systemic lupus erythematosus; SS = Sjögren's syndrome.

either rapid or insidious with mechanical compression.

Lumbar spondylosis is not as common a cause of myelopathy as cervical spondylosis. Asymptomatic spondylosis is so common that radiographic evidence of spondylosis does not exclude an alternative or coexistent cause of this type of dysfunction.

SLE is the most common cause of noncompressive myelopathy. In the majority of patients, the onset is acute with progressive leg weakness, paresthesias, sensory level deficits, and urine retention. Myelopathy in SLE is often associated with other neurologic manifestations. Myelography is normal. In the cerebrospinal fluid elevated protein, decreased glucose, and mild pleocytosis may be seen.

## PERIPHERAL NERVOUS SYSTEM

The peripheral nervous system is frequently affected by the rheumatic diseases. The distinction among the different types of neuropathy is based partially on clinical grounds, such as the nerves involved (e.g., pure motor, pure sensory, mixed), the anatomic distribution of nerve dysfunction, and the timing of evolution.

## Radiculopathies

The vast majority of radiculopathies are caused by focal nerve root compression in the spine. These root compressions are usually caused by some combination of spondylosis (discogenic degenerative disk disease) and degenerative facet joint arthritis.

Radiculopathy can occur in patients with RA, ankylosing spondylitis, and rarely vasculitis. Meningoradiculitis classically occurs in the second stage of Lyme disease. Patients with Lyme disease may have painful multifocal radiculopathies. Studies of the cerebrospinal fluid (CSF) show pleocytosis, increased protein levels, and intrathecal synthesis of antiborrelial antibody.

## Peripheral Neuropathies

Disease of the peripheral nervous system is a prominent feature of a number of rheumatic diseases. The neuropathy can present as mononeuritis multiplex, distal symmetric sensorimotor neuropathy, or asymmetric distal neuropathy.

### Distal Axonal Neuropathies

Symmetric distal sensorimotor neuropathy occurs frequently in a variety of rheumatic disorders.

The neuropathy may be the initial feature of some illnesses, whereas in others it rarely appears until late in the disease. In SLE, mixed connective tissue disease (MCTD), and cryoglobulinemia the incidence is approximately 5% to 10%. Distal sensory neuropathy is seen less frequently in vasculitides, RA, systemic sclerosis, and Sjögren's syndrome. Patients with RA who are being treated with gold can develop a distal symmetric peripheral neuropathy with rapid onset of progressive motor weakness associated with pain and paresthesias. The vast majority of patients with this form of neuropathy have causes other than a rheumatic disease, such as alcohol abuse or diabetes.

### Mononeuropathy

#### Entrapment Mononeuropathy

Entrapment neuropathies develop at sites where the nerves are vulnerable to compression. In rheumatic diseases, entrapment neuropathies develop at sites where there is increased surrounding pressure, typically by local joint and tendinous sheath synovial inflammation. Tarsal tunnel syndrome is the most common entrapment neuropathy of the lower extremity. The posterior tibial nerve is compressed as it passes through the tunnel beneath the flexor retinaculum on the medial side of the ankle. Patients often present with aching, burning, numbness, and tingling involving the plantar surface of the foot. Tinel's sign may be positive over the course of the nerve posterior to the medial malleolus.

Compression of the sciatic nerve or peroneal nerve by a Baker cyst in the popliteal fossa or knee joint inflammation can occur. Compression of the peroneal nerve can cause footdrop with weakness of the extensors of the toes and evertors of the foot.

#### Cutaneous Mononeuropathy

A mononeuropathy of a cutaneous nerve can cause a patch of sensory disturbance such as pain, paresthesias, or dysesthesia. The most common example of a cutaneous neuropathy of the lower extremity is meralgia paresthetica. The pain and paresthesias occur at the anterior lateral aspect of the thigh and are caused by compression of the lateral femoral cutaneous nerve as it emerges from beneath the inguinal ligament to enter the thigh. Rapid weight gain or loss, tight corsets or belts, and prolonged periods of hip flexion are common aggravating factors.

#### Ischemic Mononeuropathy

An ischemic mononeuropathy may occur in any disease that can manifest vasculitic neuropathy. Ischemic mononeuropathies typically begin suddenly and painfully and are often associated with dysesthesia, hyperesthesia, and sensory loss. Muscle weakness can occur as well. Proximal rather than distal limb involvement is typical.

### Mononeuropathy Multiplex

Mononeuropathy multiplex is disease of multiple individual peripheral nerves. Rheumatic diseases, especially with vasculitic involvement, are a common cause. The occurrence of mononeuropathy multiplex is often a sign of disease activity and usually an indication for more aggressive treatment of the underlying disease. Patients who develop mononeuropathy multiplex without an established rheumatic disease should be evaluated to search for other evidence of systemic vascultitis.

### Ascending Paralysis

Vasculitic neuropathy can also cause acute ascending paralysis (Guillain-Barré syndrome). Clues favoring vasculitic neuropathy rather than Guillain-Barré syndrome are that the former is more likely to cause axonal destruction, demonstrable by EMG, and that it is less likely to involve elevated CSF protein. Patients with rheumatic diseases have also been reported to present with an illness that is indistinguishable from chronic inflammatory demyelinating polyneuropathy.

## Sensory Neuronopathy

Sensory neuronopathy is a distinct syndrome characterized by severe sensory dysfunction caused by lymphocytic infiltration in the dorsal root ganglia. Sensory symptoms develop acutely or insidiously. This presentation has a specific association with primary Sjögren's syndrome.

## Neuropathic Arthropathy

Neuropathic arthropathy or Charcot's joint is a severe destructive arthropathy that is a consequence of impaired joint sensation. Initially the joint involvement may mimic osteoarthritis, but later the joint is swollen and enlarged with joint effusion and/or hypertrophic osteophytes followed by further destruction and instability. Diabetes mellitus and tabes dorsalis are the most common causes in the lower extremity. In diabetes, the forefoot and midfoot joints are the most commonly involved extremity joints. In tabes, the knee is often involved. X-ray examination is almost always diagnostic,

demonstrating extensive hypertrophic changes, subchondral bone fragmentation, and general disorganization of the joint.

## MYOPATHY

### Connective Tissue Disease

Myalgias occur frequently in patients with connective tissue disease. True inflammatory myositis can occur in all the connective tissue diseases as well. In addition to the usual clinical stigmata of the connective tissue diseases, those with associated myositis involve proximal muscle weakness and pain in association with elevated creatine phosphokinase and variable elevations of aldolase, serum glutamic-oxaloacetic transaminase, and serum glutamic-pyruvic transaminase. The electromyogram often demonstrates typical myopathic changes and the muscle biopsy reveals typical changes of polymyositis.

### Drug-Induced Myopathy

Several medications used to treat rheumatic diseases can be associated with myopathy. Patients treated with corticosteroids may develop proximal muscle weakness that is gradual in onset. The serum enzymes are normal, although urinary excretion of creatine is increased. EMG and muscle biopsy changes are usually nonspecific. The myopathy is usually reversible on withdrawal of corticosteroids.

Prolonged use of chloroquine, used in the treatment of RA and SLE, has also been known to produce a myopathy. D-Penicillamine, used in the treatment of RA and systemic sclerosis, can induce both myasthenia gravis and typical polymyositis.

## DISEASE MANAGEMENT

A thorough discussion of the management of this complex group of diseases is beyond the scope of this book. The decision to use corticosteroids and cytotoxic agents in a patient with a diagnosed connective tissue disease depends, in general, on the overall severity of the disease and the associated neurologic and nonneurologic clinical features.

The vast majority of patients with neurologic manifestations of a systemic vasculitis require cytotoxic therapy, as with cyclophosphamide, in addition to corticosteroids. Occasionally, a vasculitis (e.g., Churg-Strauss) is quite steroid responsive and can be treated with corticosteroids alone.

# 9

# Movement Disorders of the Lower Extremities

*Stephen M. Gollomp*

For health care professionals interested in the neurologic problems of the lower extremities, motor disorders affecting these limbs represent a significant portion of the infirmities that may be presented to them in the course of clinical practice. A disordered gait is readily apparent to the layperson and prompts a search for a solution to this problem via consultation with a professional. Even if treatment of these problems is not within the purview of the medical professional, it is incumbent upon that individual to recognize the problem, consider a differential diagnosis, initiate an appropriate evaluation, offer the patient insight into the problem, and make a referral to physicians who typically treat these problems.

These disorders are most common at the two extremes of the human life span, namely childhood and old age, but can present at any age. Disordered gait is a common problem among the elderly, affecting approximately 15% of the population between 65 and 74 years of age and 50% of the population older than 85 years. Gait disorders of any type are far less common in childhood, but at either end of the age spectrum, disordered gait represents a serious risk to the patient's well-being. Recognition and intervention are the keystones to prevention of serious injury and exaggeration of disability.

The movement disorders that affect the lower limbs can be broadly divided into three categories: disorders that induce disordered walking through loss of learned gait patterns, disorders in which walking is impaired because of abnormal leg posturing, and disorders of motor restlessness. This chapter discusses key issues related to these disorders. Most important, it emphasizes their recognition and differential diagnosis. The chapter cannot be exhaustive and reviews only the more common disorders, as the wealth of information concerning these entities would easily fill the entire contents of this volume.

## DISORDERS OF PATTERNED GAIT FUNCTION

### Idiopathic Parkinson's Disease

The prototypical disorder involving loss of the ability to perform skilled gait function is idiopathic, or Lewy body, Parkinson's disease. The disorder, first described in relatively modern time by James Parkinson in 1817, consists of three primary elements: rigidity, bradykinesia, and resting tremor. Typically, the diagnosis of idiopathic Parkinson's disease (IPD) is made when the patient manifests two of the three criteria. Among the many secondary signs of the disease is impaired patterned gait function with a resulting stooped, shuffling, festinating stride and compromised postural righting reflexes. Patients frequently display other signs of the disorder, including micrographia, hypophonia, seborrhea, olfactory impairment, and cognitive dysfunction (Table 9–1).

The majority of patients with IPD present with a unilateral resting tremor of the fingers or hand. The patient and the family frequently report the concurrent development of general slowing of motor activity, stooping of posture, shortening of stride, deterioration of the legibility of handwriting, softening of the voice, drooling, and unsteadiness of gait. Increasing difficulty with dressing, particularly buttoning a collar or a shirt sleeve; difficulty turning in bed; or deterioration of other skilled activity, such as a golf or tennis swing, typing, or assembling small objects, is frequently reported. Upon direct query, the patient usually reports that the senses of smell and taste have been impaired for years before the onset of these other symptoms. Typically, the presenting symptoms have been present for approximately 6 to 12 months but have initially been so mild as to be ascribed, by both patient and family, to normal aging. The mean age of onset is approximately 60 years.

IPD is one of the most common neurologic dis-

Table 9–1  **Signs of Idiopathic Parkinson's Disease**

| Primary Signs | Secondary Signs |
|---|---|
| Rigidity | Micrographia |
| Bradykinesia | Hypophonia |
| Tremor | Seborrhea |
| | Olfactory impairment |
| | Gait dysfunction |
| | Cognitive dysfunction |

orders, affecting 1% of the population older than the age of 60. It is estimated that there are well over one million patients with the disorder in the United States. The disorder is slightly more common among men. It occurs equally in all ethnic groups and has a worldwide distribution. The disorder is sporadic in its occurrence, although approximately 10% of cases appear to have a familial incidence in an autosomal dominant pattern. The genetic marker for autosomal dominant IPD was determined to be on chromosome 4 in one Italian family, but the gene has not yet been isolated. No specific etiology has been determined for the disorder, although a variety of environmental and genetic predispositions are suspected. The disorder is slowly progressive, but pharmacotherapy can relieve many of the symptoms of the disorder, and these patients have a life expectancy quite similar to that of age-matched control subjects.

As suggested to this point, the physical findings of IPD are readily demonstrable, although not all of the signs are present in each patient. It is often said that each patient has his or her own IPD, as permutations of symptoms and signs, with their complications, vary tremendously between patients. Nonetheless, 70% of these patients have a rest tremor of a limb, typically maximal unilaterally. In fact, it believed by most parkinsonologists that rest tremor is present, at some time in the clinical course, in virtually all patients with the disorder. Rigidity, the steady resistance to passive motion throughout the full range of motion of a joint, is present in virtually all patients, particularly with reinforcing maneuvers. Cogwheel rigidity refers to the superimposition of the tremor rhythm on the rigidity. This sign is frequently, but not uniformly, present. Bradykinesia, or slowing of motor activity with loss of dexterity, is nearly always present, although it may be quite subtle. There is a breakdown of the performance of rapid fine movements of the fingers, hand, and foot. A flexed, stooped posture with a shortened stride, loss of arm swing, and impairment of balance is generally readily observed. Postural righting reflexes can easily be assessed by posteriorly displacing the patient with the legs held together and the eyes open. Eighty percent of patients demonstrate inability to perceive common aromas when presented to them. At some point in the course of the disease, approximately 30% of patients develop dementia. More detailed assessment of verbal fluency reveals subtle impairments in this sphere in up to 85% of patients. In many patients, some oral pooling of saliva is noted. Loss of facial expression and a facial stare are present. The voice is noted to be soft and lacking in expression and inflection. Subtle oculomotor abnormalities can be noted in these patients, consisting of

mild slowing of pursuit eye movements. The inability to suppress eye blinking with tapping of the brow, the glabellar tap or Myerson's sign, can be elicited in many of the patients. The more conventional features of the neurologic examination, such as sensation, motor power, and reflexes, should all be normal in these patients.

With effective pharmacotherapy, many of the signs of the disease can be reversed, but generally some physical stigmata of the disorder persist. In about 20% of patients at the end of 2 years and 50% at 5 years, choreic involuntary movements are detectable. These are dancelike movements, usually of the limbs, that are a direct consequence of the dopaminergic therapy of IPD. In the same population, the effects of dopaminergic therapy become more unpredictable as the medication effect wears off after several hours, whereas previously the medication was effective for many hours without any apparent waning of effect.

There are no routinely available laboratory studies for confirmation of the diagnosis of IPD, although there are features detectable on positron emission tomography (PET) and single photon emission computed tomography (SPECT) scanning and on magnetic resonance (MR) imaging that are confirmatory of the diagnosis in the proper clinical setting. The diagnosis can be absolutely confirmed only at postmortem examination when the characteristic degeneration of the pigmented nuclei of the brain stem, namely substantia nigra, locus ceruleus, dorsal vagal nucleus, and nucleus basalis of Meynert, with the associated eosinophilic intracytoplasmic inclusions, Lewy's bodies, is demonstrated. As a consequence of the degeneration of the cells of the pars compacta of the substantia nigra, there is loss of the dopamine neuronal projections to the striatum, which directly correlates with much of the motor dysfunction noted with the disorder.

The differential diagnosis of IPD involves other disorders that result in an akinetic rigid state (Table 9–2). The most common alternative diagnosis is drug-induced parkinsonism related to the use of dopamine receptor antagonist drugs. These agents are most commonly the traditional antipsychotic

**Table 9–2  Differential Diagnosis of Parkinsonism**

Drug-induced parkinsonism
Toxin-induced parkinsonism: manganese, MPTP
Cerebral anoxia
Carbon monoxide intoxication
Cyanide poisoning
Carbon disulfide poisoning
Postencephalitic
Parkinson-plus syndromes
Multi-infarct state (vascular parkinsonism)
Normal pressure hydrocephalus

medications, but one must be cognizant that many antiemetic compounds are also dopamine receptor antagonists and thereby can induce parkinsonism. Parkinsonism can also be induced by various toxins, such as manganese and the meperidine analogue MPTP, but in routine clinical practice these exposures are extraordinarily rare. An akinetic rigid state can be seen after cerebral anoxia, carbon monoxide intoxication, cyanide poisoning, and carbon disulfide poisoning. These states can be seen rarely after encephalitides, although after World War I a worldwide pandemic occurred that resulted in many cases of postencephalitic parkinsonism. Other neurodegenerative disorders, frequently referred to as the Parkinson-plus syndromes, induce an akinetic rigid syndrome that must be differentiated from IPD. These entities are discussed briefly later in this chapter, but it is beyond the scope of this volume to discuss these entities in detail.

The cornerstone of the medical treatment of IPD is dopaminergic therapy with levodopa, combined with a peripheral decarboxylase inhibitor, either carbidopa or benserazide. Carbidopa is the only peripheral decarboxylase inhibitor available in the United States. Treatment with the decarboxylase inhibitor reduces the required pharmacologic dose of levodopa by 300% and substantially reduces the side effects of the treatment, including nausea and orthostatic hypotension. Levodopa or carbidopa therapy is necessary for the majority of patients for alleviation of the symptoms of IPD at some point in their disease course, but the decision to initiate this therapy is highly individualized. This decision requires considerable clinical judgment with collaboration between the patient, the patient's family, and the physician. For many patients, particularly those with fluctuations of medication effect, the use of controlled-release levodopa or carbidopa may be appropriate.

There are various adjunctive medications for the treatment of IPD that, not infrequently, may be the primary treatment in individual circumstances. For the patient whose principal problem is tremor, treatment with an anticholinergic drug, such as trihexyphenidyl or benzatropine, can be quite effective. For patients with early, mild disease, use of the monoamine oxidase B inhibitor selegiline or the dopamine-releasing agent amantadine may be appropriate and effective. For some of these early patients, particularly those younger than 50, the use of dopamine agonists, such as bromocriptine, pergolide, pramipexole, or ropinirole, can be quite effective. As depression is a frequent complication of the disease, antidepressants, both the older tricyclics such as amitriptyline and imipramine and the newer selective serotonin reuptake inhibitors such as fluoxetine, paroxetine, and sertraline, can be useful.

With progression of IPD, the use of multiple antiparkinson medications is the rule rather than the exception. Frequently, levodopa or carbidopa is combined with selegiline to extend the pharmacologic efficacy of levodopa. Controlled-release levodopa or carbidopa is used frequently. Dopamine agonists are also frequently required and can be useful. Occasionally, amantadine can be of assistance in this setting. Although not yet available, the catechol *O*-methyltransferase inhibitors telcapone and entocapone seem to be useful for extending the duration of the levodopa effect in patients with wearing off of the drug effect.

Surgical therapy also has a place in the management of IPD and has experienced a resurgence in the past 6 years, largely because of refinement of localization and imaging technology and greater understanding of the physiology of the basal ganglia. VIM thalamotomy can be effective for pharmacologically refractory tremor contralateral to the side of the lesion. In some instances, use of deep brain stimulation of this nucleus, rather than lesioning, is appropriate. For patients with severe choreic movements secondary to the dopaminergic treatment, lesioning of the contralateral ventroposterolateral globus pallidus interna can be effective for enhancing the quality of life. Although its use is still limited and fraught with many ethical limitations, fetal neural implantation in the caudate nuclei shows considerable promise for the treatment of severe IPD. Deep brain stimulation of the globus pallidus interna or of the subthalamic nucleus also seems to hold considerable promise in the treatment of selected patients.

In spite of the many strategies for the treatment of IPD that I have outlined, medication and surgery are not sole means for alleviation of the symptoms of the disease. Although it is more difficult to maintain than many of us would care to admit, a program of regular structured physical activity is vital for maintenance of function in this disorder. The program must be tailored to the capabilities of the individual, preferably with the assistance of a therapist skilled in the management of patients with IPD. The program should consist of stretching activities, muscle strengthening, and aerobic exercise on a thrice-weekly basis.

In summary, IPD is the most common motor disorder. Diagnosis is on a clinical basis. Management is complicated, holistic, and multimodal. With proper intervention, these patients have a nearly normal life expectancy, although disability can be a major problem as the disease progresses.

## Parkinson-Plus Syndromes

The term Parkinson plus refers to several akinetic rigid disorders that are generally resistant to medi-

**Table 9–3   The Parkinson-Plus Syndromes**

Progressive supranuclear palsy
Multisystem atrophy
Diffuse Lewy body disease
Corticobasal ganglionic degeneration

cal interventions and have a grave prognosis (Table 9–3). These disorders share the features of rigidity and bradykinesia with IPD but rarely involve tremor and have a number of other clinical features that are not seen in IPD. Their neuropathology, which is not covered in this chapter, is also different and much more extensive than that seen with IPD. The presence of cerebellar dysfunction, myoclonus, profound autonomic dysfunction, abnormal ocular motility, bulbar dysfunction, axial hypertonicity, lower motor neuron signs, unilateral dystonia, cortical sensory loss, limb apraxia, or profound, early dementia should prompt the consideration of one of these entities (Table 9–4). The failure of a patient to respond to dopaminergic therapy at a levodopa equivalent dose of 1 g/day for 1 month should lead to consideration of one of these syndromes. It is important to recognize these entities, as they respond poorly to the conventional treatment of IPD, are associated with a shortened life expectancy, and result in considerable disability fairly quickly.

The most common of these disorders is progressive supranuclear palsy. This disorder is distinguished by a gait impairment that consists of a wide-based, retropulsive, imbalanced stance with a nearly normal stride. The disorder is also characterized by prominent axial rigidity, supranuclear ophthalmoparesis, dementia, and lack of tremor. Recurrent falling is a common, serious cause of morbidity with this disorder. Early in the disease, patients may respond transiently to dopaminergic therapy.

The next most common of these disorders is multisystem atrophy. Multisystem atrophy refers to a heterogeneous disorder that may be characterized by an akinetic, rigid syndrome and even some tremor but also includes, to widely varying degrees, severe autonomic dysfunction, cerebellar signs, and

**Table 9–4   Signs of Atypical Parkinsonism**

Cerebellar dysfunction
Myoclonus
Profound autonomic dysfunction
Abnormal ocular motility
Bulbar dysfunction
Axial hypertonicity
Lower motor neuron signs
Unilateral dystonia
Cortical sensory loss
Limb apraxia
Profound dementia

pyramidal tract signs. Neuropathologically, this disorder, with protean clinical manifestations, begins to make more sense, as there is a common histologic hallmark of oligodendroglial cytoplasmic inclusions.

The next disorder in this group is diffuse Lewy body disease. This disease is thought to be rare but is probably more common than generally suspected. It is characterized by early, profound, cognitive dysfunction, including psychotic behavior, and the presence of an akinetic, rigid syndrome. Neuropathologically, there is diffuse distribution of Lewy's bodies through the cerebral cortex as well as in the pigmented nuclei of the brain stem, as seen in IPD.

The final disorder in this group that is mentioned here is corticobasal ganglionic degeneration. This disorder is characterized by unilateral limb rigidity with apraxia, unilateral cortical sensory loss, an alien limb syndrome, aphasia, cortical reflex myoclonus, and hyperreflexia with extensor plantar responses. Neuropathologically, there is profound cortical degeneration with typical swollen, ballooned, achromatic degeneration of the cerebral pyramidal neurons.

## Vascular Parkinsonism and Multi-Infarct State

In elderly patients, failure of gait function with akinesia and rigidity occurs commonly in the setting of multiple subcortical infarcts involving either the basal ganglia or the subcortical white matter. This entity has various appellations, including vascular parkinsonism, lower body parkinsonism, and gait predominant parkinsonism. The underlying pathology is readily demonstrated to be vascular with present MR imaging technology. As would be expected, this entity is usually poorly responsive to medication therapy but can be responsive to physical therapy modalities.

This disorder typically presents abruptly with inability to ambulate with preservation of the ability to move the legs in the seated or supine position. The patient finds that the legs appear to be "glued" to the floor. There are associated retropulsion, start hesitation, and festination, much as are seen with advanced IPD. There are varying degrees of rigidity and bradykinesia, typically confined to the legs, an unusual pattern for IPD. There is a history of vascular risk factors, including hypertension, diabetes, hyperlipidemia, and peripheral vascular disease. The cerebral imaging is confirmatory, as already indicated. Generally, these patients improve after the ictus with the passage of time and use of therapeutic modalities, as is typically the case with other presentations of acute cerebral ischemia.

## Normal Pressure Hydrocephalus

Normal pressure hydrocephalus (NPH) is a disorder physicians take pleasure in diagnosing, for it seemingly has a straightforward pathophysiology and simple, effective treatment. As with many things in life, this could not be further from the truth. This is a rare disorder, except in the setting of prior subarachnoid hemorrhage, meningitis, or head trauma.

The classic triad of cognitive dysfunction, urinary incontinence, and gait dysfunction was first described in 1965. Unfortunately, patients may present with only one or two elements of the triad, making the clinical diagnosis exceedingly difficult. One need not be reminded that this clinical triad is not specific for NPH. The gait disorder has not been precisely delineated, although it has been described as wide based with a shortened length of stride, marked impairment of tandem walking, reduced height of the step, feet seeming to be "firmly attached to the ground," unsteadiness, and difficult turns. In the recumbent position, the legs function normally. There may be some spasticity of the legs. Patients have no involvement of the upper extremities and no tremor, rigidity, or bradykinesia.

Pathophysiologically, the disorder is attributed to compression of descending periventricular pyramidal leg fibers by a dilating ventricular system. There is a greater than chance association with systemic hypertension, which suggests that the ischemic effects of chronic hypertension alter the compliance of the periventricular tissues, resulting in ventriculomegaly and symptomatic NPH.

Cerebral imaging, either computed tomographic (CT) or MR scanning, is confirmatory of ventriculomegaly with preservation of the cortical mantle, but the dynamics of cerebrospinal fluid flow can only be inferred with these techniques. Various techniques are used to assess cerebrospinal fluid dynamics, but none of the procedures adequately predicts response to treatment.

Treatment of this disorder involves the insertion of a ventricular shunt. When it is successful, the results of this operative intervention can be gratifying. Unfortunately, only 50% of the patients respond to shunt placement, even with the best of screening techniques, although one study suggests that cerebrospinal fluid stroke volume measurements may be predictive of a successful outcome with shunting. Of the patients treated with shunting, more than 30% suffer complications of the procedure, with severe complications in 15% of those treated. Therefore, treatment of this disorder involves considerable restraint and circumspection on the part of the physician, patient, and family.

## GAIT DISORDERS CAUSED BY ABNORMAL POSTURING OF THE LOWER EXTREMITIES

### Dystonia

Dystonia is a term used to describe abnormal posturing of a body part and refers to syndromes or disease entities that are manifest predominantly through abnormal posturing. The Dystonia Medical Research Foundation consensus definition of dystonia is a syndrome dominated by sustained muscle contractions that frequently cause twisting and repetitive movements or abnormal postures. Unless dystonia affecting the lower extremities is present, the syndromes and entities that have elements of dystonia do not particularly alter lower extremity function. This discussion is confined to the subset of dystonias that affect lower limb function.

Childhood-onset idiopathic torsion dystonia (ITD) typically begins with involuntary spasms of the musculature of a leg with action. Onset of the disorder is usually around the age of 10. Over time, the disorder gradually progresses with increased severity of the involuntary spasms of the affected limb and their presence at rest. The dystonia spreads to other body sites, becoming generalized in distribution after several years. The dystonic spasms of the legs eventually markedly hamper ambulation to the point of leaving the child wheelchair bound in many instances. Other activities of daily living become impaired, rendering the individual dependent. This disorder, fortunately rare, has an autosomal dominant inheritance with a penetrance of only 30%. The genetic locus of the disorder, termed *DYT1,* has been traced to chromosome 9, although the gene has yet to be isolated and cloned. The genetic locus for another form of the disorder with associated parkinsonism and X-linked inheritance, termed *DYT3,* has also been delineated.

Another form of childhood-onset dystonia has great sensitivity to medical intervention. This disorder is dopa-responsive dystonia (DRD) or diurnally fluctuating dystonia. Careful questioning about variation of the severity of dystonia through the day must be undertaken, as this is the clinical hallmark of the disorder. Typically, in this disorder, the patient is nearly normal after awakening in the morning but the dystonia worsens as the day progresses. DRD has been traced to a defect of GTP cyclohydrolase I on chromosome 14. Unfortunately, this defect is quite polymorphic, making genetic analysis difficult in an individual case.

On examination, these patients demonstrate normal conventional neurologic findings. Intellect is well preserved. The examination is striking for the uncontrollable spasmodic movements of the limbs, trunk, and face, exacerbated by attempts at action. In the case of DRD, one may have the opportunity to observe directly the marked variation in the patient's dystonic spasms through the diurnal cycle.

As with all the other movement disorders reviewed so far, neuroimaging and the laboratory are of little help in the diagnosis of this disorder. The major differential diagnoses include secondary causes of dystonia related to congenital encephalopathy, such as cerebral palsy, and rare metabolic disorders, such as Wilson's disease and GM$_1$ gangliosidosis. These diagnostic alternatives can be excluded with the appropriate neuroimaging, usually MR imaging, and metabolic studies of serum copper and of leukocyte enzymes. In appropriate families, screening for the *DYT1* and *DYT3* polymorphic markers can be useful for confirmation of the diagnosis of dystonia. Testing for the DRD gene is more difficult because of its polymorphisms between families.

Treatment of ITD is difficult, although up to 40% of patients respond to high-dose anticholinergic therapy. The benzodiazepine clonazepam can also be useful in the treatment of these patients. Occasionally, baclofen, dopamine receptor antagonists, and dopamine-depleting agents can be useful. Focal injections of botulinum toxin can be used for localized sites of dystonia. In selected patients, ventrolateral thalamotomy can be helpful in reducing dystonia on the contralateral side of the body. However, bilateral surgical treatment is associated with a 15% complication rate of severe bulbar dysfunction. Physical and occupational therapy modalities can be of considerable assistance to patients with some aspects of ITD, although the underlying disorder is not ameliorated. Biofeedback sometimes provides temporary alleviation of symptoms.

In contrast to ITD, DRD can be gratifying to treat, which is why it must be assiduously sought. The disorder is usually exquisitely sensitive to dopaminergic therapy, typically at a levodopa or carbidopa dose equivalent of 300 to 600 mg/day. This treatment frequently allows nearly complete normalization of function.

## Painful Legs and Moving Toes Syndrome

Although it is a most unusual entity, painful legs and moving toes syndrome (PLMTS) is a disorder with which the lower extremity specialist must be acquainted, as, in my experience, these patients almost inevitably present to physicians interested in these disciplines.

The disorder consists of constant severe pain of an affected leg and foot associated with spontaneous toe movements. Not infrequently, both lower limbs become involved. The pain is extraordinarily severe, unremitting, and poorly responsive to pharmacologic management. Onset is usually fairly abrupt. Patients describe the pain as a boring, burning, crushing, searing pain in the foot. In association, they demonstrate curious writhing, wriggling, flexion-extension, abduction-adduction toe motions that are characteristic.

Typically, this disorder develops in the setting of a prior lumbosacral radiculopathy. It is thought to be secondary to an unusual ephaptic transmission within the spinal roots. The onset is usually in patients in their mid-40s but is quite variable. The differential diagnosis is limited, as no other disorder presents in quite the same way. Rarely, PLMTS presents or in spreads to the hands and arms. Radiologic and laboratory studies are unhelpful, although electromyography and nerve conduction studies may reveal evidence of a lumbosacral radiculopathy.

Treatment of this problem is frustrating for physician and patient. There are some reports that lumbar sympathetic and peripheral nerve blocks are helpful, but I have never seen a success with that approach. Various pharmacotherapies, including opiates, anticonvulsants, antispasmodics, anticholinergics, neuroleptics, antidepressants, and steroids, are uniformly unsuccessful. Some patients report transient relief with high-dose benzodiazepines. Occasionally patients respond favorably to focal botulinum toxin injections, but this has not been the general experience. As can be imagined, this disorder can be quite disabling. It appears to be unremitting.

## DISORDERS OF LOWER EXTREMITY RESTLESSNESS

### Restless Legs Syndrome

Considering its frequency in the population, it is surprising that this disorder was not described in the medical literature until Ekbom did so in 1945. It is estimated that up to 10% of the population is affected by this disorder at some time and that prevalence gradually rises with age, reaching approximately 30% of the population older than 65. Onset can be before the age of 10, although more typically patients present to clinical attention in their later years, typically after the age of 50. This disorder is diagnosed purely on clinical grounds. In this case, the diagnosis is on a historical basis, although sleep studies can be somewhat confirmatory.

The most common presenting symptom is a recurrent, persistent urge to move, usually related to vaguely described uncomfortable, crawling, painful, grabbing sensations, primarily in the legs (Table 9–5). Probably about 20% of patients experience similar sensations in their arms. Motor activity, particularly walking, relieves these sensory symptoms. If the urge to move is ignored, the sensations become worse. The sensations worsen with relaxation, usually after some minutes, such as when the patient is attempting to fall asleep or sitting for prolonged periods, as in a movie theater. The disorder is generally worse in the evening but symptoms may be present all day long. As a consequence of this problem, patients have problems with initiation of sleep and may experience significant sleep deprivation. Frequently, these patients suffer with periodic limb movements of sleep (PLMS), which are repetitive, stereotyped, flexion and extension movements of the toes and proximal legs and, to a lesser degree, of the arms. These movements may occur at 15- to 40-second intervals during non–rapid eye movement sleep, resulting in considerable sleep disruption in some instances. There is a high correlation of PLMS with RLS. Many patients experience involuntary flexion movements of the legs while awake that appear to be the waking counterpart of PLMS. The disorder seems to be inherited in an autosomal dominant pattern in many cases. Because the diagnosis is based entirely on history, the presence of the disorder in the patient's progenitors may be grossly underestimated.

Typically, patients have a completely normal general and neurologic examination. It is quite rare for the clinician to observe any abnormal movements, except in the sleep laboratory. The disorder appears to be more common in the setting of peripheral neuropathy of any type, uremia, and anemia. If there is any evidence of a metabolic disorder, the appropriate screening serum chemistries, blood count, and anemia evaluation are in order. If there are signs of peripheral nerve or nerve lesions, an electrophysiologic study may be desirable, although it is not necessary for the diagnosis. In the setting of significant sleep disruption, a sleep study is helpful for quantitation of PLMS to assess the success of treatment.

With the appropriate history and examination, there is virtually no alternative diagnosis, although one must consider the possibility of akathisia, which is discussed later in the chapter.

**Table 9–5  Symptoms of Restless Legs Syndrome**

Uncomfortable, crawling sensation in legs, sometimes arms
Relief with motor activity
Worse symptoms with relaxation
Worse in the evening
Periodic limb movements of sleep

RLS is generally best treated pharmacologically. There is no convincing evidence that biofeedback or relaxation techniques help in this disorder and there is much to suggest that they may exacerbate it. Regular exercise, particularly before retiring, may be helpful for some patients and should always be recommended first. However, many patients who present to their physician with this problem have already exhausted the exercise approach and require more aggressive treatment.

Dopaminergic drugs are the most effective agents for the alleviation of the condition. Initiation of therapy with levodopa/carbidopa at a dose of one 25/100 mg tablet at bedtime is a good way to begin. Unfortunately, many patients begin to experience wearing off of the effect of the treatment in the middle of the night after as little as several weeks, not unlike the experience of IPD patients. This prompts the physician to change over to the controlled-release levodopa-carbidopa preparation, which can be quite helpful. The next step would be initiation of therapy with the dopamine agonist pergolide. This drug has the advantage of a significantly longer duration of action than levodopa-carbidopa. In many physicians' experience, it is the most effective agent, although it has the potential for more adverse effects.

The next tier of agents that are effective in alleviating this disorder are the benzodiazepines. Generally, most specialists prefer clonazepam for its additional effect on rapid eye movement–related sleep dysfunction, but temazepam, diazepam, and triazolam can be helpful. There are few data on the use of zolpidem, but it has been reported anecdotally to be useful. Sometimes, sedating antihistamines such as diphenhydramine can be helpful.

Various opiates have also been efficacious in suppressing this disorder. In particular, propoxyphene, codeine, and oxycodone have been useful for symptom alleviation and improvement of sleep quality. Other agents with less well defined efficacy have been utilized to treat this disorder with some success, including baclofen, carbamazepine, valproate, gabapentin, and clonidine.

## Akathisia

Akathisia is a condition in which there is a subjective sensation of inner restlessness, usually associated with inability to keep still. At first glance, this disorder may seem to be the same as RLS. However, the patient with akathisia does not experience relief with performance of the motor activity but feels compelled to perform it anyway. The most common motor activity is pacing to and fro. Although these patients may describe abnormal sensations in their limbs, this is not a dominant feature of their problem. The disorder also does not follow a diurnal pattern and is not associated with PLMS and sleep disruption. Typically, akathisia is precipitated by the use of neuroleptic medications and may be present in up 20% of patients treated with these compounds. It is also seen in patients with dementia, particularly dementia of the Alzheimer's type, and less frequently in IPD patients with dementia.

The physical examination of these patients does not yield any particular abnormalities, although there are signs of any underlying neurologic disorder, such as IPD or Alzheimer's disease. In the case of akathisia related to neuroleptic drug use, signs of drug-induced parkinsonism may be present. Laboratory studies are not helpful in evaluating akathisia, unless dictated in some way by the patient's associated medical problems.

The major differential diagnosis of this entity is psychotic agitation in the psychiatrically disturbed patient. RLS is in the differential diagnosis, but the features already described should help distinguish akathisia from RLS.

Treatment of akathisia is quite difficult. If akathisia is neuroleptically induced, reducing the dosage of or changing the neuroleptic may be helpful. The conventional treatments for drug-induced parkinsonism, such as anticholinergics, antihistamines, and amantadine, can be helpful. Sometimes benzodiazepines, β-receptor antagonists, particularly propranolol, and opiates can be helpful for this problem. There are reports of a positive effect of clonidine in some of these patients.

## Orthostatic Tremor

Orthostatic tremor (OT) is a rare disorder that is thought by some to be a variant of benign essential tremor (ET). ET is a kinetic tremor disorder, generally confined to the upper extremities, head, and voice. OT is different in that patients describe the development of tremor of the legs and trunk after standing in one place for several seconds. The tremor gradually worsens as the patient stands in place until the whole body is vibrating. It immediately terminates with walking. It is not present in the sitting position and is not associated with any inner restlessness or abnormal sensations in the limbs. It has been reported to begin in the fourth decade of life.

Once again, the conventional physical and neurologic examinations are unrevealing. However, if the patient is asked to stand with the feet together in one place for several seconds, tremulous movement of the legs and trunk are noted. Routine laboratory examinations are also unrevealing. Surface EMG analysis reveals a high-frequency tremor of the legs at approximately 15 Hz, far higher than that seen in ET.

The differential diagnosis of this disorder consists of RLS and akathisia, but both the history and the physical findings help distinguish these entities. Patients with OT do not describe the sensory symptoms of RLS and have no diurnal pattern, although they do describe worsening when they are fatigued. PLMS is not associated with OT. In contrast to patients with akathisia, those with OT do not describe an inner restlessness; they clearly demonstrate tremulousness of the legs if they stand in place, which is not present in RLS or akathisia.

Although OT is thought to resemble ET phenomenologically, it does not respond to the agents that alleviate ET, namely β-receptor antagonists. Clonazepam appears to be the most effective medication for these patients, but some patients note improvement with valproate, which is relatively contraindicated for ET. Others note responses to primidone, which is useful for many patients with ET.

## SUMMARY

Disorders of voluntary motor control are quite common, particularly when viewed in aggregate. In this chapter, the disorders that particularly affect the lower extremities were discussed at some length. These entities are likely to be encountered by the lower extremity specialist with some frequency, especially if the professional is alert to them. With the information presented, it should be possible for the physician to recognize the disorders, develop a differential diagnosis, and begin to initiate evaluation and treatment.

## BIBLIOGRAPHY

Bandmann O, Nygaard TG, Surtees R, et al: Dopa-responsive dystonia in British patients: New mutations of the GTP-cyclohydrolase I gene and evidence for genetic heterogeneity. Hum Mol Genet 5:403–406, 1996.

Baron MS, Vitek JL, Bakay RA, et al: Treatment of advanced Parkinson's disease by posterior GPi pallidotomy: 1-year results of a pilot study. Ann Neurol 40:341, 355–366, 1996.

Brans JW, Lindeboom R, Snoek JW, et al: Botulinum toxin versus trihexyphenidyl in cervical dystonia: A prospective, randomized, double-blind controlled study. Neurology 46:1066–1072, 1996.

Britton TC, Thompson PD: Primary orthostatic tremor. BMJ 310:143–144, 1995.

Burn DJ, Sawle GV, Brooks DJ: Differential diagnosis of Parkinson's disease, multiple system atrophy, and Steele-Richardson-Olszewski syndrome: Discriminant analysis of striatal [18F]-PET data. J Neurol Neurosurg Psychiatry 57:278–284, 1994.

Curran T, Lang AE: Parkinsonian syndromes associated with hydrocephalus: Case reports, a review of the literature, and pathophysiological hypotheses. Mov Disord 5:508–520, 1994.

Limousin P, Pollale P, Bennazzouz A, et al: Effect on parkinsonian signs and symptoms of bilateral subthalamic nucleus stimulation. Lancet 345:91–95, 1995.

Litvan I, Mangone CA, Mckee A, et al: Natural history of progressive supranuclear palsy (Steele-Richardson-Olsyewski syndrome) and clinical predictors of survival: A clinicopathologic study. J Neurol Neurosurg Psychiatry 61:615–620, 1996.

Mathias CJ: Autonomic disorders and their recognition. N Engl J Med 336:721–724, 1997.

Quinn N: Drug treatment of Parkinson's disease. BMJ 310:575–579, 1995.

Quinn N: Parkinsonism—Recognition and differential diagnosis. BMJ 310:447–452, 1995.

Robbins TW, James M, Owen AM, et al: Cognitive deficits in progressive supranuclear palsy, Parkinson's disease, and multiple system atrophy in tests sensitive to frontal lobe dysfunction. J Neurol Neurosurg Psychiatry 57:79–88, 1994.

Stacy M, Cardoso F, Janpovic J: Tardive stereotype and other movement disorders in tardive dyskinesias. Neurology 43:937–941, 1993.

Vidailhet M, Rivaud S, Gowder-Khouja N, et al: Eye movements in parkinsonian syndromes. Ann Neurol 35:420–426, 1994.

Walters AS: Towards a better definition of the restless legs syndrome. Mov Disord 10:634–642, 1995.

Zijlmans JC, Thijssen HO, Vogels OJ, et al: MRI in patients with suspected vascular parkinsonism. Neurology 45:2183–2188, 1995.

# Toxins Producing Clinical Effects   10

## Manifested in the Lower Extremity

*Michael I. Greenberg, Tucker Greene, and Timothy Dougherty*

An extremely wide array of toxins have been associated with peripheral neurologic manifestations. These toxic substances are of both biologic and chemical origin. Some of these materials occur naturally, whereas others are the products of synthetic processes. Careful examination of these toxins and their associated biologic effects reveals that although some have clinical effects predominantly in the lower extremities, they are seldom selective for the lower extremities. Careful clinical evaluation generally reveals the presence of at least some clinical effects in various locations in the peripheral nervous system.

This chapter describes the toxins that are most frequently recognized as having peripheral nervous system manifestations that tend to affect the lower extremities to a significant degree. Table 10–1 lists those toxins.

**Table 10–1   Toxins Affecting the Lower Extremity**

| | |
|---|---|
| Acetazolamide | Manganese |
| Almitrine | Mercury |
| Amiodarone | Methylhydrazine |
| Arsenic | Metronidazole |
| Chloramphenicol | Misonidazole |
| Cisplatin | Nitrofurantoin |
| Clioquinol | Nitrogen mustard |
| Colchicine | Nitrous oxide |
| Colistin | Perhexiline maleate |
| Cytarabine | Platinum |
| Dapsone | Phenytoin |
| Disulfiram | Procarbazine |
| Doxorubicin | Pyridoxine |
| Ethambutol | Sodium cyanate |
| Ethionamide | Strychnine |
| Gold | Sulthiame (Ospolot) |
| Hexane, 2,5-hexanedione | Taxol |
| Hexamethylmelamine | Thalidomide |
| Hydralazine | Thallium |
| Hydroxychloroquine | Tryptophan (eosinophilia- |
| Indomethacin | myalgia syndrome) |
| Isoniazid | Vinca alkyloids |
| Lead | Zimeldine |
| Lithium | |

## TRIORTHOCRESYL PHOSPHATE

In the early 1900s an ethanol and ginger root extract (ginger jake or "jake" as it was known) was popularly used as a tonic, primarily in poor rural southern areas of the United States and in the Caribbean.[1] Several drops of this mixture in tea or water were widely used as a purgative or analgesic or to improve well-being. During the era of prohibition, those not able to afford illegally produced alcoholic beverages resorted to buying several ounces of the ginger jake preparation as it often contained alcohol in quantities as high as 70% to 80%. The popularity of this preparation resulted in individuals resorting to using adulterants in the preparation in an effort to increase the volume of a batch of jake and thus their bottom-line profit. One such adulterant was triorthocresyl phosphate (TOCP), an organophosphate compound.

TOCP is an oily, viscous substance that is an excellent heat-stable lubricant often used in hydraulic fluid applications in the jet aircraft industry. TOCP is somewhat unusual in that it does not induce the cholinergic symptoms typical of exposure to insecticide organophosphates. Rather, the toxic effects are the result of direct neuronal toxicity manifested as the organophosphate-induced delayed neurotoxicity syndrome.[2, 3] The precise toxic metabolite has not been elucidated. The pathologic process resulting from TOCP exposure involves a wallerian-type dying-back axonal degeneration with secondary demyelination of the long tracts as well as destruction of anterior horn cells. TOCP-induced neuropathy is considered to be the classic isolated lower extremity neuropathy of toxic origin.

Early symptoms include nausea, vomiting, weakness, and crampy pains. Later, footdrop, gait disturbances, and diminished reflexes appear. Then symmetric motor paresis, hip girdle paralysis, spasticity, increased reflexes, and finally irreversible loss of motor function occur. Some individuals with minimal exposure to TOCP recovered. However, many others developed a typical staggering gait with footdrop now known as jake leg. The gait associated with jake leg was distinctive and was made famous by hillbilly and blues singers who both drank jake and sang of its effects on their lives. The more chronic symptoms tend to be permanent, but discontinuation of exposure diminishes or halts progression of symptoms.

## ALMITRINE

Almitrine bismesylate is an orally administered triazine derivative that has been used to treat hypoxia in some patients suffering from chronic obstructive pulmonary disease.[4] The drug has been used widely in Europe and Asia and in experimental protocols in the United States. It functions as a peripheral chemoreceptor agonist stimulating afferent carotid nerves, as in hypoxemia. This causes an increase in minute ventilation that increases oxygen delivery to alveoli. Blood gas oxygen tension is improved. It is not clear whether ventilation/perfusion versus minute ventilation effects are responsible for the increased oxygen.

Doses of 100 to 200 mg in clinical trials have resulted in reversible peripheral neuropathy characterized by an insidious onset and producing a distal sensory neuropathy primarily affecting the lower limbs.[5] This has been confirmed by both electrophysiologic and histologic evidence of axonopathy. One study indicated that 14.5% of subjects experienced paresthesias.[5] Discontinuation resulted in resolution of symptoms in substantial numbers of patients.

## AMIODARONE

Amiodarone is a class III antiarrhythmic agent that is structurally similar to thyroxine. The drug exhibits weak α- and β-adrenergic antagonist activity. The development of a demyelinating distal polyneuropathy with bilateral lower extremity weakness has been associated with this compound.[6] The development of this neuropathy has been followed by the development of various lower extremity dysesthesias. This is frequently seen in conjunction with a painless, proximal "autophagic" myopathy with elevated creatinine kinase. Nerve biopsies indicate anoxopathy with demyelination, a mixed phenomenon.

## ARSENIC

Arsenic poisoning is the most common form of acute heavy metal poisoning in the United States.

Accidental exposure to insecticides and weed killers causes the majority of cases of fatal arsenic poisonings. Chronic exposure may lead to the development of peripheral neuropathy manifest as a burning sensation in the extremities in a stocking-glove distribution with concomitant loss of plantar reflexes. British antilewisite (BAL) may be helpful in the treatment of early recognized neuropathy and may be used in chronic exposures to prevent further deterioration. Another significant lower extremity manifestation of chronic arsenic poisoning is the development of so-called *blackfoot disease.* The pathology of this entity involves a local vasculitis that can result in tissue destruction primarily in the lower extremity.

Finally, it is important to remember that arsenic intoxication can mimic Guillain-Barré syndrome. Consequently, whenever Guillain-Barré syndrome is being considered as a primary diagnosis, arsenic intoxication should be ruled out.

## LEAD

Lead is responsible for the majority of cases of chronic heavy metal poisoning in the United States today. Chronic poisoning by inorganic lead leads to anemia, colic, and neuropathy. Lead toxicity is caused by disruption of cellular enzymes by lead binding to sulfur groups. In chronic exposure neuropathy progresses gradually, and in mild cases recovery is usually complete. The neuropathy is entirely motor and affects predominantly the most exercised muscles such as finger and wrist extensors, but the lower extremity plantar extensors may also be effected. Weakness is commonly bilateral, but one side is usually affected earlier than the other. Neuropathy reaches maximal intensity within weeks. Removal of exposure in conjunction with treatment with an appropriate chelating agent usually results in complete recovery.

## CISPLATIN

Cisplatin is an antineoplastic agent often used in the management of metastatic testicular, ovarian, and bladder carcinomas. Cisplatin exerts its effects by binding across strands of DNA and thereby inhibiting RNA transcription in meiotic phases G and S1. The initial toxic effects reported with its use were primarily nausea, vomiting, and renal dysfunction. However, there has been an increase in reports of neurotoxicity.[6] Factors that affect the neuropathy induced by cisplatin include coadministration of other neuropathy-inducing antineoplastics, the dosage of cisplatin, and the presence of preexisting illnesses. There is a definite relationship between the onset of neuropathy and the total cisplatin dose to which the patient has been exposed.

Symptoms begin as numbness, tingling, and paresthesias of the hands or feet. As therapy continues, paresthesias tend to spread proximally and may progress to include altered vibrational and proprioceptive sense.[7] Ankle reflexes diminish and gait disturbances that affect walking or climbing may occur. Less often reported symptoms include diminished pain and temperature sense. Cessation of therapy may result in partial resolution of paresthesias, but this compound may have permanent effects on renal function.

## COLCHICINE

Colchicine is a naturally occurring alkaloid derived from the autumn crocus plant and is used in the treatment of gouty arthritis, familial Mediterranean fever, Behçet's disease, and alcoholic cirrhosis. Its effects are mediated through inhibition of microtubule formation by interfering with the alpha and beta subunits, ultimately inhibiting axonal flow. This activity then prevents polymorphonuclear infiltration and release of lactic acid and enzymes that mediate inflammation. Colchicine causes a mild distal, sensory axonopathy that can be accompanied by necrotizing myopathy and renal failure.[8] Cessation of therapy usually results in complete recovery.

## EOSINOPHILIA-MYALGIA SYNDROME

In 1989 several hundred cases of illness and several deaths were reported to the Centers for Disease Control after individuals ingested large quantities of L-tryptophan (150 to 2400 mg/day). This led to the development of diagnostic criteria for a disorder that has come to be known as eosinophilia-myalgia syndrome. This disorder is characterized by eosinophilia with more than 1000 eosinophils per mm³ along with generalized myalgias in the absence of infection or neoplasia. A contaminant in the L-tryptophan was found to be the causative compound rather than megadoses of L-tryptophan itself.[9] The neuropathy associated with this outbreak was similar to that in Guillain-Barré syndrome, with distal paresthesias and muscle weakness that progressed proximally. Cessation of the use of L-tryptophan usually results in resolution of symptoms.

## HEXANE AND METHYL BUTYL KETONE

Neurotoxicity has been associated with hexacarbon solvents.[10] Because of their high lipid solubility, they have a high affinity for neuronal tissues. Exposure to these agents has primarily involved occupational exposure to glues that contain these compounds in their formulation. Other significant exposures have occurred in individuals who deliberately inhale the glue vapors from within a closed space such as a small bag in order to "get high," a practice known as huffing.[11] The common metabolite of these two solvents, 2,5-hexanedione, is implicated in the development of symptoms of peripheral neuropathy. Studies by Billmaier and associates showed that 8% of 1157 workers at a coated-fabrics plant exhibited symptoms of distal, symmetric, sensorimotor polyneuropathy manifested as loss of Achilles tendon reflexes, pelvic girdle weakness, and sensory loss in the lower extremities. Pathologic studies in animals showed distal axonal degeneration and formation of neurofilament-filled axonal swellings consistent with central peripheral distal axonopathy. This suggests that descending motor pathways are affected.[12] Resolution of symptoms largely depends on the duration of exposure, but removal of the individual from exposure is essential to prevent continuing deterioration.

## MANGANESE

Manganese is present in many alloys and its compounds are used in pharmaceuticals, fertilizers, dyes, and welding equipment and as antiknock compounds in gasoline. Two forms of manganese, manganese dioxide and methylcyclopentadienyl manganese, are implicated in toxic neuropathies. Chronically exposed patients have weakness of the lower extremities with muscle cramps. Treatment with ethylenediaminetetraacetic acid (EDTA) may be helpful in eliminating manganese.

## MERCURY

Mercury is a cellular poison with multiple-system toxicities whose effects have been known for thousands of years. Mercury exists in many forms, but mercuric salts used as fungicides and organic mercury fixed in nature by bacteria are the toxic species. Elemental mercury is toxic only if inhaled; it is not toxic when enterally ingested. The neurotoxic effects are primarily peripheral, resulting in both motor dysfunction and painful dyesthesias of the leg.[13] These effects were noted during the Minamata Bay incident in Japan in the 1960s, in which methyl mercury (organic) was the toxin. Chelation with BAL is useful in eliminating mercury, but long-term exposure may result in permanent motor and sensory defects.

## STRYCHNINE

Strychnine is a naturally occurring alkaloid from the tree *Strychnos nux-vomica.* It is an odorless, tasteless, colorless crystalline compound. It exerts its effects by competitively inhibiting glycine at the postsynaptic receptor in the spinal cord. This results in opisthotonoid seizures in awake individuals. Peripheral lower extremity effects involve increased deep tendon reflexes secondary to spinal cord and central nervous system excitability. Treatment is supportive, with muscle relaxants and avoidance of central nervous system stimulation.

## THALLIUM

Thallium is a heavy metal whose compounds are used in rodenticides and rocket booster fuel. Thallium exerts its toxic effects via enzymatic sulfide binding. Acute thallium poisoning is characterized by gastrointestinal symptoms, followed by numbness and weakness of the extremities within 2 to 5 days. Seizures, cranial nerve palsies, and blindness may also occur. In chronic poisoning, alopecia, optic neuritis, and generalized polyneuritis are the most common symptoms. Paresthesia in the lower extremities, motor weakness, and loss of reflexes without or with minimal cutaneous sensory impairment are characteristic. Complete recovery from the generalized neuritis after removal of exposure predominates.

## ZIMELDINE

Fagius and colleagues[14] reported on a randomized, double-blind, placebo-controlled study in which 9 of 20 patients treated with zimeldine for chronic pain developed Guillain-Barré syndrome. This occurrence required the withdrawal of the agent in the study. The exact mode of action of zimeldine is unknown, but withdrawal of the agent resulted in resolution of symptoms.

## CHLORAMPHENICOL

Chloramphenicol is an antibiotic that exerts a bacteriostatic effect on a wide spectrum of gram-negative and gram-positive bacteria. It is particularly effective against *Salmonella typhi, Vibrio cholerae, Rickettsia,* and *Haemophilus influenzae.* Its mode of action is inhibition of or interference with bacterial protein synthesis. Serious and fatal blood dyscrasias, including aplastic anemia, limit the use of chloramphenicol. Although chloramphenicol is usually administered orally or intravenously, aplastic anemia has been associated with ophthalmologic chloramphenicol (Chloromycetin). Premature and newborn infants are susceptible to many of chloramphenicol's side effects, including a fatal toxic reaction known as gray baby syndrome. Optic neuritis, retinal toxicity, headache, delirium, and a mild sensory peripheral neuropathy have been reported, usually after long-term therapy. Some patients complained of burning paresthesias of the feet and lower legs. Their distal deep tendon reflexes were decreased, but they showed no signs of muscle weakness.[15] Patients with chloramphenicol-induced sensory neuropathy improve slowly with drug cessation.

## CHLOROQUINE

Chloroquine is 7-chloro-4-(4-diethylamino-1-methlybutylamino)quinoline. This compound is a highly active antimalarial and amebicidal agent. It is effective in treating the erythrocytic forms of *Plasmodium vivax, P. malariae,* and most stains of *P. falciparum* and has long been used in the treatment of rheumatoid arthritis and systemic lupus erythematosus. Although its exact mechanism is not known, it is believed to be related to inhibition of certain enzymes. Chloroquine may be administered orally, intramuscularly, or intravenously. Side effects associated with this drug include mild headache, tinnitus, pruritus, skin rash, abdominal cramps, anorexia, nausea, vomiting, diarrhea, and blood dyscrasia. Irreversible retinal damage and corneal deposits are common in long-term therapy. The main neuromuscular toxic side effect is a myopathy, which presents as mild, painless proximal weakness months to years after the onset of treatment.[16] The myopathy may be accompanied by a slight elevation of creatine kinase. Neurophysiologic and pathologic evidence indicates that damage to the Schwann cells with resultant demyelination is the cause of chloroquine-induced neuropathy. Although the majority of affected individuals suffer from a purely motor myopathy, a mixed sensorimotor polyneuromyopathy has been reported.[17] All patients receiving long-term therapy should be monitored periodically for evidence of distal muscular weakness. If any weakness is detected, discontinuation of the drug usually results in resolution of the symptoms.

## DAPSONE

Dapsone (4,4'-diaminodiphenylsulfone) is used as a primary treatment for dermatitis herpetiformis and as a bactericidal or bacteriostatic drug for susceptible cases of leprosy. It has also been used in the treatment of pneumocystis pneumonia and brown recluse spider bites. Dose-related hemolysis is the most common adverse side effect. Fatalities resulting from aplastic anemia and other blood dyscrasias have been reported. Other side effects include fever, psychosis, insomnia, headache, phototoxicity, blurred vision, tinnitus, exfoliate dermatitis, hepatitis, nephrotic syndrome, and male infertility.[18] Peripheral neuropathy is a rare complication of dapsone treatment after several months of therapy. A vast majority of the patients demonstrate distal motor neuropathy. Patients suffer from weakness, muscle wasting, and loss of deep tendon reflexes in both hands and feet. In rare instances, as their distal motor neuropathy continues, patients may also have mild sensory complaints (paresthesias). Neurophysiologic findings are consistent with a distal, predominantly motor, axonal neuropathy. If muscle weakness appears, dapsone should be discontinued. Recovery is seen over several months in the majority of cases and is reportedly due to axonal regeneration.

## DISULFIRAM

Disulfiram (tetraethythiuram disulfide; Antabuse) has been used for years as an aid in the management of chronic alcoholism. It blocks the oxidation of alcohol at the acetaldehyde stage. The accumulation of acetaldehyde results in the highly unpleasant Antabuse-alcohol reaction symptoms of nausea, vomiting, and flushing. Other side effects include a sulfa or garlic taste, rash, tachycardia, hypotension, abdominal pain, hepatitis, agranulocytosis, and thrombocytopenia.

Patients can also suffer from a broad range of neurologic side effects including confusion, encephalopathy, ataxia, headache, lethargy, optic neuritis, impotence, and peripheral neuropathy.[19, 20] Disulfiram-induced peripheral neuropathy appears to be dose related (500 mg/day). Patients complain of distal paresthesia and diminished sensation in the feet, progressing to the legs and hands. Sensory loss mild distal weakness, and wasting have been reported. Deep tendon reflexes are absent in the ankles and in the upper extremities. Neurophysiologic studies are consistent with axonal degeneration. There appear to be two hypotheses about how the nervous system is affected. One is based on the ability of disulfiram and its metabolite, diethyldithiocarbamate, to chelate polyvalent metal icons and disturb the homeostasis of copper and zinc ions in the tissues. The other hypothesis is based on reactions leading to chronic depletion of pyridoxal phosphate as a biochemical cofactor. Administering the higher

dosages (500 to 1000 mg/day) for no more than 2 weeks appears to be the best way to avoid the peripheral neuropathy. Most patients who do develop neuropathy show significant improvement with drug cessation.

## GOLD

Gold (gold sodium thiomalate) has been used for years in the treatment of both adult and juvenile rheumatoid arthritis. The mode of action is unknown. Gold appears to have a suppressive effect on the synovitis of active disease. Because it cannot repair previous damage, its greatest benefit occurs in the early stages of the disease. Adverse reactions occur most frequently after a total accumulation of 400 to 1000 mg. Dermatitis and stomatitis are the most common side effects. Other side effects include flushing, headache, seizures, iritis, corneal ulcer or deposits, nausea, vomiting, nephrotic syndrome, and hepatitis. Peripheral neuropathy is a rare complication of chronic use. Patients usually present with complaints of painful burning paresthesia or decreased distal sensation. Later symptoms can include asymmetric weakness, fasciculations, muscle wasting, loss of deep tendon reflexes, and complete loss of sensation. Patients may also have Guillain-Barré syndrome, trigeminal sensory neuropathy, facial palsies, and elevation of cerebrospinal fluid protein. The majority of neurophysiologic studies are consistent with segmental demyelination, with axonal degeneration being seen less commonly. Patients' symptoms usually resolve over weeks to months upon discontinuation of gold therapy. Unfortunately, some are left with permanent deficits.

## ISONIAZID

Isoniazid (isonicotinic hydrazide [INH]) has been used for years in the treatment of tuberculosis. It is rapidly absorbed, readily diffuses into the tissues, and is excreted mainly in the urine. Isoniazid is metabolized primarily by acetylation and dehydrazination. The efficiency of hepatic acetylation appears to be a genetically determined autosomal recessive trait. The majority of Eskimos and Asians are "fast acetylators." Approximately 50% of whites and blacks are "slow acetylators." Depending on the rate of acetylation, the half-life of INH can be from 30 minutes to 5 hours. The rate of acetylation is thought to affect directly the patient's risk of developing neurologic complications. INH acts against actively growing tubercle bacilli by inhibiting the phosphorylation of pyridoxine. Administration of pyridoxine (50 mg/day) has a prophylactic effect against the neuropathy. In addition to neuropathy, other side effects include fever, rash, psychosis, optic neuritis, tinnitus, nausea, vomiting, hepatitis, hyperglycemia, and blood dyscrasias. Peripheral neuropathy is the most common toxic effect. It appears to be directly related to the duration of treatment, total dosage received, and the patient's ability to acetylate. Patients present with distal sensory complaints of paresthesias of the hands and feet, followed by a stocking-glove loss of sensation. Some patients also suffer from distal weakness and muscle wasting. Studies in rats have revealed axonal degeneration without evidence of significant axonal demyelination.[21] If INH therapy is discontinued at the onset of symptoms, patients usually make a full recovery within weeks. If the symptoms are allowed to progress, recovery may take months. Good results have also been obtained with higher dose pyridoxine (100 to 150 mg/day).

## METRONIDAZOLE

Metronidazole (5-nitromidazole) is an antiprotozoal and antibacterial agent used to treat a variety of infections including trichomoniasis, vaginitis, amebic dysentery, peritonitis, skin infections, meningitis, brain abscesses, and endocarditis. The side effect profile of metronidazole includes a metallic taste, *Candida* overgrowth, reversible neutropenia and thrombocytopenia, electrocardiographic T-wave flattening, nausea, vomiting, skin rash, darkened urine, and incontinence. Two other serious adverse reactions are convulsive seizures and peripheral neuropathy. These uncommon side effects are seen in patients chronically treated with metronidazole (e.g., for inflammatory bowel disease). Patients complain of progressive burning pain starting in the feet and hands. As the peripheral neuropathy progresses, patients suffer distal dysesthesias in a stocking-glove distribution. Neurophysiologic studies are consistent with axonal degeneration.[22] Discontinuation of metronidazole should reverse the neuropathy within a year.

## MISONIDAZOLE

Misonidazole (2-nitromidazole) is structurally similar to metronidazole. It is an electron affinity agent used to sensitize hypoxic cancer cells in radiotherapy. Side effects include dizziness, gastrointestinal distress, seizures, and encephalopathy. Several weeks after completion of misonidazole therapy (doses greater than 16 to 18 g), patients complain of severe distal burning pain progressing in a stocking-

glove distribution. Like metronidazole, misonidazole causes a distal, predominantly sensory axonal neuropathy. Limiting the dose to less than 18 g and administration to no more than once a week decreases the incidence and severity of neuropathy.

## NITROFURANTOIN

Nitrofurantoin is an antibiotic used in the treatment of urinary tract infections. Major side effects include chronic, subacute, or acute pulmonary hypersensitivity reactions, hepatitis, blood dyscrasia, erythema multiforme, optic neuritis, headache, vertigo, and psychosis. Patients with impaired renal function are at greatest risk for these side effects. An axonal peripheral neuropathy occurs within weeks to months after initiation of therapy. Symptoms begin with mild distal numbness, followed by rapidly progressive distal motor weakness and muscle wasting. Discontinuation of nitrofurantoin at the first sign of neuropathy is usually followed by resolution of the symptoms in a few weeks. Although nitrofurantoin is still a second-line therapeutic agent, it should be avoided in patients with renal dysfunction.

## PHENYTOIN

Phenytoin (5,5-diphenyl-2,4-imidazolidinedione) is structurally related to barbiturates but has a five-membered ring. It is an antiepileptic that appears to stabilize the motor cortex by promoting sodium efflux from the neurons. Phenytoin is indicated for generalized grand mal and temporal lobe seizures. The most common side effects are usually dose related. These include ataxia, nystagmus, slurred speech, gingival hyperplasia, nausea, vomiting, hepatitis, dermatologic manifestations, hypertrichosis, blood dyscrasias, and a hypersensitivity reaction. Almost all patients chronically treated with phenytoin demonstrate decreased deep tendon reflexes and mild sensory loss in the feet.[23] They may also suffer from a peripheral neuropathy characterized by stocking-glove dysesthesias and mild weakness. As the dose is increased above 300 mg/day, with resultant serum levels over 25 mg/dL, the risk of neuropathy increases. Reducing the dosage or choosing an alternative antiepileptic reverses the symptoms in a majority of cases.

## PYRIDOXINE

Pyridoxine (vitamin B$_6$) is a cofactor involved in a variety of enzymatic processes. As discussed previously, pyridoxine deficiency can lead to isoniazid-induced peripheral neuropathy. However, in high megadoses (2 to 5 g/day), pyridoxine can cause its own neuropathy. Other side effects include headache, seizures, nausea, vomiting, hepatitis, and decreased serum folate levels. Several months after megadose therapy, a peripheral axonal neuropathy begins with acral numbness, sensory ataxia, and diminished deep tendon reflexes. This is followed by involvement of predominantly large-fiber proprioception, producing gait disturbances. Neurophysiologic studies show diminished sensory action potentials but the motor fibers appear to be spared. The majority of patients recover within months of cessation of pyridoxine.

## PACLITAXEL (TAXOL)

Paclitaxel (Taxol) is used in the treatment of renal cell carcinoma, breast cancer, non–small cell lung carcinoma, melanoma, epithelial ovarian cancer, and acute leukemia. It is an antimicrotubule agent that prevents mitotic function in rapidly dividing neoplastic cells. Side effects of paclitaxel include bradycardia, atrioventricular conduction disturbances, hypotension, optic neuritis, perioral numbness, neutropenia, leukopenia, gastrointestinal disturbances, alopecia, myalgia or arthralgia, and a hypersensitivity reaction. The principal neurologic manifestation of paclitaxel is a peripheral sensory neuropathy. The onset of symptoms is usually rapid, with patients complaining of numbness and burning paresthesias in a stocking-glove distribution. Loss of deep tendon reflexes and distal weakness have also been reported. The peripheral neuropathy appears to be related to the dose (greater than 200 mg/m$^2$) and cumulative dose. Neurophysiologic studies suggest axonal degeneration as the main cause, although demyelination has also been reported. Cessation of paclitaxel therapy reverses the peripheral neuropathy in the majority of cases. It appears that keeping the dosage below 200 mg/m$^2$ and increasing the dosage interval to 3 to 4 weeks may decrease the risk of neuropathy.

## THALIDOMIDE

In the early 1960s, thalidomide (3-phthalimidoglutarimide) was thought to be a safe sedative agent without any significant side effects. Unfortunately, it was not until its use became widespread and chronic that two devastating complications were reported. The first was severe teratogenic effects on fetuses resulting in multiple limb anomalies. The second was a peripheral neuropathy. After taking thalidomide for several months, patients com-

plained of distal painful paresthesia, with loss of sensation in a stocking-glove distribution. Patients also suffered from muscle cramps and weakness of the proximal muscles. Neurophysiologic data demonstrated severely decreased sensory nerve action potentials with relatively normal conduction velocities, consistent with an axonal peripheral neuropathy. Although a few patients recovered quickly after drug cessation, the rate of recovery was usually slow. Many continued to have painful paresthesias for years.

## VINCA ALKALOIDS

Vinca alkaloids, which include vincristine, vinblastine, and vindesine, are chemotherapeutic agents. They have been used for years to treat a variety of leukemias, particularly in children. The mechanism of action appears to be related to inhibition of microtubule formation in the mitotic spindle, resulting in arrest of dividing cells at the metaphase stage. Vincristine has the highest chemotherapeutic potency, followed by videsine and vinblastine, respectively. In general, the incidence of side effects appears to be related to dosage and potency. Leukopenia, alopecia, and constipation are the most common side effects. Other adverse reactions include headache, seizures, nausea, vomiting, gastrointestinal bleeding, hypertension, and arthralgias. Early neurotoxic symptoms, seen with vicristine in particular, begin with the hands and then the feet. Distal paresthesias and loss of deep tendon reflexes are followed by weakness.[24] The weakness is initially more marked in the upper extremities. Neurophysiologic findings are consistent with a mixed sensorimotor axonal neuropathy. In general, the motor abnormalities, which dominate the neuropathy, resolve slowly after discontinuation of therapy. Close monitoring for symptoms and careful control of dosing are also advised.

## REFERENCES

1. Morgan JP: The Jamaica ginger paralysis. JAMA 248:1864–1867, 1982.
2. Baron RL (ed): Pesticide-Induced Delayed Neurotoxicity: Proceedings of a Conference Co-Sponsored by the Environmental Protection Agency and the National Institute for Environmental Health Sciences, February 19–20, 1976. EPA-600/1-76-025.
3. Johnson MK: The delayed neuropathy caused by some organophosphorus esters: Mechanism and challenge. Crit Rev Toxicol 3:289–316, 1975.
4. Bardsley PA: Chronic respiratory failure in COPD: Is there a place for a respiratory stimulant? Thorax 48:781–784, 1993.
5. Winkleman BR, Kullmer TH, Kneissl DG, et al: Low dose almitrine bismesylate in the treatment of hypoxemia due to chronic obstructive pulmonary disease. Chest 105:1383–1391, 1994.

6. Pollera CF, Pietrangeli A, Giannarelli D: Cisplatin-induced peripheral neurotoxicity: Relationship to dose intensity. Ann Oncol 2:212, 1991.

7. Siegal T, Hains N: Cisplatin-induced peripheral neuropathy. Cancer 66:1117–1123, 1990.

8. Kuncl RW, Duncan O, Watson D, et al: Colchicine myopathy and neuropathy. N Engl J Med 316:1562–1568, 1987.

9. Daniels SR, Hudson JI, Horowitz RI: Epidemiology of potential association between L-tryptophan ingestion and EMS. J Clin Epidemiol 48:1413–1427, 1995.

10. Couri D, Milks MM: Hexacarbon neuropathy: Tracking a toxin. Neurotoxicology 6(4):65–71, 1985.

11. Oryshkevich RS, Wilcox R, Jhee WH: Polyneuropathy due to glue exposure. Arch Phys Med Rehabil 67:817–828, 1986.

12. Scelsi R, Poggi P, Fera L: Toxic polyneuropathy due to n-hexane. J Neurol Sci 47:7–19, 1980.

13. Levine SP, Cavender GD, Langolf GD, et al: Elemental mercury exposure: Peripheral neurotoxicity. Br J Ind Med 39:136–139, 1982.

14. Fagius J, Osterman PO, Siden A, et al: Guillain-Barré syndrome following zimeldine treatment. J Neurol Neurosurg Psychiatry 48:65–69, 1985.

15. Snavely SR, Hodges GR: The neurotoxicity of antimicrobial agents. Ann Intern Med 101:97–104, 1984.

16. Kunze K, Kauerz V, Scholdt A: Drug induced myopathy by hydroxychloroquine. Vet Hum Toxicol 29(Suppl 2):59–60, 1987.

17. Wilkenson R, Mahatane J, Wade P, et al: Chloroquine poisoning. BMJ 307:504, 1993.

18. Woodhouse KW, Henderson DB, Charlton B, et al: Acute dapsone poisoning: Clinical features and pharmacokinetic studies. Hum Toxicol 3:905–906, 1983.

19. Peters HA, Levine RL, Matthews CG, et al: Extrapyramidal and other neurologic manifestations associated with carbon disulfide fumigant exposure. Arch Neurol 45:537–540, 1988.

20. Laplane D, Attal N, Sauron B, et al: Lesions of basal ganglia due to disulfiram neurotoxicity. J Neurol Neurosurg Psychiatry 55:925–929, 1992.

21. Biehl JP, Nimitz HJ: Studies on the use of a high dose of isoniazid: I. Toxicity studies. Am Rev Tuberc 69:759–765, 1965.

22. Thomas RJ: Neurotoxicity of antibacterial therapy. South Med J 87:869–874, 1994.

23. Curtis DL, Pirbe R, Ellenhorn MJ, et al: Phenytoin toxicity: A review of 94 cases. Vet Hum Toxicol 31:164–165, 1989.

24. Jackson DV, Wells HB, Atkins JN, et al: Amelioration of vincristine neurotoxicity by glutamic acid. Am J Med 84:1016–1022, 1994.

# Metabolic and Endocrine Disorders 11

*Lubna M. Zuberi and Jeffrey L. Miller*

Many systemic diseases cause muscle weakness and various forms of neuropathies. The clinical manifestations of any endocrine disorder may result from either overproduction or underproduction of an essential hormone. Myopathy and neuropathy are frequently manifest as part of the clinical syndrome. This chapter describes the clinical presentation of neuropathies and myopathies affecting the lower extremity and discusses screening for an underlying endocrinopathy.

## DIABETES MELLITUS

Diabetes mellitus is the most common metabolic disorder, estimated to affect more than 5 million people in the United States. Of the many complications, neuropathy is the most frequent. A large prospective study, consisting of mostly older patients with type 2 diabetes mellitus (non–insulin dependent), revealed an 8% prevalence of clinical polyneuropathy at the time diabetes was diagnosed. This prevalence rose to 50% after 25 years of follow-up. Of type 2 patients free of neuropathy at the time of diagnosis, the risk of developing neuropathy is estimated to be 4% by 5 years and 15% by 20 years.[1]

The diagnosis of diabetes is confirmed by either a fasting plasma glucose level greater than 140 mg/dL on two occasions or a random plasma glucose value greater than 200 mg/dL with classic symptoms of polyuria and polydipsia. The diabetic neuropathies closely resemble neuropathies caused by numerous other conditions and therefore require careful and extensive evaluation and differentiation. Several other conditions prevalent in older individuals, such as anterior disk protrusion, malignant nerve root infiltrations, spinal cord tumors, and vascular or inflammatory neuropathies, must be excluded by further studies.

Several classification schemes have been proposed. A major division into symmetric and asymmetric (or focal) is now generally accepted, with the understanding that overlapping syndromes are frequently seen.[2,3] These can further be subdivided into sensory, sensorimotor, and motor neuropathies.

## Distal Symmetric Neuropathy

This form is the most common diabetic neuropathy. Although it is always bilateral and of distal onset, its symmetry may be disturbed by concomitant vascular insufficiency. It is a predominantly sensory disturbance with varying degrees of autonomic and relatively little motor involvement. It can be subdivided in ascending order of frequency into large-fiber, small-fiber, and mixed variants.

The large-fiber variant is the least common. Patients may be completely asymptomatic or present with either sensory ataxia (particularly notable in the dark or with the eyes closed) or distal paresthesia. Pain is not present. A tight bandlike sensation around the feet and ankles and an electric tingling sensation may be reported. Examination reveals distal sensory loss predominantly affecting vibration and proprioception, diminished or absent reflexes, distal weakness, and sensory ataxia.

The small-fiber variant presents with spontaneous pain, prominent dysesthesias, and symptoms of autonomic dysfunction. Contact hypersensitivity is often prominent, and a common complaint is that the patient cannot tolerate sheets or blankets and sleeps with socks even in warm weather. There is distal sensory loss, which, when severe, allows unsuspected trauma to go unnoticed, resulting in the development of Charcot's joints. On examination, strength and deep tendon reflexes are typically preserved. Absent temperature and pain sensation is noted. Autonomic signs of orthostatic hypotension, resting tachycardia, distal anhidrosis, and miotic pupils with sluggish light response may be present.

The mixed large- and small-fiber variant is the most common one and represents an overlap of the preceding variants.

## Asymmetric (Focal) Neuropathies

Diabetic amyotrophy was a term first used by Garland in 1955 as a descriptor for a syndrome of asymmetric proximal lower extremity weakness seen in middle-aged, or older diabetics. On the basis of an analysis of clinical and electrodiagnostic data, Bastron and Thomas suggested calling this disorder diabetic polyradiculopathy. It is characterized by an acute or subacute onset of moderate to marked weakness and wasting of pelvifemoral muscles, accompanied by back, hip, and thigh pain with preserved sensations in the region of pain. The distribution is typically although not invariably asymmetric. The maximum weakness and atrophy usually occur within a few weeks, and the condition then remains stable for weeks to months. Slight weight loss may occur in some patients. This disorder is usually seen in patients in their 50s and 60s, although younger individuals may be infrequently affected. The prognosis for recovery is fairly good, with spontaneous improvement in 12 to 24 months.

Entrapment mononeuropathy, also a form of asymmetric neuropathy, affects the upper extremity more commonly. In the lower extremity, nerves at risk of compression are the peroneal nerve at the fibular head and the lateral cutaneous nerve at the thigh. No consistent relationship is seen between the onset of this neuropathy and the duration of diabetes, the age and sex of the patient, or the degree of control.

## Treatment

Effective therapy for diabetic neuropathy is not yet available. The Diabetes Control and Complications Trial (DCCT) has clearly demonstrated that effective and early treatment of hyperglycemia is the only important factor in delaying early progression of neuropathy.

The asymmetric and focal neuropathies either are self-limited or do not respond to any treatment modality. Attempts at treatment are largely symptomatic and directed toward distal symmetric sensorimotor polyneuropathies. Several classes of medications have been used, including tricyclic antidepressants, anticonvulsants, phenothiazines, intravenous lidocaine, and topical capsaicin. Not only are there associated side effects, but also the response has been disappointing. Some other classes of medications, such as α-lipoic acid and acetyl-L-carnitine, are undergoing further clinical trials. Severe incapacitating painful neuropathies unresponsive to conventional treatment may benefit from therapy in a multidisciplinary pain center.

## HYPOTHYROIDISM

Hypothyroidism develops when there is an inadequate effect of thyroid hormone on body tissues. In more than 98% of patients it is caused by thyroid disease (primary hypothyroidism). In the remaining 2% it may be caused by pituitary or hypothalamic disease (secondary hypothyroidism). Rarely, it may be due to failure of tissues to respond to normal or elevated levels of thyroid hormone (thyroid hormone–resistant syndromes). Central nervous system manifestations include lethargy, fatigue, dementia, decreased attention span, memory loss, impaired hearing and taste, and cerebellar ataxia. Paresthesias occur in 50% of overtly hypothyroid patients, and slow reflex relaxation is elicited on physical examination in half of the patients. Muscle pain and at times gait impairment are also noted. The diagnosis of primary hypothyroidism in most instances can be made on the basis of an elevated level of thyroid-stimulating hormone (TSH).

Polyneuropathy, when it involves the lower extremity, is predominantly distal, sensorimotor, or sensory in nature. Its prevalence is estimated to be 718 per 1000 hypothyroid patients.[4] Most of these patients complain of paresthesias and pain. In distal segments of peripheral nerves, a conduction abnormality can frequently be demonstrated before clinical symptoms. A review of electrophysiologic studies of 39 hypothyroid patients found that polyneuropathy was present in 72% of patients but only 64% were symptomatic.[4] The most common sites of abnormal nerve conduction were the sensory nerves, particularly the sural nerve (in 69%). The duration of hypothyroidism, etiology of this disorder, and duration of disease were not predictive of peripheral nerve involvement. There have also been occasional case reports of peroneal nerve palsy leading to footdrop. This has been shown to respond to L-thyroxine therapy.

Myopathy is seen in 30% to 80% of patients with hypothyroidism.[5] Myopathy is usually seen in cases of long-standing hypothyroidism, in which the severity of myopathy parallels the duration and degree of hypothyroidism. Not infrequently, it is also seen in association with acute transient hypothyroidism. One third of these patients present with stiffness and cramping pain, the latter being more common. Proximal muscle weakness, when present, develops insidiously over months. Creatinine kinase levels elevated 10- to 100-fold are seen. When these are present with painful myopathy, a misdiagnosis of polymyositis may be made.[6, 7]

## HYPERTHYROIDISM

Of the several varieties of hyperthyroidism, the most common is Graves' disease, an autoimmune disease in which thyroid-stimulating hormone receptor antibodies bind to and stimulate the thyroid gland. This results in excessive secretion of thyroxine ($T_4$) and triiodothyronine ($T_3$) or both, resulting in clinical manifestations of hyperthyroidism. Graves

(1835) and Basedow (1840) were the early observers who recognized muscle weakness associated with hyperthyroidism. Thyrotoxic myopathy occurs in 60% to 80% of patients with hyperthyroidism. It is usually a proximal myopathy, but occasional involvement of only the distal muscles is seen. In the lower extremity, hip flexors are predominantly affected. Ten percent of patients present with muscle aches confined to the thighs and calves that are associated with the onset of muscle weakness.[8] Muscle fasciculations, seen in 12% of patients, do not occur in the lower extremities. Serum creatinine phosphokinase activity is always normal, reflecting the paucity of muscle fiber damage seen in muscle biopsies. In 40% of the patients tendon reflexes are brisk in the lower limbs. This myopathy is reversible with treatment, and partial improvement is noted initially with propranolol.

Peripheral nerve involvement in hyperthyroidism is rarely reported but is a possible manifestation. It affects mostly the lower extremity (Basedow's paraplegia)[9] and is associated with areflexia. A few patients even have pyramidal tract signs, producing a clinical picture easily mistaken for that of amyotrophic lateral sclerosis.

Hypokalemic periodic paralysis is a well-known although not common complication of hyperthyroidism. It is seen more commonly in patients of Chinese or Japanese ancestry, in whom its incidence is 8% to 30% in males and 0.2% in females.[10] Weakness appears first in the proximal leg muscles and becomes generalized in a course of several hours, with possible respiratory involvement. The episode may last up to 12 hours, with distal muscles recovering first. The serum potassium level is normal between episodes. Recovery may be hastened with administration of 80 to 100 mEq of potassium over 4 to 6 hours. Propranolol may prevent further attacks, and these episodes resolve after patients are rendered euthyroid. Myasthenia gravis occurs in fewer than 0.1% of patients with hyperthyroidism, but about 5% of myasthenia patients have hyperthyroidism.[11] Because of its neuromuscular blocking properties, propranolol should be used cautiously for myasthenic patients, although in practice it does not seem to cause much difficulty.

## ACROMEGALY

Hypersecretion of growth hormone in adults leads to acromegaly, with enlargement of facial features, hands, and feet. The effects of chronic hypersecretion of growth hormone are mediated through insulin-like growth factor 1 (somatomedin C). The changes that result are subtle, slow, and progressive for years and lead to the dramatic clinical syndrome.

Increased mortality is attributed to cerebrovascular, cardiovascular, and pulmonary diseases. In addition, there appears to be an increased incidence of colon polyps and cancer in these patients.

Generalized weakness may be a part of the presenting syndrome in 80% to 90% of patients, with overt myopathy in 40%. Proximal muscle weakness and atrophy were first recorded in patients with acromegaly in 1886. Of 17 consecutive patients with acromegaly, three fourths reported easy fatigability and half had proximal muscle weakness.[11, 12] Symptoms began 8 to 12 years after acral enlargement. After pituitary surgery, improvement of strength was slow and was still incomplete 12 to 21 months later.

Peripheral neuropathy in patients with acromegaly, first reported in 1891, is still poorly understood. Whereas polyneuropathy involving the lower extremities is uncommon, acroparesthesias are frequently seen. Of the 77 patients with acromegaly seen at the Neurological Institute of New York, 16 complained of acroparesthesias. In 7 of the 16, the paresthesias involved the lower extremity. Distal symmetric polyneuropathy of sensorimotor type may also be seen, severe cases of which may present as footdrop. Jamal and colleagues[13] studied 24 patients with acromegaly, 8 of the 24 patients had generalized peripheral nerve dysfunction, with either diminished or absent knee and ankle jerks. All 8 patients had distal sensory changes bilaterally, in a stocking distribution, involving diminished sensation to light touch, pinprick, and vibration. In 10 of the 24 patients, ulnar and/or popliteal nerves were thought to be enlarged clinically.[13]

Sural nerve biopsies show segmental demyelination and in advanced cases onion bulb formation. Growth hormone levels that are markedly elevated over a short period of time or moderately elevated over a longer period are associated with these changes. The presence of onion bulb formation marks the development of end-stage neuropathy.[14]

## CUSHING'S SYNDROME

The clinical syndrome is due to excessive production of steroid hormone by the adrenal glands (endogenous) or to sustained administration of glucocorticoids (exogenous). Endogenous Cushing's syndrome may occur as a result of (1) pituitary adenoma (68%), in which case it is also known as Cushing's disease; (2) adrenal adenoma or hyperplasia (17%); or (3) ectopic adrenocorticotropic hormone production (15%).

Common clinical features include central obesity, hypertension, glucose intolerance, plethoric facies, purple striae, hirsutism, menstrual irregularities, easy bruising, and osteoporosis. Muscular weakness (seen in 60% of the patients) and wasting are among the cardinal signs. Proximal lower extremity weakness is present in almost half of the patients as the presenting clinical symptom. Muscle wasting and weakness begin in the pelvifemoral muscles, especially the quadriceps, and spread to the trunk, anterior neck, shoulders, and upper arms. Patients complain of a mild ache; severe pain does not occur. The onset is usually subacute. On examination, the affected muscles are flabby and wasted, but no fasciculations are seen and tendon reflexes are well preserved. Creative phosphokinase and other muscle enzyme levels are typically normal.[15]

## Exogenous Cushing's Syndrome

Myopathy can result from treatment with all commonly used glucocorticoids, regardless of the medical condition being treated. There is a marked variation in individual susceptibility to development of steroid-induced myopathy, although in general larger doses are more likely to produce myopathy. It may take a few weeks (as early as 3 weeks) to a few months for the myopathy to become manifest. Once myopathy develops, it tends to worsen rapidly.[16] For treatment it is safer to decrease the dose (by half). Complete recovery can be expected in 2 to 3 months after discontinuation of glucocorticoids.

Neuropathies are not a common part of this syndrome. Rarely, the development of spinal epidural lipomatosis may lead to compression of the spinal cord or cauda equina and cause peripheral neuropathy.

The first step in diagnosis is confirmation of hypercortisolemia, done by screening a 24-hour urine collection for urinary free cortisol or with an overnight dexamethasone suppression test. This is followed by further work-up aimed at differentiating the three forms of Cushing's syndrome and localization procedures.

## HYPERPARATHYROIDISM

Before routine determinations of serum calcium were initiated in the early 1970s, primary hyperparathyroidism was an infrequent diagnosis. In the 1990s it has been diagnosed in 1 per 1000 population. The male:female ratio is 1:2 to 1:3. Most patients are older than 50 years. It is caused by parathyroid adenoma in 80%, hyperplasia of parathyroid glands in 20%, and parathyroid carcinoma in less than 1%.

The classical myopathic syndrome of primary hyperparathyroidism (described by Vicale in 1949), with symmetric muscular weakness and atrophy,

gait abnormalities, and hyperreflexia, is now rare. In a study by Turken and colleagues,[17] 22 of 42 patients with primary hyperparathyroidism had neuromuscular symptoms consisting of muscle cramps (45%), paresthesias (45%), or both (18%). Of these 22 patients, 10 had normal findings on examination. Twelve had abnormal findings, including mild loss of pain sensation and diminished vibration sensation with absent reflexes. These symptoms subsided quickly after successful parathyroid surgery.[18–20]

Proximal muscle weakness is uncommon but, when present, improves within a few days to weeks after parathyroid surgery.

## HYPOPARATHYROIDISM

Hypoparathyroidism is seen most commonly postoperatively, after injury to the parathyroid glands during neck surgery. The various causes of hypoparathyroidism are listed in Table 11–1. Whatever the cause, patients present with hypocalcemia and may have symptoms of tetany secondary to peripheral nerve hyperexcitability. They may complain of pedal spasms, muscle pain, and paresthesias of lower extremities. Mild proximal muscle weakness is seen in association with hyporeflexia or areflexia.

## ADRENOCORTICAL INSUFFICIENCY

Inadequate adrenal function is due to destruction of the adrenal cortex (primary adrenal insufficiency or Addison's disease) or adrenocortical atrophy caused by adrenocorticotropic hormone deficiency (secondary adrenal insufficiency). In the latter case, mineralocorticoid function is preserved. There must be greater than 90% destruction of the adrenal gland before Addison's disease is clinically manifest.

Eighty percent of cases of Addison's disease are caused by autoimmune destruction of the adrenal glands, which is sometimes associated with other forms of polyglandular failure. Other causes include

**Table 11–1  Causes of Hypoparathyroidism**

Surgical hypoparathyroidism
HAM syndrome (hypoparathyroidism, Addison's disease, and mucocutaneous candidiasis)
Acquired hypoparathyroidism
  Deposition of metals (e.g., Fe in transfusion-dependent thalassemias, Cu in Wilson's disease)
  Radiation
  Infiltrative processes (e.g., breast cancer, amyloidosis, sarcoidosis, tuberculosis)
Functional (e.g., hypomagnesemia)
Neonatal syndromes (e.g., DiGeorge's syndrome)
Pseudohypoparathyroidism

granulomatous diseases (tuberculosis, histoplasmosis, sarcoidosis), infiltrative diseases (amyloidosis, lymphomas, hemochromatosis, and metastatic diseases), acquired immunodeficiency syndrome, and bilateral adrenal hemorrhage (resulting from anticoagulants, coagulopathy, trauma). Other cases are congenital (adrenal leukodystrophy, familial glucocorticoid deficiency).

Clinical features of chronic adrenal insufficiency include weakness, fatigue, anorexia, nausea, vague abdominal pain, and vomiting. Weight loss, hyperpigmentation (seen only in Addison's disease), and hypotension are generally found. Only 6% of patients complain of muscular or joint pains. Painful flexion contractures of the lower extremity may occur and are often preceded by episodes of violent muscle cramps, mostly affecting thigh muscles. In between these painful paroxysms, patients may have continuous muscle rigidity, rendering examination extremely difficult.

Hyperkalemia is commonly seen on laboratory assessment. Hyperkalemic periodic paralysis, however, is a rare complication. Peripheral neuropathy is also rare and occurs together with the onset of other symptoms. When present, it is more severe in the lower extremities and responds to glucocorticoid replacement therapy.

## HYPERALDOSTERONISM

Hyperaldosteronism has received much attention as a potentially treatable cause of hypertension. Muscular weakness is the most frequent symptom (aside from hypertension), occurring in 73% of cases. Periodic hypokalemic paralysis and tetany each occurred in 20% of cases. The myopathy and periodic paralysis are caused by potassium deficiency, whereas tetany is caused by associated alkalosis.

## OSTEOMALACIA

In Western countries this is rarely seen, other than in nursing home patients or those with malabsorptive syndromes. The affected patients present a distinctive picture of bone pain and slowly progressive proximal muscle weakness (93%) and atrophy that is more severe in the lower extremity. More than half the patients have a waddling gait on examination, and one fifth are unable to walk. A similar myopathy is seen in patients with chronic renal failure who have uremic osteodystrophy.

The diagnosis is suggested by the presence of pseudofractures and biconcave vertebrae. Serum alkaline phosphatase is increased in 80% to 93% of cases. Low serum calcium and phosphorus concentrations are found in 40% of patients. Low serum levels of vitamin D and its metabolites are also found. The response to therapy is variable.

Neuromuscular involvement of the lower extremity in an endocrinopathy is not uncommon. Thus, part of an initial evaluation of a lower extremity neuropathy or myopathy, in addition to electromyographic studies for anatomic localization, should include screening serum glucose, thyroid-stimulating hormone, and calcium levels. Further endocrine evaluation should then be based on any clinical signs and symptoms.

## REFERENCES

1. Ross MA: Neuropathies associated with diabetes. Med Clin North Am 77:111, 1993.
2. Harati Y: Diabetes and the nervous system. Endocrinol Metab Clin North Am 25:325, 1996.
3. Horowitz SH: Diabetic neuropathy. Clin Orthop 296:78, 1993.
4. Beghi E, Delodorici ML, Bogliun G, et al: Hypothyroidism and polyneuropathy. J Neurol Neurosurg Psychiatry 52:1450, 1989.
5. Evans RM, Watanabe I, Singer PA: Central changes in hypothyroid myopathy: A case report. Muscle Nerve 13:952, 1990.
6. Mastalgia FL, Sarnat HB, Ojeda VJ, et al: Myopathies associated with hypothyroidism: A review based on 13 cases. Aust N Z J Med 18:799, 1988.
7. Torres CF, Moxley RT: Hypothyroid neuropathy and myopathy: Clinical and electrodiagnostic longitudinal findings. J Neurol 237:271, 1990.
8. Puvanendran K, Cheah JS, Nagunathan N, et al: Thyrotoxic myopathy, a clinical and quantitative analytic electromyographic study. J Neurol Sci 42:441, 1979.
9. Feibel JH, Campa JF: Thyrotoxic myopathy (Basedow's paraplegia). J Neurol Neurosurg Psychiatry 39:491, 1976.
10. Guan R, Cheah JS: Hyperthyroidism with periodic paralysis, acropachy, pre-tibial myxedema, transient atrial fibrillation and myopathy. Postgrad Med J 58:507, 1982.
11. Layzer RB: Neuromuscular manifestations of systemic diseases. Contemp Neurol Ser 25:98, 1985.
12. Mastaglia FL, Barwick DD, Hall R: Myopathy in acromegaly. Lancet 2:907, 1970.
13. Jamal GA, Kerr DJ, McLellan AR: Generalized peripheral nerve dysfunction in acromegaly: A study by conventional and novel neurophysiological techniques. J Neurol Neurosurg Psychiatry 50:886, 1987.
14. Stewart BM: The hypertrophic neuropathy of acromegaly. Arch Neurol 14:107, 1966.
15. Olafsson E, Jones RH, Guay AJ, et al: Myopathies of endogenous Cushing's syndrome: A review of clinical and electromyographic features in 8 patients. Muscle Nerve 17:692, 1994.
16. Khaleeli AA, Edwards RHT, Gohil K, et al: Corticosteroid myopathy, a clinical and pathological study. Clin Endocrinol 18:155, 1983.
17. Turken SA, Cafferty M, Silverberg SJ, et al: Neuromuscular involvement in mild, asymptomatic primary hyperparathyroidism. Am J Med 87:553, 1989.
18. Gentric A, Jezequel J, Pennec YL: Severe neuropathy related to primary hyperparathyroidism cured by parathyroidectomy. J Am Geriatr Soc 41:759, 1993.
19. Becker KL: Principles and Practice of Endocrinology and Metabolism, 2nd ed. Philadelphia, JB Lippincott, 1995.
20. Felig P, Baxter JD, Frohman LA: Endocrinology and Metabolism, 3rd ed. New York, McGraw-Hill, 1995.

# Neuroimmunology

# 12

*Richard A. Sater and Abdolmohamad Rostami*

Many neurologic disorders are due to disturbances in the immune system. Neuroimmunologic disorders may be classified according to their anatomic targets. Immunologic diseases affecting the lower extremities may be secondary to pathology in the central nervous system, nerve, neuromuscular junction, or muscle. In general, the physical examination and electrophysiologic tests provide sufficient clues to locate the lesion. The history and additional laboratory tests help to determine the nature of the disorder. Treatment for these diseases includes a combination of medical care and immunomodulation. After a brief overview of immunology, transverse myelitis, chronic inflammatory demyelinating polyneuropathy, myasthenia gravis, and polymyositis are discussed.

## OVERVIEW OF IMMUNOLOGY

The primary function of the immune system is to protect the individual against infectious agents in the environment. To accomplish this in an effective manner, humans have developed a complex network of cells and humoral factors that cooperate to eliminate or disable microorganisms. To direct an immune response, self must be distinguished from nonself. Failure of tolerance to self-antigens can lead to autoimmune disorders. Adaptive immunity is manifested by B and T lymphocytes and becomes more specific with time. In addition, lifelong immunity frequently follows an adaptive immune response. Most autoimmune disorders occur because of breakdowns in the regulation of the adaptive immune response. A detailed review of immunology is beyond the scope of this chapter. However, familiarity with the components of the immune system and core principles of immunology is critical to understanding inflammatory disorders that lead to neurologic impairment.

## Cellular Components of the Immune System

Different cells are responsible for the cognitive and effector mechanisms of the immune system. Immune cognition, recognition of self versus nonself, is primarily a function of the B and T lymphocytes. B cells differentiate into antibody-secreting cells. They also present antigen to T cells, enabling them to promote the further proliferation and differentiation of specific B cells. T lymphocytes direct other immune cells through secretion of cytokines and cell-cell contact. T helper cells, expressing CD4 on their surface, are further divided into Th1 and Th2 cells. Th1 lymphocytes release interferon-γ, a potent macrophage activator, and interleukin-2 to enhance cell-mediated immune responses. This process appears important in polymyositis and Guillain-Barré syndrome. Th2 cells release factors, such as interleukin-4 and interleukin-10, that promote humoral immunity through B cells and mast cells. A subset of T lymphocytes expressing CD8 on their surface is capable of destroying cells that are intracellularly infected by viruses or bacteria. Under certain circumstances, they also destroy self-reactive B lymphocytes and activated T lymphocytes.

Phagocytes, such as macrophages and neutrophils, are part of the effector arm of the immune system. By themselves, they are potent weapons against many bacteria. They become much more effective when directed by cytokines produced by T lymphocytes and antibodies produced by B lymphocytes. Macrophages and related cells, such as microglia in the central nervous system (CNS), also present antigen to lymphocytes to increase the efficiency of the adaptive immune response.

Other cells that are not leukocytes play important roles in the immune response. Endothelial cells constitute the blood-brain and blood-nerve barriers that give an element of immune privilege to parts of the nervous system. In addition, in response to stress or inflammation, they secrete cytokines that attract and activate immune cells. Astrocytes and Schwann's cells may also participate in inflammatory responses by presenting antigen to T cells.

## Humoral Components of the Immune System

Soluble proteins play important roles in immune responses. Antibodies are complex molecules with several functions. The antibody molecules have two functional domains. The Fab domain is quite variable and is specific for epitopes on the antigen. Rearrangement of the immunoglobulin variable regions allows millions of antibodies with unique specificities to be produced. These rearranged, but unmutated, antibodies are immunoglobulin M (IgM) of low affinity. They predominate during the primary antibody response. Further exposure to antigen results in a longer lasting secondary antibody response consisting predominantly of IgG. The variable regions of the antibody are somatically mutated to generate high-affinity Fab domains.

The second functional domain of the antibody molecule is the constant region, Fc. The constant region of the antibody interacts with other components of the immune system. Secreted antibodies have one of four major distinct constant domains: M, G, A, or E. IgM is a large pentameric protein that is produced during the primary antibody response. In certain immunologic and pathologic states, it is produced for extended lengths of time. IgG constitutes the bulk of circulating antibody. It tends to have high affinity and a long half-life and crosses the placenta, offering protection to newborns. IgA is present at low levels in serum but much higher levels in secretions and in the gut. IgE, bound to mast cells and basophils, binds antigen, causing degranulation and histamine release. Paraproteins are greatly increased quantities of specific antibodies in the serum.

Antibodies can bind to and inactivate certain soluble proteins. However, their main purpose is to help guide interactions between cells of the immune system and pathogens. Antibodies can coat the surface of microbes. Then macrophages and neutrophils bind the antibody through the Fc portion and phagocytose and destroy the pathogen in a process known as opsonization.

Complement refers to a group of serum proteins that, upon activation, promote opsonization, attract leukocytes, and lyse target cells. The complement cascade is initiated by antibody binding or by a foreign cell membrane alone. Both pathways converge to activate other complement components forming a complex that inserts pores in target cell membranes, which can cause cell death. Along the way, certain active fragments of complement serve as opsonins that promote phagocytosis and as chemokines that attract leukocytes. Only IgM and some subsets of IgG are capable of activating the classical cascade. The activation of complement by antigen-bound antibody is of major significance in several neuroimmunologic diseases such as myasthenia gravis (MG) and dermatomyositis.

## Blood-Brain and Blood-Nerve Barriers

Several mechanisms produce an immunologic barrier between the CNS and capillaries. Capillary endothelium excludes large proteins (including immunoglobulin) from passage into the CNS parenchyma. The endothelial tight junctions also prevent passage of most immune cells. Astrocyte foot processes form an additional barrier that further limits interaction between the brain and blood. In addition, many CNS cells, including neurons, do not express basal levels of major histocompatibility complex on their surface. This prevents direct interactions between neurons and T cells.

Inflammation caused by infection, vascular disturbances, or ongoing neuroimmune processes cause the blood-brain barrier to leak, allowing some passage of cells and proteins. Nerves and muscles have barriers that are similar to, although less complete, than the blood-brain barrier.

Most pathologic neuroimmunologic processes are caused by one or more hypersensitivity reactions. Antibody-dependent cytotoxic hypersensitivity (type II) is caused by recognition of self by antibodies and subsequent complement activation or opsonization. Cells can be killed or damaged by the resulting cytotoxic action. MG and dermatomyositis are caused by this type of hypersensitivity. Immune complex disorders such as systemic lupus erythematosus are type III hypersensitivity disorders. Delayed-type hypersensitivity (type IV) involves cell-mediated immune reactions. In many delayed-type hypersensitivity responses, activated T cells choreograph an inflammatory reaction and activate macrophages. Diseases such as Guillain-Barré syndrome and polymyositis, in which activated macrophages are guided to their target by antibodies and complement, probably involve combinations of type II and type IV hypersensitivities.

## CLINICAL NEUROIMMUNOLOGY

### Transverse Myelitis and Multiple Sclerosis

Transverse myelitis (TM) is a general term for localized inflammation of the white matter of the spinal cord that leads to motor, sensory, and autonomic symptoms and signs. The etiology may be primarily inflammatory, infectious, or vascular. Idiopathic TM and multiple sclerosis (MS) are the two primary causes of inflammatory demyelinating TM. Idiopathic TM can be restricted to the spinal cord or also involve the white matter of the brain. TM is sometimes the first manifestation of MS and also occurs in patients with established MS. Devic's disease is a rare variant of MS consisting of TM and optic neuritis with relative sparing of the remainder of the CNS. MS lesions in the brain also cause lower extremity symptoms. Both cellular and humoral immunities have been implicated in TM.

Idiopathic TM characteristically follows an upper respiratory infection, varicella, or rubeola. Idiopathic TM also occurs after rabies or other vaccinations. New rabies vaccines manufactured in diploid cells rather than grown in rabbit spinal cord have greatly reduced the incidence. Typically, the patient presents with weakness in the legs and decreased sensation below a thoracic level. Symptoms increase over a period of hours to days and begin to resolve after one to several weeks. Bladder dysfunction and back pain are common. Other CNS involvement occurs and may lead to dysphagia, seizures, and altered vision. In the case of TM secondary to MS, the progression is typically slower and back pain and fever are uncommon.

On physical examination, a sensory level is often found by pinprick testing. Leg weakness varies from minimal to complete paralysis. Depending on the extent and level of TM, the arms may also be involved. Deep tendon reflexes are brisk and the plantar responses can be extensor. A resolving skin rash may be observed in postinfectious TM.

The differential diagnosis of TM is extensive. Correct and rapid diagnosis is important because treatment for inflammatory TM is quite different from treatment for the many processes that mimic demyelinating TM. Spinal magnetic resonance imaging (MRI), with and without contrast, should be promptly carried out to rule out compressive or intrinsic spinal cord lesions. If MRI is unavailable or the patient cannot tolerate MRI, computed tomographic (CT) scan is of value. Typically, with MRI, white matter lesions of increased intensity are seen on T2-weighted images. Despite the name, transverse myelitis usually extends much farther vertically than it does transversely. Cerebrospinal fluid should be obtained and analyzed for cell count, protein, glucose, oligoclonal bands, and culture. Cerebrospinal fluid cytology must be carried out to test for carcinomatous meningitis. Second-line diagnostic tests include brain MRI, brain stem auditory evoked responses, somatosensory evoked responses, and visual evoked responses to determine whether MS is a more likely diagnosis. Blood tests for syphilis, Lyme disease, antinuclear antibodies, erythrocyte sedimentation rate, and vitamin $B_{12}$ help rule out other causes of spinal cord disease that mimic inflammatory TM.

As with other neuroimmunologic processes, treatment is directed on two fronts: supportive medical care and immunomodulation. Some of the more seriously affected patients become bedridden and are at risk of developing deep venous thromboses, contractures, and decubitus ulcers. In these patients, subcutaneous heparin (5000 units every 12 hours) and thromboembolic disease stockings (or pneumatic calf compression) help prevent thrombophlebitis. Physical therapy and splinting should be used early in the course of TM to preserve range of motion and to prevent contractures. If spasticity becomes painful, baclofen is often beneficial. The typical starting dose is 10 mg/day. The dose can be slowly increased to 10 to 20 mg three or four times a day, if tolerated. If the urinary residuals after voiding are high, intermittent catheterization may be necessary. Proper bowel regimen with bisacodyl and psyllium helps to prevent severe constipation. Most patients benefit from being moved to a comprehensive rehabilitation facility when medically stable.

Corticosteroid therapy remains the mainstay of immunomodulatory therapy in TM. A typical schedule is intravenous methylprednisolone at 15 mg/kg/day for 3 days followed by oral prednisone at 1 mg/kg/day for 7 days. After this, steroid tapering over 1 to 3 weeks is completed. Patients receiving high-dose corticosteroids should take concurrent medications for gastric prophylaxis such as ranitidine or sucralfate. In addition, glucose levels should be followed and hyperglycemia treated with a sliding-scale regular insulin regimen.

The prognosis for TM is variable. About one third of patients recover fully. Most of the remaining patients have mild or moderate residual neurologic deficits. TM rarely recurs in patients with idiopathic or postvaccinal TM. More frequently, TM recurs in the same or a different distribution in MS patients.

## Chronic Inflammatory Demyelinating Polyneuropathy

Several peripheral neuropathies are caused by immunologic processes (Table 12–1). Chronic inflammatory demyelinating polyneuropathy (CIDP) refers to progressive symmetric sensorimotor neuropathies that take more than 1 month to develop. Although most cases of CIDP are idiopathic, some patients have underlying disorders such as systemic lupus erythematosus (SLE), human immunodeficiency virus infection (HIV), hepatitis, or paraproteinemias. The existence of paraproteins necessitates a more extensive evaluation and has therapeutic consequences. In most cases, the myelin antigens targeted for immune attack are unknown. However, some patients have IgM paraproteins directed against myelin-associated glycoprotein (MAG). Sural nerve biopsies often show an onion bulb appearance on electron microscopy resulting from repeated rounds of demyelination and remyelination.

Most patients present with distal paraesthesias and motor weakness that develops over a period of months. There is seldom a prodromal infectious or vaccinal association. The disease takes three forms. Idiopathic CIDP is occasionally monophasic over a period of months to several years. Most patients,

Table 12–1  **Neuroimmunologic Disorders**

Central nervous system
  Multiple sclerosis
  Transverse myelitis
    Demyelinating, idiopathic (postinfectious, postvaccinal)
    Demyelinating, multiple sclerosis
    Vasculitic (systemic lupus erythematosus)
    Infectious (human immunodeficiency virus, human T-cell
      lymphotropic virus, herpes, Lyme, syphilis, tuberculosis)
Root or nerve
  Acute inflammatory demyelinating polyradiculoneuropathy
    Classic Guillain-Barré syndrome
    Variants (acute motor axonal neuropathy, Miller-Fisher
      syndrome)
  Chronic inflammatory demyelinating polyneuropathy
  Monoclonal gammopathy of unknown significance
  Anti–myelin-associated glycoprotein (anti-MAG)
  Multifocal motor neuropathy with conduction block
  Cryoglobulinemia
  Idiopathic lumbosacral plexopathy
  Vasculitis
  Sarcoid
Neuromuscular junction
  Myasthenia gravis
  Lambert-Eaton myasthenic syndrome
Muscle
  Polymyositis
  Dermatomyositis

however, have a remitting-relapsing course. Some idiopathic and many paraprotein-associated cases are more chronic and progressive in nature. Fewer than 15% of patients develop cranial nerve symptoms or signs. Respiratory failure is even more rare. Patients with anti-MAG CIDP may have only a sensory neuropathy that causes a gait disturbance.

On physical examination, distal sensory loss is universal with varying degrees of motor weakness. Results of the sensory and motor examinations are nearly symmetric. The legs are usually much more involved than the arms. Proximal weakness is frequent and does not occur in the absence of distal weakness. Deep tendon reflexes are decreased or absent. Distal atrophy and contractures are often seen in long-standing cases

The differential diagnosis of CIDP includes metabolic neuropathies associated with uremia and diabetes mellitus. Genetic diseases such as Charcot-Marie-Tooth type I and porphyria may mimic CIDP. Heavy metal poisoning and hexacarbon abuse are toxic causes of chronic progressive neuropathies. Carcinomatous meningitis, usually secondary to lung cancer, lymphoma, or breast cancer, sometimes presents in a similar fashion.

Additional diagnostic procedures should be performed to confirm the diagnosis and to test for possible underlying processes. Nerve conduction studies demonstrate demyelination manifested by reduced velocities, prolonged distal latencies, temporal dispersion or conduction block, and prolonged or absent F-wave latencies. Needle electromyography often demonstrates distal chronic denervation. As with Guillain-Barré syndrome albuminocytologic

dissociation is usually found on cerebrospinal fluid examination. Cerebrospinal fluid should also be sent for cytopathology. Patients should have blood tests for HIV, hepatitis B and C, glucose, blood urea nitrogen, and antinuclear antibodies. A serum sample should be analyzed by serum protein electrophoresis with assurance from the laboratory that negative samples are further analyzed by immunofixation. If porphyria and heavy metal poisoning are suspected, urine should be analyzed to rule them out. In atypical cases or in cases with mixed axonal features on electromyography, a sural nerve biopsy should be performed to determine whether vasculitis or amyloidosis is present. If a paraprotein is discovered, a radiologic skeletal survey may demonstrate lesions consistent with osteosclerotic multiple myeloma. A bone marrow biopsy helps evaluate the possibility of a lymphoproliferative disorder.

Treatment must be individualized with judicious use of immunomodulatory therapy for more severely affected patients. Many patients with the anti-MAG paraprotein have mild sensory neuropathies and do not require treatment. In patients with CIDP with moderate or severe symptoms who are able to tolerate corticosteroids, a typical starting dosage is 1 mg/kg/day. If patients improve, the prednisone is tapered and switched to an alternate-day regimen. If no improvement is observed within 2 or 3 months, a second therapy such as azathioprine, intravenous immunoglobulin (IVIG), or plasma exchange should be started. Severely affected patients and those who are unable to tolerate steroids may benefit from IVIG or plasmapheresis at the outset. Cyclophosphamide or cyclosporine is used in patients who have progression despite steroids and IVIG. In general, patients who require long-term high-steroid dosing should be started with azathioprine to reduce the prednisone dose. If a lymphoproliferative disorder is discovered, chemotherapeutic treatment under the supervision of an oncologist may be necessary. A single osteosclerotic myeloma lesion is often treated with radiation therapy.

The prognosis for patients with CIDP depends on the underlying cause of the disease. Patients with idiopathic CIDP and patients with IgG paraproteins are usually well controlled with steroids and/or IVIG. These patients often have few or no neurologic deficits. In general, patients with a chronic progressive course do not respond as well to immunomodulation as patients with a relapsing-remitting course. Only about 3% to 5% of patients die directly of CIDP. Relapses are common with aggressive tapering or discontinuance of steroids.

## Myasthenia Gravis

MG is an autoimmune disorder of the neuromuscular junction (NMJ). Transmission across the NMJ is disrupted because of a decrease in absolute numbers of acetylcholine receptors and a breakdown in the usual architecture of the NMJ. Autoantibodies against the acetylcholine receptor activate complement at the NMJ, contributing to the destruction.

MG is characterized by weakness and rapid fatigue. Although the extraocular muscles and eyelids are most frequently involved, proximal limb muscles are often weak and are the predominant or only complaint in about 10% to 20% of patients. In more severe MG, respiratory and swallowing weakness may lead to a life-threatening myasthenic crisis. The disease often remits and recurs. However, most patients never have a period totally free of weakness. MG is sometimes associated with other autoimmune disorders, especially rheumatoid arthritis and thyroiditis. In addition, about three fourths of MG patients have either thymic hyperplasia (85%) or thymoma (15%).

Ocular findings of ptosis and/or diplopia are present in more than 85% of patients on initial physical examination. Of these, about one half have generalized weakness. Of the patients with only limb weakness as their presenting complaint, most eventually develop ocular symptoms. Objective sensory examination is normal and deep tendon reflexes are normal in muscles capable of voluntary motion. In moderate or severe MG, the vital capacity is often reduced.

Classical MG is rarely mistaken for other processes. However, in patients who present without ocular findings, inflammatory myopathies and late-onset genetic muscle diseases can be considered. Mild MG with negative confirmatory tests is easily confused with hypothyroidism or neurasthenia. The Lambert-Eaton myasthenic syndrome (LEMS) and botulism are also disorders of the NMJ with weakness as a primary complaint.

The diagnosis must be firm before initiating treatment. More than 80% of patients with generalized myasthenia and more than 50% of patients with ocular MG have increased titers of anti–acetylcholine receptor antibodies at presentation. This test is fairly sensitive, with false positives rarely found in patients with LEMS or amyotrophic lateral sclerosis. An edrophonium (Tensilon) test is useful when performed by experienced personnel. For this test, edrophonium is injected and clinically weak muscles are observed for improvement over the next several minutes. A decrement of more than 15% during repetitive nerve stimulation of clinically weak or proximal muscles is diagnostic of an NMJ disorder. Abnormal blocking or increased jitter in single-fiber electromyography is a sensitive test for MG. However, false-positive results are found with partially denervated muscles and in some elderly patients. Thyroid function, antinuclear antibodies, and rheumatoid factor tests are useful. Mediastinal CT or MRI is necessary to image the thymus. A tuberculin test should be performed before initiating corticosteroid therapy.

Anticholinesterases such as pyridostigmine (Mestinon) are first-line therapeutic agents. The absorption is rapid, with onset of action occurring within 20 minutes, peaking at about 2 hours, and declining over the next several hours. Patients can be started with 60 mg every 4 hours while awake and the dose increased, if necessary, to 90 to 120 mg every 3 to 4 hours. Patients who awaken with weakness often benefit from an extended-release form of pyridostigmine (Timespan). Diarrhea is common and easily reduced with atropine or loperamide. Most patients require further therapy. Corticosteroids are the most used second-line agents. Because steroids sometimes increase weakness in the short term, patients with moderate or severe MG should have initial therapy in the hospital. In milder cases of MG, doses of prednisone start at 20 mg/day and are increased as necessary. As with other diseases, a gradual change to an alternating-day regimen is preferred when clinical improvement is noted. The dose is then gradually reduced, but rarely discontinued, as tolerated. Other immunosuppressive agents such as azathioprine or cyclosporine are used for refractory patients or those who do not tolerate corticosteroids. Hospitalized patients with severe MG often benefit from the rapid, but transient, effects of plasmapheresis. Some patients benefit from chronic IVIG therapy. Patients with thymic masses should have a thymectomy. Thymectomy in patients without known thymic masses may lead to improvement or remission of weakness. Thus, this procedure is considered for medically healthy patients with generalized MG. Many drugs increase weakness in MG and should be avoided (Table 12–2).

The prognosis is generally good for patients with mild to moderate generalized symptoms. These

**Table 12–2  Drugs to Avoid in Myasthenia Gravis**

| Class | Drug |
| --- | --- |
| Antibiotics | Aminoglycosides (all) |
| | Lincomycin |
| | Clindamycin |
| | Chloroquine |
| Cardiovascular | β-blockers |
| | Quinidine |
| | Procainamide |
| Ophthalmic | β-blockers |
| Rheumatologic | D-Penicillamine |
| | Chloroquine |
| Other | Succinylcholine |
| | Curare |

patients usually respond to pyridostigmine and prednisone. Patients with severe weakness are at increased pulmonary risk and treatment is often less effective. Patients with thymomas and older patients may have less favorable outcomes.

## Polymyositis and Dermatomyositis

Polymyositis (PM) and dermatomyositis (DM) are the two most common inflammatory myopathies, occurring with an annual incidence of 1 per 100,000. These diseases occur by themselves or overlap other autoimmune disorders such as scleroderma, rheumatoid arthritis, systemic lupus erythematosus, mixed connective tissue disorder, or MG. D-Penicillamine, used for the treatment of rheumatoid arthritis, increases the risk of inflammatory myopathy. PM is rare in children but a variant of DM is more prevalent.

The weakness in PM is progressive and develops over several weeks to months in a fairly symmetric fashion. The proximal limb and trunk muscles are most involved. Pain is rare in PM but is more common in the overlap syndromes. Although involvement of the pharyngeal muscles is common, the ocular muscles are always spared. A similar, but often more rapid, pattern of weakness occurs in DM. These patients also have characteristic skin changes that may accompany, precede, or follow the muscle weakness. An erythematous rash often develops over the neck, back, and chest as well as over the extensor surfaces of the knees, elbows, and finger joints. In addition, a heliotrope (lilac) rash may occur over the eyelids and the bridge of the nose. Periorbital edema is common.

On physical examination, weakness is most pronounced in the hip girdle, thighs, and shoulders. Atrophy is rare early in the disease course. Deep tendon reflexes should be present, although the responses are often reduced. Often, skin and joint changes are seen in patients with an overlap syndrome.

Several other diseases mimic PM and DM. Genetic myopathies such as adult acid maltase deficiency and limb-girdle dystrophy develop more slowly than PM or DM. The history usually distinguishes patients with a drug-induced myopathy. Sarcoid myopathy and HIV–associated myopathy also resemble PM and DM. Inclusion body myositis is similar to PM in superficial histology but is usually more insidious and may have neuropathic features as well. Inclusion body myositis is often intractable to immunomodulatory therapy.

Additional laboratory tests help to confirm the diagnosis before embarking on potentially harmful therapy. The creatine kinase activity in serum is elevated 2- to 50-fold in 85% of the patients. Most patients have a myopathic electromyographic pattern. Specifically, many short-duration, small-amplitude polyphasic voluntary units are seen in proximal muscles. These units recruit to an early full interference pattern. Increased spontaneous activity consisting of fibrillation potentials and positive sharp waves is commonly observed. A muscle biopsy, of a muscle not tested by electromyography, should be performed before initiating corticosteroid therapy. In PM, $CD8^+$ cytotoxic T cells and macrophages surround individual muscle fibers. In stark contrast, DM biopsies show a perifascicular infiltrate of B cells, $CD4^+$ T cells, and few $CD8^+$ T cells. Special stains reveal antibody and complement bound to damaged endothelial cells. Perifascicular atrophy is a result of microinfarction.

Despite significant differences in the pathophysiology of DM and PM, treatment is similar. Both diseases usually respond to corticosteroid therapy. Patients should have tuberculin skin testing before initiation of steroids. A typical regimen would begin with oral prednisone at 1 mg/kg/day until the patient begins to improve or until several months have passed. Improvement in strength typically takes several weeks to several months to occur. Then the prednisone dose is slowly switched to an alternate-day dose of 1.5 to 2 mg/kg. At this point, the alternate-day dose is decreased by 5 to 10 mg/kg per month as tolerated. Vitamin D, calcium, and ranitidine (or sucralfate) should be given concurrently with prednisone. Although the alternate daily dose regimen reduces side effects, many patients still develop cataracts, hypertension, glucose intolerance, and osteoporosis. Avascular necrosis is a rare but serious side effect of prednisone therapy. For patients with severe prednisone side effects or those with steroid-resistant weakness, azathioprine, methotrexate, cyclosporine and IVIG are alternative immunomodulatory agents.

The prognosis for PM and DM is generally favorable. The majority of patients are stabilized with corticosteroid therapy. Remissions, however, are rare and treatment is usually lifelong. Patients with overlap syndromes are often less responsive and have worse prognoses. There is an increased risk of solid tumors of the lung, gastrointestinal tract, ovaries, and breast in patients with DM. These patients should have periodic cancer screening.

## BIBLIOGRAPHY

Roitt I, Brostoff J, Male D: Immunology, 3rd ed. St. Louis, CV Mosby, 1993.
Paul W (ed): Fundamental Immunology, 3rd ed. NewYork, Raven Press, 1995.

Dalakas MC: Clinical, immunopathologic, and therapeutic considerations of inflammatory myopathies. Clin Neuropharmacol 15:327–351, 1992.

Drachman DB: Medical progress: Myasthenia gravis. N Engl J Med 330: 1797–1810, 1994.

Dyck PJ, Prineas J, Pollard J: Chronic inflammatory demyelinating polyneuropathy. *In* Dyck PJ, Thomas PK (eds): Peripheral Neuropathy, 3rd ed. Philadelphia, WB Saunders, 1993.

Engel AG, Hohlfeld R, Banker, BQ: The polymyositis and dermatomyositis syndromes. *In* Engel AG, Franzini-Armstrong C (eds): Myology, 2nd ed. New York, McGraw-Hill, 1994.

Sanders DB, Scoppetta C: The treatment of patients with myasthenia gravis. Neurol Clin North Am 12: 343–368, 1994.

Tyor WR: Post infectious encephalomyelitis and transverse myelitis. *In* Johnson RT, Griffin JW (eds): Current Therapy in Neurologic Disease. St. Louis, CV Mosby, 1995.

# Soft Tissue Injuries

of the Lower Extremity

# 13

*Bruce Vanett*

The muscles, fascia, cartilage, and nerves are commonly injured in both sports and work activities. Contusions, overuse tendinitis, strains, compartment syndrome, stress fractures, and chondromalacia patellae make up the bulk of these injuries and are covered in this chapter. Because of the position of the bones in the lower extremity, contusions of bone or muscle are frequently seen. If the area is well padded by muscle (e.g., femur), muscle contusions predominate; if the bone is less protected (e.g., pelvis, tibia), the bone bruises more easily. It is incumbent upon the treating physician to distinguish between a more serious underlying bone injury and a deep contusion, and radiographs and scanning are employed routinely. The common thread of treatment, which includes rest, compression, ice, anti-inflammatories, stretching, and protective padding, is emphasized. The goal of all treatment modalities is to relieve pain, restore function, and prevent reinjury in the healing process.

## CONTUSIONS

Contusions, or bruises, are results of a direct blow to the area. This can result from an object, from trauma, or from a sports-related injury. As mentioned previously, pelvic and shin bones (tibia, fibula) are subcutaneous and prone to injury. The femur is enveloped by large thick muscles and is less prone to direct trauma; therefore, muscle contusions are the rule in the thigh. The iliac crest at the junction of abdominal oblique and gluteal muscle attachment is susceptible to injury and, when injured, is called a "hip pointer" (Fig. 13–1). Contact sports such as football or soccer can also lead to thigh contusions; fortunately, the thick muscles around the femur can absorb significant trauma without apparent damage. Aching and soreness accompanied by pain on passive stretch are characteristic of a thigh contusion. No hematoma or bleeding is seen because the contusion is quite often deep. Treatment consists of rest, ice, and gentle stretching. Padding to prevent reinjury during healing is helpful. There

is no place for heat or massage in this regimen—these measures increase blood flow, increase swelling, and increase the risk of myositis ossificans or bone formation in the hematoma. This bone growth can be quite disabling and can even be misdiagnosed as tumor. Tibial contusions are seen frequently because of the subcutaneous position of this bone with lack of anterior muscle protection; on occasion, the collections of blood in this area are large and painful enough to warrant aspiration and, rarely, surgical excision.

## STRAINS AND TENDINITIS

Strains are muscle pulls or partial tears, whereas sprains are ligament injuries. Any imbalance between strength and flexibility can lead to muscle strain or tendinitis. One cannot easily differentiate between tendinitis and a partial tear, so these entities are grouped together. Improper warm-up, especially of weekend athletes, and improper training techniques lead to these types of muscle injuries. It is foolish to think that middle-aged men or women can go out on a weekend and play basketball, racquetball, or softball without properly stretching the muscles used in the sport, yet overuse tendinitis is the most common injury seen in any sports physician's office. Muscles do not respond readily to sudden changes in tension or length, and the result of these stresses is inflammation or tearing.

Many of these injuries are preventable by proper preparation for the sport by stretching before the season, stretching before the event, and "cooling down" by stretching after the sport to relax the muscle fibers. Ice and an anti-inflammatory also help when the muscle is irritated. Improper training technique is seen commonly in all athletes. Even professional players often suffer groin pulls, hamstring strains, or rotator cuff tendinitis when they do not maintain a balance between muscle-strengthening exercises (weight machines and free weights) and muscle-stretching exercises. It is always more fun to work out with weights in a gym than to do

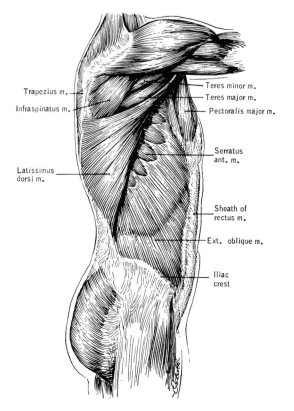

**Figure 13–1.** Iliac crest, site of "hip pointer." Note subcutaneous position of bone with muscles above and below. (From O'Donoghue DH: Treatment of Injuries to Athletes, 4th ed. Philadelphia, WB Saunders, 1984, p 408.)

ning surface, or running direction often have significant shin, calf, and knee symptoms; pitchers, tennis players, or swimmers who increase their playing time often complain of muscle symptoms. Muscles can adapt to new stresses, but gradual changes are tolerated better than rapid ones. Treatment is similar to that for all soft tissue injuries—rest from the inciting activity temporarily, ice, aspirin or other anti-inflammatory, and then a carefully progressive stretching and endurance muscle exercise program. If true muscle weakness is found, strengthening exercises can be added later.

## OVERUSE SYNDROMES

Specific tendon groups are quite sensitive to overuse tendinitis. Groin, hamstring, and quadriceps tendinitis is often caused by repetitive stress or microtrauma. Patients do not recall one traumatic incident but simply complain of pain after a lengthy activity session. Iliotibial band tendinitis, with either hip or lateral knee pain, is seen especially in runners (Fig. 13–2). With excess hip or knee rotation, stress is placed on the lateral thigh and snapping or pain is felt where the tendon crosses the greater trochanter, lateral femoral condyle, or its insertion on Gerdy's tubercle of the tibia. Injection can be added to the usual conservative regimen, and on rare occasion Z-plasty surgical lengthening of the tendon may be required. Patellar tendinitis or "jumper's knee" is seen in running, jumping, or skiing athletes and is easily diagnosed by point tenderness over the painful site of the tendon with negative radiologic findings. The same rules of treat-

hamstring stretches and towel pulls, but the boring stretching is probably the more important of the two in preventing injuries. Also, any change in the intensity or duration of a sport can lead to overuse tendinitis. Runners who change mileage, shoes, run-

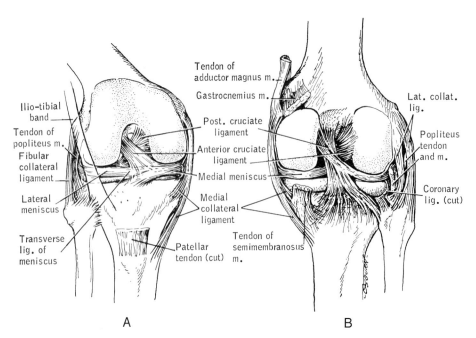

**Figure 13–2.** Iliotibial band at knee, a common cause of knee tendinitis. (From O'Donoghue DH: Treatment of Injuries to Athletes, 4th ed. Philadelphia, WB Saunders, p. 477.)

A                                    B

ment apply, and a special knee sleeve with a counterpressure strap is often beneficial (Fig. 13–3).

Shin splints are the bane of serious runners. The exact etiology is unclear—most believe it is tendinitis of a specific muscle group, some ascribe the syndrome to microtearing of the muscle, and still others think it is a periostitis or tendon-bone irritation. In any case, it is often associated with abnormal foot anatomy (e.g., pes planus) or abnormal foot biomechanics (e.g., equinus contracture, limited subtalar motion). Changes in training technique, as described earlier, such as changes in mileage, frequency, duration, surface, or footwear, can often be traced as the inciting cause. The pain is usually diffuse over the shin, with anterior, posterior, or lateral predominating. Shin splints are often bilateral. One caveat: if the pain localizes to one point unilaterally, look closely for a stress fracture. Many feel that shin splints and stress fractures are on a continuum and that untreated or persistent tendinitis can go on to a hairline fracture. The cornerstone of treatment is rest. The inciting activity or sport must be temporarily stopped; other aerobic activities that do not entail axial loading (bicycling, swimming, Nordic track) can be substituted if they do not cause pain. Stretching followed by strengthening exercises helps. Correction of abnormal foot anatomy and/or biomechanics by shoe modification or orthotics can result in a significant improvement in the patient's symptoms. Anterior tibial, posterior tibial, and peroneal tendinitis is treated in similar fashion, with appropriate site-specific stretching coupled with shoe adjustments to relieve the pain caused by these conditions. Rarely, the pain is severe enough to warrant casting to rest the involved area completely; occasionally, bracing may also be beneficial.

## COMPARTMENT SYNDROME

Certain conditions can increase the amount of tissue or free fluid in a closed space; if the pressure is raised high enough, a compartment syndrome can ensue. Most muscles have a fascial covering and this fascia encloses the muscle in a fixed compartment. Normally, the tissue pressure in a muscle compartment is 0 mm Hg; if this pressure rises to within 10 to 30 mm Hg of the patient's diastolic pressure, the diagnosis of compartment syndrome is made.

Pain out of proportion to the severity of the injury is the hallmark of this problem. Direct trauma, crush injuries, long-bone fractures, burns, and arterial injury are classic causes, but anterior, posterior, and peroneal compartment syndromes can also be seen with overuse or exercise. The five Ps of pain, pallor, paresthesias, passive stretch pain,

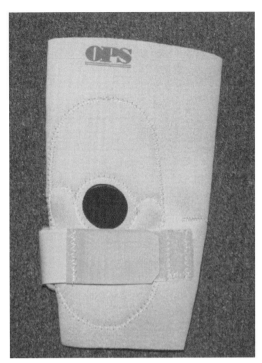

**Figure 13–3.** Jumper's knee sleeve.

and pulselessness, are classic, but the presence of a distal pulse can be misleading as the pulse may never be totally obliterated even with full-blown compartment syndrome. It is the local ischemic effect of pressure on small arteries and veins that causes muscle and nerve damage. In an alert patient, clinical complaints suggest this syndrome to the treating physician; in an unconscious patient, a high index of suspicion coupled with compartment pressure monitoring is needed to make the correct diagnosis. Early diagnosis and early surgical fasciotomy to decompress the involved compartment are needed because watchful waiting and conservative treatment play no role in this condition—the muscle and nerve damage is irreversible if it occurs and can lead to amputation! Whitesides and colleagues first described a manometer wick catheter for measuring compartment pressures (Fig. 13–4); Bourne and Rorabeck have modified these techniques (Fig. 13–5), and several commercial units are now available.

When the diagnosis is made, surgical decompression is immediately indicated—all involved compartments must be released. In the acute setting, fractures must be stabilized, fasciotomies done, and the wound left open for later closure, often with skin grafting. In chronic cases, subcutaneous procedures can often be employed. Care must be taken to differentiate compartment syndrome from deep vein thrombophlebitis, cellulitis, arterial occlusion, neuropraxia, or fracture pain itself, which can mimic the problem.

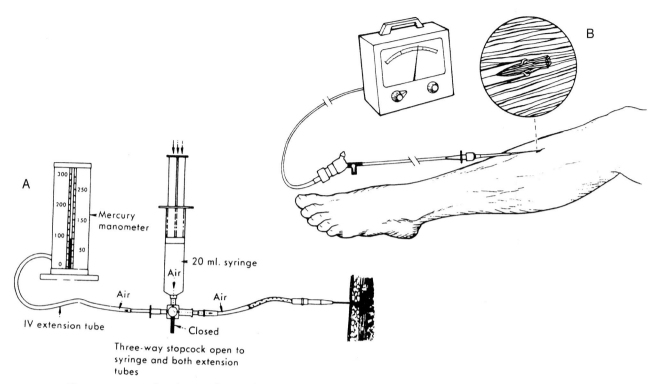

**Figure 13–4.** Wick catheter technique for measuring intracompartment pressure. (From Whitesides TE, Haney TC, Morimoto K, Harada H: Tissue pressure measurements as a determinant for the need of fasciotomy. Clin Orthop 114:43–51, 1975.

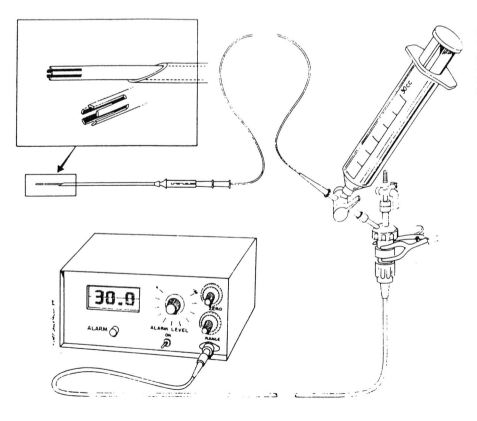

**Figure 13–5.** Slit catheter modification of original compartment pressure measuring system. (From Bourne RB, Rorabeck CH: Compartment syndromes of the lower leg. Clin Orthop 240:97–104, 1989.)

## STRESS FRACTURES

Repetitive stress on a bone can eventually result in a hairline or stress fracture of the bone. As mentioned earlier, shin splints, tendinitis, and stress fractures are on the same continuum of overuse injuries. When shin, foot, thigh, or groin pain localizes to one area and does not relent, a stress fracture must be considered. Plain radiographs are most often normal in the early stage and may show nothing until there is evidence of bone healing and periosteal reaction 14 to 21 days later. The bone scan and now the magnetic resonance imaging scan can provide a definitive diagnosis, with increased uptake or a hot spot being visualized on the films. My treatment for these injuries is rest from the inciting activity; if the patient has pain with a particular sport but not with walking, I recommend stopping the sport. If the patient has pain with the sport and walking, then casting or crutch walking is indicated. For a true stress fracture, sports are stopped for 3 to 4 weeks; then a stretching, endurance, and strengthening program is instituted. The recurrence risk is high and the patient must be aware of this fact. Some change in training, technique, or activity is often needed. Females are more prone to this disorder because of their decreased bone mass in proportion to their muscle density.

## CHONDROMALACIA PATELLAE

Anterior knee pain in the athlete or worker is probably the second most common soft tissue injury, next to contusions. The knee is used in all sports and working activities because of our upright stance. Significant forces cross the patellofemoral joint, with a force of four times body weight often involved in stair climbing activities. Even though some differentiate all causes of this problem, I like to group them into one diagnosis, chondromalacia patellae, with several different contributory causes. Chondromalacia patellae actually means softening of the cartilage of the kneecap, and this is a pathologic diagnosis. It is not always seen in this problem, and I, therefore, think of this more as a clinical syndrome.

Radiographs are often negative, and even direct arthroscopy in the more severe cases often does not show significant pathologic changes. The diagnosis is then based on history and physical examination. Classical complaints include pain on kneeling, squatting, and using stairs. Catching and giving way, not true locking, are seen. Swelling is common. Pain and stiffness after inactivity, such as sitting in a movie, car, or at a desk, have led to a symptom of a "positive movie sign." Many patients have crepitus,

or noise in the knee. Even though patients look for a definitive traumatic incident that brings the symptoms on, most incidents have an insidious onset or patients notice the symptoms the night of, or day after, performing some activity. Physical findings localize the tenderness to the kneecap and surrounding prepatellar tissues. These patients do not have joint line tenderness, ligamentous laxity on stress testing, or bone tenderness. They can have an effusion, or "water on the knee," caused by synovitis—it is always serous or yellow in color and is not bloody. The patellar compression test is usually positive (picture patellar tracking) An increased Q angle and abnormal patellar tracking are often seen (Fig. 13–6). Lateral patellar tracking caused by an abnormally high Q angle (greater than 15 degrees) and lateral muscle overpull are a common cause of this syndrome and can be severe enough to cause subluxation or true dislocation of the patella. This abnormal tracking pattern is one of the few indications for surgical intervention in this syndrome. A helpful analogy for the patient is to visualize the underside of the patella as similar to a baby's buttocks—it is normally quite smooth and articulates easily with the femur below. When pa-

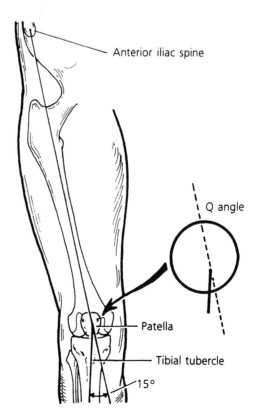

**Figure 13–6.** The Q angle is the angle intersected by a line measured from anterior superior iliac spine to midpatella and from midpatella to tibial tubercle. Any value greater than 15 degrees may lead to abnormal tracking of the patella and symptoms related to subluxation or dislocation. (From Ellison AE, et al (eds): Athletic Training and Sports Medicine. Chicago, American Academy of Orthopaedic Surgeons, 1984.)

thology occurs, it becomes more like the moon with smooth areas interspersed with pits and craters; when these "craters" rub against the femur, they cause pain, swelling, and giving way—the classical symptoms of this syndrome.

The treatment of chondromalacia patellae is nonsurgical. Because we do not know the true etiology of this disease, we do not know the true cure. Patients should be told early that there is no reliable cure and that this conservative program can help to relieve and quiet their symptoms. The natural history of this disease is quite variable; the symptoms never truly go away in adults, although growing children can sometimes regenerate articular cartilage if there is damage. Normal activities of daily living, such as walking, using stairs, arising from chairs, and kneeling, can exacerbate the symptoms even if the patient stops doing a sport or activity. Weather changes often initiate symptoms. Still, the first tenet of treatment is to avoid the inciting activity—runners must at least temporarily stop running, carpenters must stop kneeling, and line workers must stop climbing poles. This treatment of avoidance of inciting activities can relieve symptoms in 80% of patients. I let pain be the warning guide to activity—when pain free, the patient can go back to a usual activity, but recurrence of pain indicates that the activity must be stopped again to prevent further damage. Second, ice and aspirin should be used for symptomatic treatment. Ice for 15 minutes four times a day, when needed, helps decrease pain and inflammation. No heat in any form—whirlpool, hot packs, methyl salicylate–menthol (Ben-Gay), or massage—should be used, as that treatment increases inflammation. Aspirin or any anti-inflammatory can be taken every 4 hours, as needed, for similar reasons. Acetaminophen (Tylenol) has no anti-inflammatory action and is not as helpful. Third, stretching, not strengthening, of quadriceps and hamstrings is beneficial. These exercises, isometric or limited arc, do not change the bone or cartilage itself but they can improve patellar tracking and decrease secondary muscle spasm and inflammation. They can also help to stabilize the patella in the femoral groove and can stop some of the giving way or weakness of the leg. Do not allow full range of motion or isotonic exercises for this problem, as bending of the knee past 30 to 45 degrees causes a significant increase in the patellofemoral contact stresses and increases the patient's symptoms of pain and crepitus. Lastly, a knee sleeve or support sometimes is used (Fig. 13–7). The support should have a patellar cutout to avoid direct pressure on the kneecap and a horseshoe or straps, if indicated, to keep the kneecap centered on motion. Many different brands are available, with neoprene rubber and cotton being the most popular. These

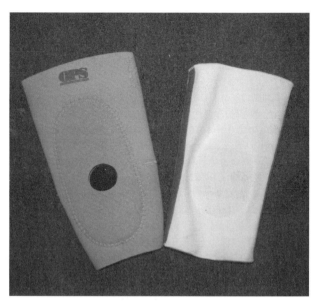

**Figure 13–7.** Commercially available knee sleeves.

knee pads do not require metal bars on the sides or lace-up straps as in braces used for other knee problems (Fig. 13–8). The sleeve can help decrease symptoms when used in conjunction with the preceding measures. In summary, routine treatment for chondromalacia patellae includes the following:

1. Avoidance of inciting activities
2. Symptomatic treatment with and without aspirin
3. Isometric and limited-arc home exercise program
4. An altered knee sleeve with patellar cutout.

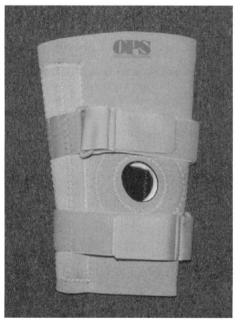

**Figure 13–8.** Patellar stabilizing brace—can be used for recurrent dislocating patella.

On occasion, surgical intervention can be used if conservative treatment fails. There is no role for arthroscopic shaving of the patella—this procedure simply thins the remaining cartilage layer and decreases the effectiveness of the shock absorption. Lateral release and patellar realignment can be done to correct abnormal tracking of the patella and work well in selected cases. Some patients with refractory pain undergo a Maquet tibial osteotomy to elevate the tibial tubercle and patella to decrease the contact forces. The last resort is patellectomy or removal of the patella, but this is a mildly disabling procedure and permanently weakens the quadriceps muscle.

## SUMMARY

It is important to recognize, diagnose, and treat soft tissue injuries of the lower limb. Although not as dramatic as fractures, they are much more common and can be just as painful and disabling. History and physical examination point to the problem, and conservative treatment with rest, ice, aspirin, stretching, and padding often leads to a successful outcome. Understanding these entities and their treatment allows the treating physician to make the correct choices for the patient and speed the patient's recovery.

## BIBLIOGRAPHY

Bourne RB, Rorabeck CH: Compartment syndromes of the lower leg, Clin Orthop 240:97–104, 1989.

Elleson AE, et al (eds): Athletic Training and Sports Medicine. Chicago, American Academy of Orthopaedic Surgeons, 1984.

O'Donoghue DH: Treatment of Injuries to Athletes, 4th ed. Philadelphia, WB Saunders, 1984.

Whitesides TE, Naney TC, Morimoto K, Harada H: Tissue pressure measurements as a determinant for the need of fasciotomy. Clin Orthop 114:43–51, 1975.

# Paraneoplastic Syndromes

# 14

*Robert D. Aiken*

Paraneoplastic syndromes (PNSs) consist of several conditions that affect the central and peripheral nervous systems and, by definition, are not due to a direct invasive or metastatic property of the tumor itself. Although the mechanism of most of these disorders has not been established, PNSs are thought to be caused by endocrine and autoimmune mechanisms. Endocrine PNSs are caused by hormone or prohormone production by the tumor tissue.[1] The resultant syndrome is produced by the active hormone on the target tissue. Four endocrine paraneoplastic syndromes have been defined and are discussed in this chapter: (1) Cushing's syndrome caused by precursor adrenocorticotropic hormone (ACTH) or ACTH production, (2) hypercalcemia caused by parathyroid hormone production, (3) syndrome of inappropriate antidiuretic hormone (SIADH) secretion, and (4) hypoglycemia caused by production of insulin-like growth factors.

The nonendocrine PNSs are a heterogeneous group of disorders that are thought to be the consequence of autoimmune mechanisms.[2] According to the prevailing theory, an immune response with antibody production is generated against many epitopes on the tumor cells. If one or more of these epitopes are shared with normal neural tissue, an autoimmune attack may develop against the normal neural tissue, producing the characteristic PNS. Evidence for this mechanism has been persuasively presented for Lambert-Eaton myasthenic syndrome[3] (LEMS) with small cell lung cancer and myasthenia gravis (with thymoma), but strong evidence exists for paraneoplastic cerebellar degeneration, sensory neuronopathy, retinal degeneration, and encephalomyelitis (e.g., limbic, bulbar). The paraneoplastic disease is, therefore, a consequence of a normal immunologic defense against the tumor tissue that cross reacts with normal neural antigens. Small amounts of the tumor tissue can produce this response. The clinical syndrome produced may lead to a strong suspicion of the presence of an underlying malignancy.

In this chapter, endocrine and nonendocrine PNSs are discussed in which trunk and lower extremity symptoms and findings predominate.

## ENDOCRINE PARANEOPLASTIC SYNDROMES

### Cancer-Related Production of Adrenocorticotropic Hormone and Related Peptides

Cushing's syndrome associated with cancer was the second hormonal syndrome to be described in cancer.[4] Pro-opiomelanocortin (POMC) is the precursor molecule of ACTH and also contains the amino acid sequences of several other hormones including endorphins, enkephalins, and melanocyte-stimulating hormone.[5] Humans have a single POMC gene. Three promoter regions control transcription of the gene: P1, P2, and P3. Normal ACTH levels are maintained by a relative check of these three promoters on the POMC gene.[6] However, in cancer-related ACTH production, there is altered promoter control that results in excessive ACTH or POMC production. Cancers of the lung (small cell variety mainly), cancers of the thymus and pancreas (including islet cell and carcinoid), and medullary carcinoma of the thyroid are the most common cause of this syndrome. It is less commonly seen with cancers of the ovary, prostate, breast, kidney, testis, esophagus, and appendix and in acute myeloblastic leukemia. The consequences of excess hormone production are psychiatric disturbances, truncal fat deposition, and proximal pelvic and shoulder girdle weakness caused by myopathy.

### Cancer-Related Production of Parathyroid Hormone–Related Protein

Hypercalcemia in the cancer patient is usually due to osseous metastases. A minority of cases of cancer-related hypercalcemia are due to the elaboration of a parathyroid hormone–related protein.[7] Two different proteins produced from a single gene by alternative splicing are responsible for this syndrome.[8] Cancers of the lung, kidney, and ovary most commonly produce this syndrome. Multiple myeloma and T-cell lymphoma produce hypercalcemia by producing a bone-resorbing substance similar to osteoclast-activating factors.

Hypercalcemia is the common consequence of these hormonal schemes and may result in anorexia, impaired arousal (from somnolence to coma), and diminished or absent deep tendon reflexes. Treatment is usually a medical emergency requiring intravascular volume expansion with normal saline and furosemide. Occasionally, calcitonin and biphosphonate therapy is required. Curative therapy of cancer-related hyperparathyroid-related protein is rarely possible and consists of curative resection of the inciting neoplasm.

## Syndrome of Inappropriate Antidiuretic Hormone

Excessive production of ADH has been reported to occur in a wide variety of cancers and Hodgkin's disease. Small cell lung cancer is the cancer that most commonly causes the syndrome of inappropriate antidiuretic hormone (SIADH) (up to 40% of cases).[1] Manifestations of SIADH are confusion (with Na <125 mEq/L), seizures (with Na <110 mEq/L), and water retention. SIADH has been suggested as a contributing cause in central pontine myelinolysis.[9]

## Cancer-Related Hypoglycemia

A small group of neoplasms, mainly sarcomas, cause hypoglycemia by excessive production of insulin-like growth factors I and II.[10] The hypoglycemia may be severe and life threatening. Neuropsychiatric manifestations, disturbances in arousal from somnolence to coma, and irreversible brain damage may occur.

## NEUROLOGIC PARANEOPLASTIC SYNDROMES

Except for LEMS, treatment of neurologic PNS is ineffective. LEMS is generally amenable to treatment with plasmapheresis. It is hypothesized that the rapid onset of disabling neurologic signs and symptoms combined with the difficulty in making a certain diagnosis results in irreversible neuronal damage and a poor result with existing therapy. There is limited evidence that early treatment may be beneficial.[11]

## Paraneoplastic Cerebellar Degeneration

Subacute cerebellar degeneration is the most common and best characterized of these rare neurologic PNSs. It is characterized pathologically by extensive loss of the Purkinje cells of the cerebellar cortex. Deep cerebellar nuclei, basket cells, and tangential fibers are usually preserved.[12] It may be present in patients without cancer, but it is most often associated with cancers of the lung (especially small cell lung cancer), breast, and ovary and both Hodgkin's and non-Hodgkin's lymphomas.

The disorder generally begins with mild gait incoordination but evolves over weeks to months. Appendicular and axial ataxia, dysarthria, nystagmus, and oscillopsia are prominent. Patients usually lose the ability to walk or sit without support. Severe dysarthria may preclude speech being clearly understood. Oscillopsia and diplopia may preclude the ability to read. A mild to moderate dementia is often present. In about 50% of patients, other neurologic abnormalities point toward more diffuse involvement: extrapyramidal signs, pathologic reflexes with or without extensor plantar reflexes, sensorineural auditory dysfunction, and peripheral neuropathy. Early in the disorder, computed tomographic and magnetic resonance images of the brain may be normal. As the disorder progresses, cerebellar atrophy with prominence of the cerebellar folia is usually seen. Cerebrospinal fluid may contain an increased number of lymphocytes (from 8 to 20 white blood cells per mm³). Oligoclonal banding is often positive. Protein is often moderately increased from 60 to 120 mg/dL but may be normal.

Paraneoplastic cerebellar degeneration has been found in association with several autoantibodies. The most commonly found are polyclonal immunoglobulin G anti–Purkinje cell autoantibodies, termed anti-Yo antibodies, which are present in high titers.[13] The titers are usually much higher in cerebrospinal fluid than in serum, suggesting active synthesis within the central nervous system. These autoantibodies are largely found in female patients with paraneoplastic cerebellar degeneration between 26 and 85 years old who have cancers of the ovary, breast, or female genital tract.[14] In spite of their high association with paraneoplastic cerebellar degeneration, proof is lacking that these autoantibodies actually cause the clinical syndrome.

Other patients do not have anti-Yo antibodies. Paraneoplastic cerebellar degeneration associated with Hodgkin's disease may present with less specific autoantibodies, namely type 1 antineuronal antibodies, anti-Hu antibodies, and anti-Ri antibodies. Anti-Hu antibodies are more prevalent in paraneoplastic encephalomyelitis or sensory neuronopathy.

In summary, the cerebellar disease is usually rapid in onset, progressing over weeks to months, and then reaches a plateau. Patients generally become quite disabled because of limb and truncal ataxia, nystagmus, oscillopsia, and dysarthria. When the syndrome reaches a plateau, neurologic function may not change significantly and patients may remain disabled for years before they die of recurrent cancer or another illness.

## Paraneoplastic Encephalomyelitis

Paraneoplastic encephalomyelitis occurs in different forms. Subacute limbic encephalitis is a rare complication of small cell lung cancer,[15] but is also seen with other cancers. Patients typically develop the subacute onset of personality and mood difficulty (over weeks to months) associated with progressive and often severe impairment of memory, retrograde and antegrade amnesia, agitation, confusion, hallucinations, and seizures. The disorder is characterized pathologically by loss of neurons in the amygdala, hippocampus, and insular cortex, but there may also be involvement of deep gray matter structures.

Brain stem encephalitis may occur as an isolated neurologic syndrome or as a manifestation of a more diffuse neurologic process.[16] Patients develop subacute onset of nausea, vertigo, and dysphagia. Disturbances of articulation, facial and sensory involvement, and cranial neuropathies are also often present.

Subacute sensory neuronopathy is a rare paraneoplastic disorder that presents with sensory loss in the limbs. It occurs in the setting of cancer but may be present in persons with autoimmune conditions such as Sjögren's syndrome.[17] Most patients with the paraneoplastic syndrome have small cell lung cancer.

Initial symptoms are numbness, tingling, and dysesthesias in the hands and feet. The sensory symptoms progress over weeks to involve all limbs and may ascend to the trunk and face, causing a severe sensory ataxia that may resemble cerebellar degeneration. All sensory modalities are affected; this distinguishes it from cis-platinum neuropathy, which preferentially affects vibration and proprioception. Deep tendon reflexes are diminished or absent, but power is spared.[18]

The pathologic findings consist of loss of primary sensory neurons in the dorsal root ganglia and gasserian ganglia. There may be a variable lymphocytic infiltrate in the ganglia and secondary loss of white matter tracts in the posterior columns of the spinal cord.

## Myelitis and Necrotizing Myelopathy

Necrotizing myelopathy is a rare syndrome that occurs with lymphoma or leukemia more than with other cancers. Patients develop a rapidly ascending flaccid paraplegia[19] in association with back pain or radicular symptoms. The syndrome may precede the discovery of cancer and the process may lead to respiratory paralysis and death. Cerebrospinal fluid is typically inflammatory and neoplastic cells are absent. Treatment is usually unsuccessful.

Nonnecrotizing myelitis more commonly occurs in the spectrum of brain stem–limbic encephalomyelitis.[20] Patients present with progressive weakness and sensory loss and may progress to respiratory paralysis and death. It may resemble amyotrophic lateral sclerosis early in its course. The cerebrospinal fluid formula is usually inflammatory. Pathologic evaluation of the spinal cord shows an intense inflammatory reaction and loss of neurons in the anterior and posterior horns. In small cell lung cancer, paraneoplastic myelitis is often associated with the anti-Hu antibody.[16]

## Stiff-Man Syndrome

Stiff-man syndrome is a rare condition characterized by painful cramps in association with generalized or segmental continuous muscle fiber activity.[21] It may occur in association with brain stem or limbic encephalomyelitis. The condition may be ameliorated by treatment with corticosteroids.

## Subacute Motor Neuronopathy

Subacute motor neuropathy is a rare complication of Hodgkin's disease and non-Hodgkin's lymphomas.[22] It is characterized by subacute progressive lower motor neuron–type weakness of the legs without sensory loss. The arms are less affected than the legs. The process is usually independent of the activity of the underlying neoplasm and usually does not incapacitate the patient. Occasionally, a full recovery can occur over months to years. The condition is characterized pathologically by patchy degeneration of neurons in the anterior horns of the spinal cord.

## PERIPHERAL NERVOUS SYSTEM DISORDERS

### Paraneoplastic Sensorimotor Neuropathy

Combined motor and sensory neuropathies are common in patients with cancer. They may be caused by several mechanisms including metabolic disorders, neurotoxic chemotherapy, and malnutrition and may not be paraneoplastic per se.[23]

Subacute sensorimotor neuropathy causes a distal symmetric polyneuropathy that is more marked in the legs than the arms, with weakness, stocking-glove sensory impairment, and loss of deep tendon reflexes. There is pathologic and electrophysiologic evidence of an axonal neuropathy, although some patients have slowing of motor conduction consistent with demyelination.

## Peripheral Neuropathies and Plasma Cell Dyscrasias

Patients with neuropathy and paraproteinemia present subacutely with progressive, symmetric, distal sensorimotor and autonomic neuropathies. Monoclonal immunoglobulin M proteins have been found that react with antigens on peripheral nerve myelin including myelin-associated glycoprotein (MAG) and $GM_1$ ganglioside.[24] Plasmapheresis may produce clinical improvement in some patients. Peripheral neuropathy is also a rare complication of multiple myeloma and is present in less than 5% of patients. It occurs in four clinical situations[25]: (1) associated with osteolytic multiple myeloma without amyloidosis, (2) associated with osteolytic multiple myeloma and systemic amyloidosis, (3) in association with osteosclerotic multiple myeloma, and (4) in association with the POEMS syndrome (polyneuropathy, organomegaly, endocrinopathy, M protein, and skin changes). Surgical resection or radiation of solitary osteosclerotic myeloma may result in recovery of lost neurologic function.

## Guillian-Barré Polyradiculoneuropathy

A Guillian-Barré–like syndrome may develop in the setting of Hodgkin's disease.[26] Symptoms may develop when the lymphoma is active or in remission. The neuropathy and the neoplasm follow independent courses. Plasmapheresis may be effective.

## Lambert-Eaton Myasthenic Syndrome

This syndrome is highly associated with underlying cancer; about 60% have underlying small cell lung cancer. Patients present with proximal muscle weakness and fatigue with sparing of the bulbar musculature. Deep tendon reflexes are diminished or absent. Autonomic and anticholinergic dysfunction (e.g., dry mouth, impotence, and dysphagia) occurs in some.

Electrophysiologic study demonstrates a characteristic pattern of normal nerve conduction velocities and low-amplitude compound muscle action potentials (CMAP). With exercise the compound muscle action potentials may become normal. Repetitive nerve stimulation causes a decrement of the compound muscle action potential at low stimulation rates and an increment at high rates.

LEMS is caused by autoantibodies to the voltage-dependent calcium channels of the presynaptic terminal. The antibodies decrease calcium entry in response to an action potential, diminishing subsequent acetylcholine release from the presynaptic terminal. This syndrome has been induced in laboratory animals by passive transfer of immunoglobulin G from patients with the disorder.

Unlike most PNSs, LEMS responds to treatment with plasmapheresis or immunosuppression. Guanidine hydrochloride and 3,4-diaminopyridine are also helpful but have significant potential side effects. Cholinesterase inhibitors used in the treatment of myasthenia gravis are rarely helpful.

## Polymyositis and Dermatomyositis

These inflammatory myopathies are also probably due to underlying autoimmune mechanisms. The syndrome presents and progresses with proximal pelvic and shoulder girdle muscle weakness with or without muscle pain and tenderness. Creatine kinase is usually elevated and electromyography discloses a myopathic pattern. Muscle biopsy reveals lymphocytic infiltration of skeletal muscle fascicles. Some authorities dispute that the incidence of polymyositis or dermatomyositis is increased in patients with cancer, but most believe that in older patients, especially those with dermatomyositis,[27] the condition is likely to be paraneoplastic and not just a coincidence. The sexes are about equally affected and weakness may precede the discovery of cancer. The most commonly associated tumors consist of cancers of the breast, lung, ovary, and stomach, but many other malignancies have been reported.

The clinical disorder and underlying tumor may respond differently to treatment. Muscle and skin symptoms and signs may respond inconsistently to treatment of the underlying cancer.[28] Treatment with corticosteroids and immunosuppressant drugs is often helpful.

## Myasthenia Gravis

Myasthenia gravis is not commonly a PNS. However, it occurs in 30% of patients with thymoma. Fifteen percent of patients with myasthenia gravis have a thymoma. Proximal pelvic and shoulder girdle muscle weakness with or without bulbar muscle involvement is the hallmark feature of this disorder.

Patients commonly respond to treatment with corticosteroids, plasmapheresis, or immunosuppressant therapy.[29] Curative resection of the thymoma may render the myasthenia gravis more amenable to treatment.

Despite their rare occurrence, it is important to recognize PNSs. Neurologic symptoms and findings precede the discovery of cancer in about half of patients. Because many PNSs are associated with certain cancers, awareness of these syndromes can lead to timely discovery of the cancer and more prompt treatment. If the cancer is small, cure may be possible. In patients already known to have cancer, recognition of the syndrome may render extensive costly testing unnecessary. Unfortunately, although the cancer may be more controllable, patients are often severely disabled and may live for years considerably impaired by their neurologic handicaps.

# REFERENCES

1. Odell WD, Wolfson A, Yoshimoto Y, et al: Ectopic peptide synthesis: A universal concomitant of neoplasm. Trans Assoc Am Physicians 90:204, 1977.
2. Posner JB: Pathogenesis of central nervous system paraneoplastic syndromes. Rev Neurol (Paris). 148:505, 1992.
3. Leys K, Lang B, Johnston I, et al: Calcium channel autoantibodies in Lambert-Eaton myasthenic syndrome. Ann Neurol 29:307, 1991.
4. Liddle GW, Nicholson WE, Island DP, et al: Clinical laboratory studies of "ectopic" hormone production. Recent Prog Horm Res 25:283, 1969.
5. Nakanishi S, Inoue A, Kita T, et al: Nucleotide sequence of a cloned cDNA for bovine corticotropin-β-lipotropin precursor. Nature 278:423, 1979.
6. Clark AJ, Lavender PM, Besser GM, Rees LH: Proopiomelanocortin mRNA size heterogeneity in ACTH-dependent Cushing's syndrome. J Mol Endocrinol 2:3, 1989.
7. Li X, Drucker DJ: Parathyroid hormone–related peptide is a downstream target for *ras* and *src* activation. J Biol Chem 269:6263, 1994.
8. Mangin M, Ikeda K, Dreyer BE, et al: Two distinct tumor-derived parathyroid hormone–like peptides result from alternate RNA splicing. Mol Endocrinol 2:1049, 1988.
9. Illowsky BP, Laureno R: Encephalopathy and myelinolysis after rapid correction of hyponatremia. Brain 110:855, 1987.
10. Gordon P, Hendricks CM, Kahn CR, et al: Hypoglycemia associated with non–islet cell tumor and insulin-like growth factors: A study of the tumor types. N Engl J Med 305:1452, 1989.
11. Moll JW, Henzen-Logmans SC, Van der Meche FG, Vecht CH: Early diagnosis and IVIg in paraneoplastic cerebellar degeneration. J Neurol Neurosurg Psychiatry 56:112, 1993.
12. Brain WR, Wilkinson M: Subacute cerebellar degeneration associated with neoplasms. Brain 88:465, 1965.
13. Peterson K, Rosenblum MK, Kotanides H, Posner JB: Paraneoplastic cerebellar degeneration: A clinical analysis of 55 anti-Yo antibody positive patients. Neurology 42:1931. 1992.
14. Hammack JE, Kimmel DW, O'Neill BP, Lennon VA: Paraneoplastic cerebellar degeneration: A clinical comparison of patients with and without Purkinje-cell cytoplasmic antibodies. Mayo Clin Proc 65:1423, 1990.
15. Corsellis JA, Goldberg GJ, Norton AR: "Limbic encephalomyelitis" and its association with carcinoma. Brain 91:481, 1968.
16. Dalmau J, Graus F, Rosenblum MK, et al: Anti-Hu–associated paraneoplastic encephalomyelitis/sensory neuronopathy. A clinical study of 71 patients. Medicine (Baltimore) 71:59, 1992.
17. Moll JW, Markusse HM, Pijnenburg JJ, et al: Antineuronal antibodies in patients with neurological complications of primary Sjögren's syndrome. Neurology 43:2574, 1993.
18. Horwich MS, Cho L, Porio RS, et al: Subacute sensory neuronopathy: A remote effect of carcinoma. Ann Neurol 2:7, 1977.
19. Ojeda VJ: Necrotizing myelopathy associated with malignancy. A clinopathological study of two cases and literature review. Cancer 53:1115, 1984.
20. Scully RE, Mark EJ, McNeely WF, et al: Case records of the Massachusetts General Hospital. Case 9–1988. N Engl J Med 318:563, 1988.
21. Roobol TH, Kazzaz BA, Vecht CJ: Segmental rigidity and spinal myoclonus as a paraneoplastic syndrome. J Neurol Neurosurg Psychiatry 50:628, 1987.
22. Schold SC, Cho ES, Somasundaram M, et al: Subacute motor neuronopathy: A remote effect of lymphoma. Ann Neurol 5:271, 1979.
23. Hawley RJ, Cohen MH, Saini N, et al: The carcinomatous neuromyopathy of oat cell lung cancer. Ann Neurol 7:65, 1980.
24. Latov N: Neuropathy and anti-GM1 antibodies. Ann Neurol 27(Suppl):S41, 1990.
25. Kelly JJ Jr, Kyle RA, Miles JM, et al: The spectrum of peripheral neuropathy in myeloma. Neurology 31:24, 1991.
26. Lisak RP, Mitchell M, Zweiman B, et al: Guillian-Barré syndrome and Hodgkin's disease: Three cases with immunological studies. Ann Neurol 1:72, 1977.
27. Richardson JB, Callen JP: Dermatomyositis and malignancy. Med Clin North Am 73:211, 1989.
28. Dalakas MC: Polymyositis, dermatomyositis, and inclusion-body myositis. N Engl J Med 325:1487, 1991.
29. Verma P, Oger J: Treatment of acquired autoimmune myasthenia gravis: A topic review. Can J Neurol Sci 19:360, 1992.

# Nerve Injuries in the Lower Extremity

# 15

*Michael S. Downey*

The physician managing the lower extremity must be keenly aware of the potential for concomitant nerve trauma with virtually any soft tissue or osseous injury, whether acute or chronic in nature. If nerve injuries are not properly identified, assessed, and treated, the sequelae may remain problematic long after any associated soft tissue or osseous injuries have healed. Knowledge of these sequelae demands that the physician treating lower extremity trauma includes the immediate evaluation of the peripheral nervous system in virtually any injury.

## ETIOLOGY

Peripheral nerve injury after trauma may be either primary or secondary. Primary nerve injury results from the same mechanical trauma that injures a bone or joint. In a large study, Lyons and Woodhall[1] found that about 40% of all peripheral nerve lesions were associated with either bone or joint injury. These injuries include fractures, lacerating or penetrating wounds, crush injuries, dislocations, and sprains. In some situations, the neural injury is caused by traction, stretching, compression, therapy injury, or manipulation performed after the initial injury. Secondary nerve injury results when the nerve becomes entangled or damaged by infection, scar tissue, bone callus, or vascular complications such as hematomas. Compartment syndromes are common examples of secondary nerve injuries.

## CLASSIFICATION

A classification system of nerve injury provides the clinician who infrequently sees nerve injuries with basic guidelines for treatment. Certain types of trauma typically lead to certain patterns of nerve injury. The prognosis for full and complete recovery is typically based on the severity of the nerve injury and the timeliness and quality of the treatment provided.

The classification of nerve injuries proposed by Seddon[2, 3] is most widely accepted. He divided nerve injuries into three degrees:

1. *Neurapraxia* generally results from a minor contusion or compression of a peripheral nerve. The injury causes disruption of a localized segment of the myelin sheath of the nerve, and the transmission of nerve impulses by saltatory conduction is temporarily halted. There is no anatomic disruption of the nerve fiber in this injury. Thus, this injury is a physiologic conduction deficit without anatomic axonal disruption. Recovery from neurapraxia is usually complete with no residual effects and occurs over several hours to a few weeks.

2. *Axonotmesis* designates more significant nerve injury than neurapraxia and is defined as axonal disruption without destruction of the endoneurial tubes. Varying amounts of distal wallerian degeneration (i.e., degeneration of the axon distal to the point of injury) occur, and nerve conduction is absent distal to the injury. Because the endoneurial tubes are intact, spontaneous regeneration and complete recovery can result.

3. *Neurotmesis* indicates the most severe nerve injury with complete anatomic severance of the nerve with or without gross disruption of the epineurium. In the lower extremity, these injuries most often result from lacerating or penetrating trauma or from extensive crush or avulsion injuries. Unlike neurapraxia or axonotmesis, neurotmesis always results in imperfect recovery at best.

Each of these injuries is caused by specific types of trauma (Table 15–1). As outlined, lesser injuries without disruption of the endoneurial tubes (neurapraxia and axonotmesis) are associated with anatomic regeneration and less potential for pathologic sequelae. More extensive injuries with complete disruption of the entire nerve (neurotmesis) are more prone to loss of nerve function (Table 15–2).

Another useful classification system was de-

Table 15–1  **Causes of the Three Main Types of Nerve Injury***

| Cause of Injury | Neurapraxia | Axonotmesis | Neurotmesis |
|---|---|---|---|
| Cuts and lacerations | − | ± | + |
| Fractures | − | + | ± |
| Missiles | + | + | + |
| Traction | + | + | + |
| Compression | + (momentary) | + (prolonged) | − |
| Thermal | + | + | − |
| Ischemia | + | + | + |

*+, frequent; ±, occasional; −, infrequent.
From Downey MS: Neurologic trauma. *In* Scurran BL (ed): Foot and Ankle Trauma, 2nd ed. New York, Churchill-Livingstone, 1996, p 236.

scribed by Sunderland.[4, 5] Sunderland's classification divided nerve injuries into five degrees that incorporated and expanded Seddon's three types of injury. In this classification, peripheral nerve injuries are arranged in ascending order of severity from first-degree injury to fifth-degree injury. Each increase in the degree of injury suggests greater nerve injury, greater anatomic disruption, and a poorer prognosis for complete recovery.

*First-degree injury* corresponds closely to Seddon's neurapraxia and is a conduction deficit without axon disruption. The most common cause is compression or a mild contusion. The loss of nerve function is variable. Recovery is typically complete and occurs within hours to a few weeks. Factors predictive of the rate of recovery include the nature, intensity, and duration of the injuring or compressive forces.

*Second-degree injury* involves disruption of the axon with wallerian degeneration distal to the point of injury and proximally for one or more nodal segments. This degree of injury corresponds to Seddon's axonotmesis and is frequently caused by crushing trauma, mild traction, compression, or thermal injury.[6]

*Third-degree injury* can be considered a form of axonotmesis and neurotmesis and involves disruption of the axons and endoneurial tubes with preservation of the perineurium. Moderate to severe traction or stretching injuries are the most common causes of this injury pattern. Injury results in disorganization of the internal arrangement of the nerve and commonly heals as a neuroma-in-continuity.

*Fourth-degree injury* involves more extensive nerve impairment with disruption of some of the perineurium and epineurium but without complete severance of the nerve. Therefore, it is a form of neurotmesis. In the lower extremity, severe crush or traction injuries most frequently cause this injury.[6] Continuity of the nerve trunk is preserved in this injury, but healing ultimately results in a tangled mass of disrupted fasciculi, Schwann's cells, regenerating axons, and scar tissue. This healed injury is considered a neuroma-in-continuity. This damage is irreversible and often requires surgical intervention.

*Fifth-degree injury* is the "true" neurotmesis with complete severance of the entire nerve trunk. Lacerations, penetrating or missile trauma, severe crush injuries, or rupture resulting from severe stretch injuries may produce this degree of injury. This injury almost always requires surgical repair.[6]

Both Seddon's and Sunderland's classifications are helpful in describing a nerve injury. It should be remembered that mixed nerve injuries may occur with variations of the degrees or types outlined. In other words, different portions of the same nerve may have varying degrees of nerve injury. Classification of nerve injuries enables the traumatologist to determine the prognosis for the injury and the possible need for surgical intervention.

Table 15–2  **Differentiating Features of the Three Main Types of Nerve Injury**

| Feature | Neurapraxia | Axonotmesis | Neurotmesis |
|---|---|---|---|
| Pathologic | | | |
|   Anatomic continuity | Preserved | Preserved | May be lost |
|   Essential damage | Myelin sheath distortion | Wallerian degeneration with endoneurial tube preservation | Complete disorganization |
| Clinical | | | |
|   Motor paralysis | Complete | Complete | Complete |
|   Muscle atrophy | Very little | Progressive | Progressive |
|   Sensory paralysis | Usually spared | Complete | Complete |
|   Autonomic paralysis | Usually spared | Complete | Complete |
| Recovery | | | |
|   Quality | Perfect | Perfect | Imperfect |
|   Rate | Rapid; days to weeks | 1–2 mm/day | 1–2 mm/day (if surgically repaired) |
|   March | No order | According to order of innervation | According to order of innervation |
| Treatment | | | |
|   Surgical repair | Not necessary | Usually not necessary | Essential |

From Downey MS: Neurologic trauma. *In* Scurran BL (ed): Foot and Ankle Trauma, 2nd ed. New York, Churchill-Livingstone, 1996, p 237.

## DIAGNOSIS

The diagnosis of peripheral nerve trauma in the lower extremity begins with a complete history and physical examination. Failure to identify an acute nerve injury can result in a squandered opportunity to provide timely treatment and the best chance for recovery from the neural trauma may be lost. It should be remembered that in patients with polytrauma, the extent of nerve injury is often concealed by the state of consciousness of the patient. As soon as feasible, examination of the peripheral nervous system should be performed. The impaired motor, sensory, and autonomic function of a peripheral nerve can then be assessed.

### Motor Function

When a peripheral nerve is severed at a given level, all motor function provided by the nerve distal to that level is abolished. All muscles innervated by the nerve distal to the level of injury become paralyzed and atonic. When evaluating for a suspected injury of a nerve with a motor component, a full muscle inventory should be performed. The muscles should be evaluated individually and compared with the identical muscles in the contralateral extremity. Muscle mass should be quantitated by measuring the circumference of the injured limb and comparing it with that of the contralateral uninjured limb at various levels. Muscles may demonstrate partial paralysis or paresis (i.e., the muscle is partially denervated so that the voluntary effort is weakened) or complete paralysis (i.e., the muscle is totally deprived of innervation and disuse atrophy can occur). Denervation atrophy is muscle wasting that is due to muscle paralysis. Disuse atrophy occurs in normally innervated muscle that is rendered inactive by the nerve injury or immobilization.

In the lower extremity, the nerves with major motor components that are most commonly injured are the femoral nerve, the sciatic nerve, the common peroneal nerve, and the posterior tibial nerve. The femoral nerve is often injured by penetrating trauma to the lower abdomen or by stretching or contusion injuries to the nerve associated with pelvic fractures.[7] Sciatic nerve injuries often accompany hip trauma or dislocations of the hip. Lacerations, severe contusions, and traction injures are also common culprits in sciatic nerve injuries. In the thigh, the nerve is most commonly injured by penetrating wounds or fractures of the femoral shaft.[8] The common peroneal nerve is most often injured where it courses around the head of the fibula at the knee. Direct or indirect trauma can injure the common peroneal nerve at this level. Lacerations, severe

crush injuries, and knee dislocations can cause severe nerve injury. Furthermore, compression injuries to the common peroneal nerve are often seen when the nerve is subjected to constant pressure, such as when the patient lies with pressure against the nerve for prolonged periods (e.g., the unconscious or debilitated patient), or when a short leg cast is poorly applied, causing unnecessary pressure on the nerve. The posterior tibial nerve may be injured in many ways, with lacerations and severe crushing trauma to the medial ankle or hindfoot being the most frequently inciting incidents.

### Sensory Function

In the lower extremity, virtually every nerve has a sensory component, and sensory loss after nerve trauma usually follows a definite anatomic pattern. A thorough knowledge of the anatomic sensory distribution of the nerves in the lower extremity is therefore imperative (Fig. 15–1). It must be remembered that anatomic variants of nerve distribution are common in the foot and ankle and can result in areas of sensory overlap by adjacent nerves. Sensibility testing is the mainstay of the evaluation of peripheral nerve injuries in the lower extremity. Primary sensory qualities that can be readily evaluated include pain or sharp-dull distinction, light touch or pressure, two-point discrimination, temperature, vibration, and proprioception.

If a nerve is totally divided, the physical sensory examination distal to the area of injury finds no sensory function for which the injured is responsible. Patients with partial nerve injuries may be in enough pain to limit their cooperation and ability to respond accurately. The sensibility tests are generally subjective in nature, and the clinician must be careful to consider this in the assessment. Patients often have ill-motivated reasons (e.g., work-related injuries and compensation, active or anticipated litigation, drug dependence) for exaggerating or falsifying their pain and sensory perception. Accurate documentation of sensory findings in partial nerve injuries allows future reassessment and comparison. Subtle changes over time can be critical in determining the progression or regression of recovery.

When considering nerve injuries in the lower extremity, a simple checklist can be used to assess major motor and sensory nerve function in a timely fashion (Table 15–3).

### Autonomic Function

Any injury to a peripheral nerve is followed by autonomic dysfunction in the area of the nerve's

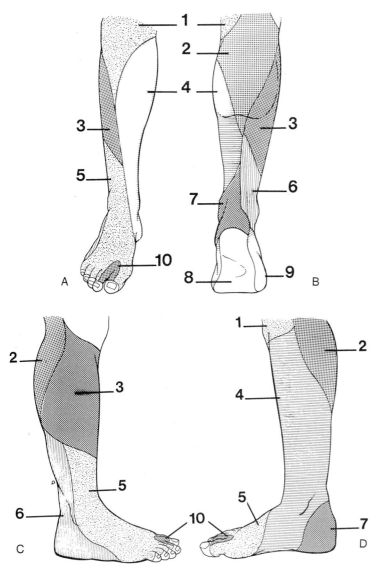

**Figure 15-1**  Anatomic sensory distribution of peripheral nerves. *A,* Anterior *B,* Posterior. *C,* Lateral. *D,* Medial. 1, Medial and intermediate femoral cutaneous nerves (L2, L3); 2, Posterior femoral cutaneous nerve (S1, S2, S3); 3, Lateral sural cutaneous nerve (L5, S1, S2); 4, Saphenous nerve (L3, L4); 5, Superficial peroneal nerve and IDCN and MDCN (L4, L5, S1); 6, Sural nerve and LDCN (L5, S1, S2); 7, Medial calcaneal nerve (S1, S2); 8, Medial plantar nerve (L4, L5); 9, Lateral plantar nerve (S1, S2); 10, Deep peroneal nerve (L4, L5). (From Downey MS: Surgical treatment of peripheral nerve entrapment syndromes. *In* Oloff LM [ed]: Musculoskeletal Disorders of the Lower Extremities. Philadelphia, WB Saunders, 1994, p 686.)

distribution. Unlike sensory findings, many of the autonomic functions can be objectively assessed. Loss of sweating and skin wrinkling, loss of pilomotor response, and vasomotor paralysis (i.e., abnormal skin color, generally mottled or purplish) are seen. In nerve injures with complete nerve interruption, the sudomotor response is lost, and this presents as an area of diminished sweating and skin wrinkling that may be slightly larger than the area of the peripheral nerves distribution. Testing for

**Table 15-3  Preliminary Checklist to Assess Lower Extremity Nerve Function**

| | Sciatic | | | | |
| | Peroneal | | Posterior Tibial | | |
| **Type** | Deep | Superficial | Medial Plantar | Lateral Plantar | **Femoral** |
|---|---|---|---|---|---|
| Motor | | | | | |
| Knee | | Flexion | | | Extension |
| Ankle | Ankle dorsiflexion | Foot eversion | Ankle and toe plantar flexion | | — |
| Toe | Great toe extension | Extensor digitorum brevis | Abductor hallicus brevis | Other intrinsic functions | — |
| Sensory | Dorsum foot first web only | Dorsum foot except first web | Great toe | Small toe | Anterior thigh and medial calf |

sudomotor function is the easiest clinical way to test an area objectively for denervation. The test to perform to check for loss of skin wrinkling is the wrinkle test described by O'Riain.[9] In this test, the injured area is immersed in warm water (40°C) for 30 minutes. Normally innervated skin shrivels or wrinkles when this is done. A denervated area does not provide similar findings. Likewise, loss of sweat production can be assessed. An area suspected of being denervated can be placed under a heat lamp for several minutes. This should be done under direct observation to avoid a thermal burn to any insensate area. Using the +20 lens of an ophthalmoscope, the presence or absence of sweat production can be carefully assessed.[10]

## Reflexes

Complete severance of a peripheral nerve results in a cessation of all reflex activity distal to the level of nerve injury. Partial nerve injuries may also result in loss of some reflexes. Therefore, although they should be assessed, reflexes should not be relied on by themselves to determine the severity of a peripheral nerve injury.

## Compartment Syndromes

Compartment syndromes in the lower extremity require rapid assessment and treatment to prevent myoneural ischemia and its pathologic sequelae. Compartment syndrome occurs when there is an increase in intracompartmental pressure within a closed fascial compartment, typically of the foot or leg. These syndromes most commonly occur after crush injuries, severe contusions, burns, or infections. Potential compartment syndromes must be evaluated by clinical examination and compartment pressure studies. Clinical findings include diminished or absent pulses, paresthesias with altered sensibility testing, trophic changes, and pain that is often unremitting and out of proportion to the underlying trauma. The "six P's" of compartment syndromes are pain, pressure, paresthesias, paresis, pain with passive stretch, and pulses.[11]

## Electrodiagnosis

Electrodiagnosis may be helpful when subjective and objective clinical testing is not definitive. Electrodiagnosis may also be used to help confirm a diagnosis. Nerve conduction velocities may reveal a decreased conduction velocity through the injured nerve, and electromyography may document motor pathology.

## TREATMENT

As with any other injury, the initial management of the patient with potential peripheral nerve injury should be aimed at protecting life and limb with a careful assessment of vital functions. Once evaluated and stabilized, a traumatized patient can be examined for any suspected peripheral nerve injury.

Any open wound with which there is potential for significant nerve injury should be thoroughly cleansed and débrided of any foreign material and/or necrotic tissue. A careful assessment is then made of the wound for any peripheral nerve damage. If nerve damage is encountered, plans for its treatment are made. Only if the patient is stable and the wound is fresh, clean, and simple in nature is immediate repair of the nerve and wound undertaken. In other situations, plans for both the nerve repair and wound coverage need to be made with the appropriate specialists. If there are suspicions regarding the quality and viability of the wound and nerve bed, the nerve repair should be delayed 2 to 4 weeks. This rationale is exemplified in the management of localized crush injuries, blast injuries, and missile injuries. In such injuries, meticulous débridement is performed and the nerve ends are only grossly reapproximated. This reapproximation lessens retraction of the nerve ends. The definitive repair of the nerve is then delayed until the wound and nerve bed are clean and viable.[7]

With a suspected closed injury to a peripheral nerve, careful assessment of the residual nerve function and any deficits should be documented. Protection of the injured extremity with appropriate splinting allows inspection and testing for neural function. After the initial pain of the injury has subsided, early active motion of the joints of the injured extremity should be started. Again, splinting should be done to support and protect the injured extremity and to prevent contractures. Other supportive measures to minimize and control associated edema are instituted. Generally, when minimally displaced, closed fractures are associated with suspected peripheral nerve injury, conservative treatment is initiated and immediate surgical exploration of the injured nerve is avoided. The progression or regression of the nerve's recovery is then scrupulously followed. If rapid recovery is not seen or regression is identified, timely exploration of the injured nerve is undertaken. With more severe injuries or closed fractures with unacceptable displacement, open exploration is performed. Open reduction and fixation of any fracture or dislocation are achieved. At the same time, the injured nerve is visualized and repaired if necessary. It should be noted that prolonged conservative observation should not be a substitute for surgical intervention when surgery is indicated, or irreversible intraneural and end-organ damage may occur.[6, 12]

## Surgical Treatment

There is no single preferred time or method for the repair of all peripheral nerve injures. When a third-, fourth-, or fifth-degree nerve injury is confirmed, surgical intervention is usually indicated. The initial surgery might consist of primary nerve repair (i.e., primary neurorrhaphy) or nerve reapproximation for later nerve repair or nerve grafting. After nerve injury of any degree, scar tissue may develop over time, resulting in significant symptoms or a conduction deficit. This scarring may be intraneural or extraneural and may require neurolysis (i.e., freeing the nerve from inflammatory adhesions or scar tissue). Other nerve injuries may result in a neuroma-in-continuity or other painful sequelae necessitating nerve resection to afford relief. If needed, this nerve resection may be accompanied by nerve grafting to attempt reconstruction of the nerve and a return of nerve function. Thus, surgery may consist of nerve suture (neurorrhaphy), nerve scar tissue resection (internal or external neurolysis), nerve resection (neurectomy), or nerve resection with grafting (nerve reconstruction).[6]

## SPECIFIC NERVE INJURIES

### Sciatic Nerve

The sciatic nerve is the largest nerve in diameter in the body and is analogous in importance in the lower extremity to the brachial plexus in the upper extremity. The sciatic nerve can be subjected to injury in a multitude of ways, and injury to the nerve can often be difficult to differentiate from lower back problems, such as disk herniation. The sciatic nerve can be primarily or secondarily injured by gunshot wounds of the thigh or buttocks, lacerations, intramuscular injections into the buttocks, posterior dislocations and/or fractures of the hip, severe contusions, or traction injuries. In the thigh, the nerve is usually injured by penetrating wounds or fractures of the femoral shaft.[8]

The extent of deficits after sciatic nerve injury depends on the level and severity of the injury. The sciatic nerve and its branches supply numerous muscles in the lower extremity. A careful muscle inventory comparing it with the contralateral extremity (if it is uninjured) is required in any suspected sciatic nerve injury. Injuries at the hip level may result in denervation of the hamstrings with profoundly weakened knee joint flexion, and more distal injuries may be associated with less motor weakness and less resultant disability. Vasomotor and trophic changes can be severe in proximal sciatic nerve injuries. An extremity in which the sciatic nerve has been divided may ultimately develop an equinus deformity of the ankle, clawing of the toes, and atrophy of the muscles innervated by the nerve.

### Femoral Nerve

The femoral nerve is most often injured by penetrating wounds of the lower abdomen. It may also be injured by operations in this area. Because of their close anatomic proximity, the iliac artery and femoral nerve may be injured together. Concern over the arterial injury and resulting hemorrhage can cause injury to the femoral nerve to be overlooked. The femoral nerve can also be contused or subjected to traction or stretching in pelvic fractures. Compression neuropathies of the femoral nerve can result from hematomas of the abdominal wall caused by trauma, anticoagulation therapy, or hemophilia. Furthermore, during operations performed with the patient prone, care must be taken to avoid compression injuries to the nerve. Other iatrogenic injuries can occur with misplaced injections during arteriography procedures, radiation for pelvic malignancies, or direct injury in surgeries near the nerve such as total hip arthroplasty, herniorrhaphy, inguinal node resection, or femoropopliteal bypass procedures.

Damage to the femoral nerve is usually associated with weakness of the quadriceps femoris and eventual atrophy of the anterior thigh musculature. Although knee extension is weakened, the patient is usually able to extend the knee enough to walk, so careful muscle examination must be performed when this injury is suspected. The patellar tendon reflex may be diminished or absent in the affected extremity. The anteromedial aspect of the thigh and the cutaneous distribution of the saphenous nerve show varying degrees of altered sensibility and hypoesthesia when the femoral nerve is injured. Electrodiagnostic testing is valuable in assessing femoral nerve function.

### Lateral Femoral Cutaneous Nerve

The lateral femoral cutaneous nerve (LFCN) is primarily a sensory nerve that innervates the anterior and lateral aspects of the thigh. Meralgia paresthetica is a compression neuropathy of this nerve. Use of a thigh tourniquet, especially for prolonged periods or with inadequate padding, can cause this condition. Similarly, tight belts, a corset, or an ill-fitted above-knee cast can cause pressure on the lateral femoral cutaneous nerve. On rare occasions, the traumatic neuropathy has been related to the removal of an iliac crest bone graft or to the use of a groin flap.

Hypalgesia and hypoesthesia are seen in varying degrees over the distribution of the lateral femoral cutaneous nerve. Tenderness is usually present over the site of maximal compression or nerve entrapment. Usually, the patient has burning pain that ranges from an annoying sensory disturbance to intractable pain.

## Common Peroneal Nerve

Traumatic injury is the most common reason for primary and secondary injuries of the common peroneal nerve. The nerve is extremely vulnerable because of its comparatively large size and superficial route around the fibular neck. Injuries around the knee including high fibular fractures (i.e., Maisonneuve's fractures) and knee joint dislocations may cause direct nerve injury or extraneural pressure via both direct osseous contact and indirect extraneural hemorrhage. Lesser injuries including blunt trauma to the lateral knee area (e.g., trauma caused by a heavy piece of luggage) may result in intraneural or extraneural hemorrhage. Traction injures to the common peroneal nerve may result from sudden ankle supination or adduction of the leg. Compression neuropathy secondary to cast pressure can at times become severe enough to result in an iatrogenic footdrop deformity.[13] Furthermore, improper positioning of a patient on an operating room table, sitting for long periods with one's legs crossed, prolonged kneeling ("Sunday morning paralysis"), decubitus pressure affecting the bedridden patient, chronic pressure in an incapacitated or unconscious patient, popliteal (Baker's) cysts, osseous tumors or traumatic ganglia of the fibular head, and even an enlarged fabella in the lateral head of the gastrocnemius muscle are possible injurious forces.

In severe common peroneal nerve injuries, the patient has profound weakness of the muscles innervated by the nerve. Weakness or paralysis of the tibialis anterior, long extensors (i.e., extensor digitorum longus and extensor hallucis longus), and peroneals (i.e., peroneus longus, peroneus brevis, and peroneus tertius) is present. In such instances, footdrop is seen that cannot be overcome or disguised by any muscle substitution or trick movement. Frequent leg cramps at night may occur in the early stages of this compression neuropathy.

Pain and altered sensation over the anterior and lateral aspects of the leg and the dorsal and lateral aspects of the foot are major complaints associated with common peroneal nerve damage. Manual muscle testing is important in the assessment of the suspected common peroneal nerve injury. In addition, and especially with lesser injuries, percussion of the nerve and elicitation of abnormal sensibility findings are often the key to the diagnosis. Electromyography or nerve conduction velocities are helpful in assessing injury of this nerve and often aid in the diagnosis.

## Saphenous Nerve

Injuries to the saphenous nerve caused by direct trauma are rather uncommon except in certain contact sports such as football.[14] Occasionally, chronic compression injuries may occur with genu valgum, medial tibial positioning, or compensatory knee changes related to faulty foot biomechanics. A small branch of the nerve innervates the medial aspect of the knee joint and can be traumatized by medial meniscus protrusion, by spurring at the joint's edge, or by meniscus surgery. In the foot and ankle, the most frequently encountered area of nerve damage is that where the nerve passes anteriorly over the medial malleolus and courses dorsomedially to the first metatarsal base. Chronic pressure by shoes or roller blade or in-line skating boots, occasionally associated with a first metatarsocuneiform exostosis, may result in chronic saphenous nerve compression. Surgeries involving the medial ankle (e.g., ankle arthroscopy), the medial arch and medial column, or the proximal first ray can cause direct or indirect trauma to the saphenous nerve.

The key diagnostic finding of saphenous nerve injury is altered sensibility testing along the anatomic course of the nerve. Careful examination and localization are needed to differentiate a saphenous nerve injury from the symptoms and findings associated with tarsal tunnel syndrome. In saphenous nerve injuries, the pain and/or altered sensibility is anterior to the medial malleolus, whereas in tarsal tunnel syndrome the abnormal findings are posterior to the malleolus.[12] The patient with saphenous nerve injury often complains of pain developing after prolonged walking and standing (especially with the knee extended).

## Superficial Peroneal Nerve

The common peroneal nerve branches into the superficial, deep, and recurrent peroneal nerves. The superficial peroneal nerve originates from the common peroneal nerve proximally and terminates distally by bifurcating into the medial and intermediate dorsal cutaneous nerves. The nerve's bifurcation occurs near the junction of the middle and distal thirds of the leg where the nerve exits the deep fascia. The bifurcation may occur after the superficial peroneal nerve emerges through the deep fascia but more often occurs deep to the fascia before the nerve appears more superficially. It is at the point of emergence through the deep fascia that the nerve or its branches often become entrapped. Compression injuries involving the superficial peroneal nerve may result from compartment syndromes in the anterior crural compartment. Contusions to the front of the leg (commonly seen in soccer or field hockey players), shin splints secondary to biomechanical pathology, fibular fractures, and tibial fractures have been reported as etiologies of anterior compartment syndrome.[12] Any athlete may develop shin splints because of faulty biomechanics, and the resultant exertional compartment syndrome may cause superficial peroneal nerve injury.[15] In addition, traction injuries to the superficial peroneal nerve can occur with plantiflexion-inversion sprains or injuries to the foot and ankle.[16]

Symptoms of superficial peroneal nerve compression or injury usually consist of hypoesthesia or altered sensibility along the course of the nerve and its terminal branches. In some injuries, sharp, burning pain along the nerve's distribution is noted. Severe involvement may disrupt motor function to the peroneus brevis and longus. In such cases, weakness of foot eversion (peroneus brevis) and active plantarflexion of the first ray (peroneus longus) are discernible with manual muscle testing. The diagnosis of superficial peroneal nerve injury may be supported by electrodiagnostic testing or, in certain situations, by a diagnostic nerve block. If compartmental syndrome is suspected, compartmental pressures should be obtained.

## Medial and Intermediate Dorsal Cutaneous Nerves, Digital Nerves

Like the saphenous nerve, the medial dorsal cutaneous nerve (MDCN) is most frequently entrapped at the level of the ankle or as it passes over the first metatarsocuneiform joint. Certain shoes can cause compression at the anterior aspect of the ankle, but more often the MDCN is compressed as it passes dorsally over the first metatarsocuneiform joint, creating the commonly known "vamp pain." Excessive hypermobility of the first ray can result in dorsal first metatarsocuneiform joint spurring, causing the symptom complex and nerve injury to occur more quickly.[17]

Conversely, the intermediate dorsal cutaneous nerve (IDCN) is rarely involved in compression neuropathies. Occasionally, shoegear causes compression of the nerve over the anterior aspect of the ankle or over the dorsum of the tarsometatarsal joint area.

Both the MDCN and IDCN are often injured by crushing injuries to the dorsum of the foot. Forklift and other occupational injuries, vehicular injuries, or injuries in which the feet are crossed by heavy objects often damage these nerves. Missile injuries and gunshot injuries, although not quite as common, occasionally cause direct or indirect MDCN and IDCN injury.

Unfortunately, iatrogenic injuries to the MDCN and IDCN are also common. These nerves are often directly injured or become secondarily entrapped after surgical approaches to the anterior ankle or midfoot area. Portals used for ankle arthroscopy surgery can cause direct trauma to these nerves. Entrapment of the MDCN and IDCN on the dorsum of the foot can occur after almost any surgical approach used in the midfoot or forefoot. Recognizing the high incidence of postincisional nerve entrapment in the dorsum of the foot, Kenzora[18] labeled the medial two thirds of the dorsum of the midfoot the neuromatous zone or N zone.

The MDCN, IDCN, and their terminal branches (the digital nerves) are primarily sensory nerves. Therefore, confirmation of suspected MDCN or IDCN nerve injury is usually based solely on sensibility testing. Occasionally, sensory nerve conduction velocities or diagnostic nerve blocks can be helpful in confirming or supporting the clinical diagnosis.

## Lateral Dorsal Cutaneous Nerve (Sural Nerve)

Lateral dorsal cutaneous nerve (LDCN), or sural nerve, injury usually results from direct trauma and can occur anywhere along the course of the nerve. Displaced fractures of the ankle, hindfoot, fifth metatarsal, or even an os peroneum can result in primary or secondary injuries to these nerves. Hematomas associated with soft tissue injuries can cause secondary extraneural compression resulting in sural nerve or LDCN damage. Surgical procedures on the Achilles tendon, the posterolateral heel, the fibular malleolus, or along the lateral column of the foot can result in inadvertent damage to the sural nerve or LDCN.

Like the MDCN and IDCN, the sural nerve and LDCN are primarily sensory nerves. In many patients, communicating branches exist between either the sural nerve or the LDCN and the IDCN. The most common variant is a small communicating branch between the LDCN and the IDCN that courses directly over the sinus tarsi and anterior beak of the calcaneus. Damage to this communicating branch can be misinterpreted as sinus tarsi syndrome.[12] As with the MDCN and IDCN, sensibility testing is the mainstay of the assessment for sural nerve or LDCN injury. Electrodiagnosis or diagnostic nerve blocks can be useful as adjuncts in the diagnosis.

## Deep Peroneal Nerve

The deep peroneal nerve, also known as the anterior tibial nerve, originates from the common peroneal nerve. The deep peroneal nerve, like the superficial peroneal nerve, can be compressed when anterior compartment syndromes occur. The nerve is much deeper in the leg than the superficial peroneal nerve and is therefore less subject to direct trauma in the leg. More commonly, the nerve is compressed at the ankle or just distal to the ankle. The deep peroneal nerve passes deep to the superior and inferior extensor retinaculum at the ankle joint and is often compressed or entrapped at this level. The resultant symptom complex has been termed the *anterior tarsal tunnel* or *anterior tarsal syndrome*.[19–21] This syndrome or entrapment typically follows injuries in the form of direct trauma or severe ankle supination. Direct trauma can also injure the nerve distal to the ankle joint. A direct blow to the dorsum of the foot injures the nerve where it passes relatively superficially over the lesser tarsus. Chronic trauma to the deep peroneal nerve can also occur. Biomechanically induced microtrauma in the cavus foot aggravated by tight shoegear and pressure on the nerve from osseous prominences over the dorsum of the foot are frequent etiologies.[12] Dellon[22] described 20 cases of chronic compression of the deep peroneal nerve in which the nerve was injured as it passed over the dorsum of the first and second metatarsocuneiform joints. The terminal portion of the deep peroneal nerve can be injured by sesamoid trauma or surgeries involving the first intermetatarsal space.

Injury or compression of the deep peroneal nerve near its origin, like compression or injury of the common peroneal nerve, can lead to denervation and paralysis of the anterior crural musculature with a resultant footdrop. Furthermore, in the foot, prolonged entrapment of the nerve can affect the extensor digitorum brevis and interosseous muscles supplied by the nerve. The diagnosis of a deep peroneal nerve injury requires a full evaluation of the nerve's function, including both its sensory and motor components. Sensory loss between the first and second toes is the classic sensory loss associated with deep peroneal nerve entrapment or injury.

Electromyography and nerve conduction studies may be helpful in localizing the level of entrapment and in confirming the suspected diagnosis. If an anterior rural compartment syndrome is suspected, compartment pressures should be obtained.

## Tibial Nerve, Posterior Tibial Nerve

The tibial nerve is a terminal branch of the sciatic nerve. It is superficial and subject to injury in three locations: just distal to the gluteal fold as a component of the sciatic nerve, in the popliteal fossa, and just above the medial aspect of the ankle where it lies over the posterior surface of the tibia before entering the tarsal tunnel. The tibial nerve is most often injured by lacerations, compression injuries, and burn injures at these sites and may be injured by fractures of the distal femur or fractures and dislocations of the distal tibia and calcaneus. The posterior tibial nerve is most frequently injured by chronic compression where it passes deep to the flexor retinaculum posteromedial to the ankle. This compression neuropathy is commonly referred to as *medial tarsal tunnel syndrome* or simply *tarsal tunnel syndrome*. Tarsal tunnel syndrome has a myriad of etiologies including direct or indirect trauma, biomechanical disorders, an accessory or hypertrophic abductor hallucis muscle belly, tenosynovitis or ganglion formation of the nerve itself or tendons in the tarsal tunnel (i.e., posterior tibial, flexor digitorum longus, flexor hallucis longus), varices or venous insufficiency of the posterior tibial venae comitantes, intraneural or extraneural tumors, and posttraumatic scarring.[12] Iatrogenic injures to the tibial nerve can also occur. These have been reported as complications after femoral popliteal bypass surgery and knee arthroscopy.[7]

Tibial nerve injury typically presents with altered sensibility over the course of the nerve. Tarsal tunnel syndrome often develops insidiously and is typically associated with altered sensation, burning pain, or numbness affecting the sole of the foot, the abductor canal in the medial arch, or the tarsal tunnel region itself. A positive Tinel's sign (i.e., a sensation of tingling felt distally over the course of a nerve when the nerve is percussed at the level of injury or compression; or more simply put, distal tingling on percussion) is often seen with percussion of the tarsal tunnel. Weakness of the posterior calf musculature may be seen in more proximal injuries, whereas wasting of the intrinsic musculature of the foot is seen only many months after an injury causing denervation. The tibial nerve also has a significant autonomic component. In fact, the majority of the sympathetic fibers to the lower extremity are in the sciatic and tibial nerves. Autonomic dysfunction may be seen with tibial nerve injuries. This often presents as altered sweat production, livedo reticularis, and other signs of vasomotor instability. These changes are most visible on the plantar aspect of the foot.

Diagnosis of tarsal tunnel injury is based on a thorough history and physical findings. The distribution of altered sensorimotor changes must be carefully assessed. Nerve conduction velocities and electromyography may be helpful in confirming the diagnosis and in monitoring conservative or surgical therapy.

## Medial and Lateral Plantar Nerves, Medial Calcaneal Nerve

The medial and lateral plantar nerves are the terminal branches of the posterior tibial nerve. Most commonly this termination and division occur beneath the flexor retinaculum or more rarely proximal to the retinaculum. Havel and colleagues[23] found that roughly 93% of the bifurcations occurred under the flexor retinaculum and 7% occurred proximal to the retinaculum. In no case was the bifurcation noted to occur distal to the retinaculum. The origin and course of the medial calcaneal nerve are much more variable. The nerve arises either within the tarsal tunnel or proximal to the flexor retinaculum from either the posterior tibial nerve or the lateral plantar nerve. Only rarely does the nerve arise from the medial plantar nerve.[23, 24]

Injuries to the medial and lateral plantar nerves are most frequently caused by puncture wounds, lacerations, or direct trauma to the sole of the foot. Hematomas or plantar space infections can cause compartment syndromes resulting in nerve injury. Chronic compression or repetitive trauma can damage these nerves and their terminal branches, the plantar digital nerves. Morton's neuroma is a common example of an entrapment neuropathy of the plantar digital nerves. Damage to the medial calcaneal nerve most often results from surgeries for plantimedial heel pain or from direct trauma, such as lacerations.

The diagnosis of medial and lateral plantar nerve injury is similar to that of the posterior tibial nerve. Abnormal sensibility testing is most frequently seen. Electrodiagnostic testing is less reliable as the nerves are deep and difficult to assess routinely and accurately. The medial calcaneal nerve is primarily sensory in nature, and the diagnosis of medial calcaneal nerve injury is based on the sensory examination, often in combination with a diagnostic nerve block.

## REFERENCES

1. Lyons WR, Woodhall B: Atlas of Peripheral Nerve Injuries. Philadelphia, WB Saunders, 1949.
2. Seddon HJ: Classification of nerve injuries. Br Med J 2:237, 1942.
3. Seddon HJ: Three types of nerve injuries. Brain 66:237, 1943.
4. Sunderland S: A classification of peripheral nerve injuries producing loss of function. Brain 74:491–516, 1951.
5. Sunderland S: Nerve Injuries and Their Repair: A Critical Appraisal. New York, Churchill-Livingstone, 1991, pp 221–232.
6. Downey MS: Neurologic trauma. In Scurran BL (ed): Foot and Ankle Trauma, 2nd ed. New York, Churchill-Livingstone, 1996, pp 233–263.
7. Aldea PA, Shaw WW: Management of acute lower extremity nerve injuries. Foot Ankle 7:82–94, 1986.
8. Lusskin R, Battista A: Peripheral neuropathies affecting the foot: Traumatic, ischemic, and compressive disorders. In Jahss MH (ed): Disorders of the Foot and Ankle, 2nd ed. Philadelphia, WB Saunders, 1991, pp 2089–2124.
9. O'Riain S: New and simple test of nerve function in hand. Br Med J 3:615–616, 1973.
10. Kahn EA: Direct observation of sweating in peripheral nerve injuries. Surg Gynecol Obstet 92:22, 1951.
11. Daly N, Dayton PD, Tafuri SA: Vascular trauma. In Scurran BL (ed): Foot and Ankle Trauma, 2nd ed. New York, Churchill-Livingstone, 1996, pp 265–285.
12. Downey MS: Surgical treatment of peripheral nerve entrapment syndromes. In Oloff LM (ed): Musculoskeletal Disorders of the Lower Extremities. Philadelphia, WB Saunders, 1994, pp 685–717.
13. Downey MS: Below-knee casting. In Kane P, Schlefman BS, Vickers NS (eds): Podiatric Office Management and Procedures, St. Louis, Mosby–Year Book, 1992, pp 283–302.
14. Kopell HP, Thompson WAL: Knee pain due to saphenous-nerve entrapment. N Engl J Med 263:351-353, 1960.
15. Garfin S, Mubarak SJ, Owen CA: Exertional anterolateral-compartment syndrome: Case report with fascial defect, muscle herniation, and superficial peroneal-nerve entrapment. J Bone Joint Surg Am 59:404–405, 1977.
16. Lerman BI, Gornish LA, Bellin HJ: Injury of the superficial peroneal nerve. J Foot Surg 23:334–339, 1984.
17. Tobin R, Krych S, Harkless LB: First metatarsal-cuneiform dorsal exostosis: Its anatomical relation with the medial dorsal cutaneous nerve. J Foot Surg 28:442–444, 1989.
18. Kenzora JE: Symptomatic incisional neuromas on the dorsum of the foot. Foot Ankle 5:2–15, 1984.
19. Adelman KA, Wilson G, Wolf JA: Anterior tarsal tunnel syndrome. J Foot Surg 27:299–302, 1988.
20. Cangialosi CP, Schnall SJ: The biomechanical aspects of anterior tarsal tunnel syndrome. J Am Podiatry Assoc 70:291–292, 1980.
21. Marinacci AA: Neurological syndromes of the tarsal tunnels. Bull Los Ang Neurol Soc 33:90–100, 1968.
22. Dellon AL: Deep peroneal nerve entrapment on the dorsum of the foot. Foot Ankle 11:73–80, 1990.
23. Havel PE, Ebraheim NA, Clark SE, et al: Tibial nerve branching in the tarsal tunnel. Foot Ankle 9:117–119, 1988.
24. Dellon AL, Mackinnon SE: Tibial nerve branching in the tarsal tunnel. Arch Neurol 41:645–646, 1984.

# 16

# Polyneuropathy

*Leo McCluskey*

The syndrome of polyneuropathy is one of the most frequently represented lower extremity neurologic disorders. As described by Schaumburg,* the term polyneuropathy or symmetric polyneuropathy "designates a generalized process producing widespread and bilaterally symmetrical effects on the peripheral nervous system. It may be motor, sensory, sensorimotor, or autonomic in its effects, and proximal, distal, or generalized in its distribution." The large number of affected patients coupled with the broad differential diagnostic possibilities makes polyneuropathy a challenging problem. However, an understanding of the anatomy and pathophysiology of neuropathic disorders along with a thorough history and neurologic examination yields a list of potential diagnostic possibilities. With the directed use of laboratory studies, an etiologic diagnosis can be made in the majority of cases and appropriate therapy can be initiated.

## FUNCTIONAL ANATOMY OF THE PERIPHERAL NERVOUS SYSTEM

The peripheral nervous system, an artificial construct, consists of the cells and their processes that extend out of the central nervous system (brain and spinal cord). The motor neurons residing within the anterior horn of the spinal cord and in brain stem motor nuclei project motor axons via the anterior roots and various cranial nerves to skeletal muscles. The primary sensory neurons residing within the dorsal root ganglia or sensory cranial ganglia project sensory axons to the peripheral sensory receptors and via the dorsal roots or cranial nerves to the spinal cord or brain stem. The autonomic neurons residing within the brain stem and spinal cord project efferent and afferent axons via cranial nerves and anterior roots to the periphery.

Peripheral mixed nerves consist of sensory, motor, and autonomic axons as well as investing connective tissue, blood vessels, and lymphatic vessels. Axons, long cytoplasmic extensions of sensory, motor, or autonomic neurons, are invested by the processes of individual supporting cells known as Schwann cells. In turn, Schwann cells lie within a

basement membrane. Myelinated axons are surrounded by concentric loops of Schwann cell cytoplasm, creating a series of alternating layers of lipid and protein constituting the myelin sheath (Fig. 16–1). Each Schwann cell myelinates only a single axon. A series of Schwann cells are longitudinally arrayed along the entire length of an individual myelinated axon, extending from just beyond the cell body to the terminal endings at the myoneural junction in the case of motor fibers or at a sensory end organ or terminal sprouts in the case of sensory fibers. Along the axon length, individual Schwann cells and their myelin sheath are separated at a site on the axon known as the node of Ranvier. Here, the axon is exposed to the extracellular space. The portion of the axon between each node of Ranvier that is completely invested by the myelin sheath is known as the internodal segment (Fig. 16–2). The integrity of the myelin sheath is dependent both on the Schwann cell and the axon it invests.

Unmyelinated axons are invested by Schwann cell processes so that they are not exposed to the extracellular space but do not possess the specialized Schwann cell–generated myelin sheath. Unlike Schwann cells of myelinated axons, individual Schwann cells often associate with multiple unmyelinated axons.

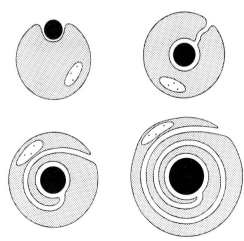

**Figure 16–1** Diagram to illustrate the changing axon–Schwann relationship leading to the development of a myelinated nerve fiber. (From Sunderland S: Nerve Injuries and Their Repair: A Critical Appraisal. New York, Churchill Livingstone, 1991, p 18.)

---

*Schaumberg HH, Berger AR, Thomas PK: Disorders of Peripheral Nerves, 2nd ed. Philadelphia, F.A. Davis, 1992, pp 1–20.

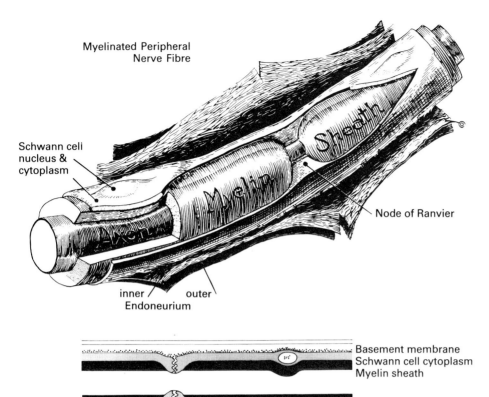

Myelinated Peripheral
Nerve Fibre

Schwann cell
nucleus &
cytoplasm

Node of Ranvier

inner / outer
Endoneurium

Basement membrane
Schwann cell cytoplasm
Myelin sheath

Inner
Outer  endoneurium

**Figure 16–2** Diagrammatic representation of the essential histologic features of a myelinated nerve fiber. (From Sunderland S: Nerve Injuries and Their Repair: a critical appraisal. New York, Churchill Livingstone, 1991, p 17.)

The cell body of the sensory or motor neuron contains the bulk of the machinery necessary for maintenance of the axon structure and function. Axonal transport away from the cell body is required to maintain the axonal membrane and cytoskeletal structures, the membrane conducting properties, and neurotransmission and to exert a trophic influence on innervated tissue (Sunderland). Axonal transport away from the cell body is usually divided into fast (40 to 500 mm/day) and slow (1 to 8 mm/day) transport. Axonal transport toward the cell body conveys material from the periphery to the cell body. Relying on the integrity of the cell body and a bidirectional transport system, the axons are extremely vulnerable to any metabolic or structural process that disrupts this cellular machinery.

Axons within a peripheral mixed nerve can be divided on the basis of function into motor, sensory, and autonomic. Axons can be further divided into various populations on the basis of diameter and, because of a direct relationship between diameter and conduction velocity, speed of conduction into A, B, and C fibers. A further division can be made into myelinated and unmyelinated fibers (Table 16–1). The presence of the insulating myelin sheath investing the sensory or motor axons also results in a marked increase in conduction velocity. The axons of alpha motor neurons subserving skeletal extrafusal muscle fibers are all myelinated and are among the largest and fastest conducting nerve fibers. Sensory axons are distributed over a broad range of fiber diameters and conduction velocities. The largest

**Table 16–1  Relationship Between Nerve Fiber Types, Diameters, Conduction Velocity, and Function**

| Nerve Fiber | Nerve Fiber Diameter (μm) | Conduction Velocity (m/s) | Function |
|---|---|---|---|
| A Alpha | 12–20 | 70–120 | Motor, extrafusal muscle fibers, proprioceptors |
| Beta | 5–12 | 30–70 | Touch, pressure |
| Gamma | 3–6 | 15–30 | Motor, intrafusal muscle fibers |
| Delta | 2–5 | 10–30 | Nociceptors, touch, temperature |
| B | 1.5–3 | 3–15 | Preganglionic sympathetic fibers |
| C | Less than 2.0 | 0.5–2 | Nociceptors, postganglionic sympathetic fibers |

From Sunderland S: Nerve Injuries and Their Repair: A Critical Appraisal. New York, Churchill Livingstone, 1991, p 22.

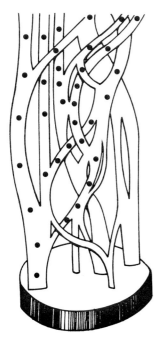

**Figure 16–3** Diagrammatic representation of the fascicular redistribution and dispersal of a branch fiber system brought about by fascicular plexuses. (From Sunderland S: Nerve Injuries and Their Repair: a critical appraisal. New York, Churchill Livingstone, 1991, p 35.)

sensory fibers subserve proprioception and discriminative touch, whereas the smaller sensory fibers subserve pain and temperature. The smallest sensory fibers are unmyelinated or only thinly myelin-

ated. The autonomic axons within the peripheral nerve are all small, slowly conducting, and unmyelinated.

The axons of a peripheral nerve are grouped together into fascicles. Each fascicle is surrounded by a connective tissue sheath known as the perineurium. Each fascicle contains within it a connective tissue network known as the endoneurium. Multiple fascicles are grouped within a connective tissue framework known as the epineurium (Fig. 16–3). The fascicles repeatedly divide and reassociate along the length of the nerve, forming a fascicular plexus (Fig. 16–4). The vascular supply of nerve (vasa nervorum) is provided by a series of nutrient arteries derived from local vessels along the length of the nerve. The arterioles are distributed within the epineurium. The vessels within the perineurium or endoneurium are with few exceptions capillaries.

## PATHOPHYSIOLOGY OF PERIPHERAL NERVE DISORDERS

Four classically described pathologic changes affect peripheral nerve axons. These are wallerian degeneration, axonal degeneration, neuronal degeneration, and demyelination.

### Wallerian Degeneration

Axonal interruption leads to a series of pathologic changes within axons known as wallerian degenera-

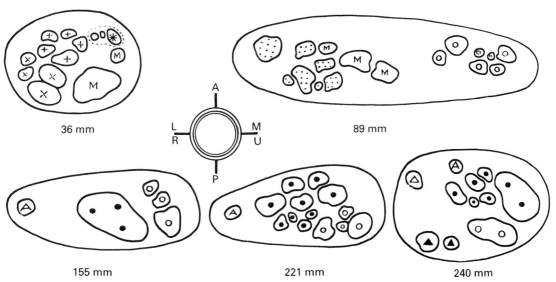

**Figure 16–4** Selected transverse sections of serially sectioned specimen of an ulnar nerve to illustrate the fascicular distribution of branch fiber systms in the limb (not to scale). They illustrate the long course of the dorsal cutaneous branch fascicular group as an independent system within the nerve though the fasciculi comprising the group engage in plexus formations among themselves. Levels are in millimeters above the tip of the radial styloid process. M, deep (muscular) division fibers;*, cutaneous fibers from hypothenar eminence; +, cutaneous fibers from the ulnar side; x, cutaneous fibers from fourth digital interspace; small dots, combined terminal cutaneous fibers; large dots, combined terminal motor and cutaneous fibers; ○, dorsal cutaneous fibers. △, flexor carpi ulnaris fibers; A, branch fibers to the ulnar artery; ▶, flexor digitorum profundus fibers. (From Sunderland S. Nerve Injuries and Their Repair: a critical appraisal. New York, Churchill Livingstone, 1991, p 35.)

tion. The axonal segment and myelin sheath distal to the site of axonal interruption disintegrate over the course of days. Conduction fails. This degeneration is usually followed by a sequence of regenerative events including sprouting from the proximal segment, longitudinal regrowth of one or more of these sprouts within bands of proliferated Schwann cells and inside each axon's appropriate basal laminar tube, and remyelination. The remyelination of the regenerated axon is notable for shorter internodal segments.

Functional recovery depends on the effective regeneration of all or at least a large percentage of the interrupted axons. In addition, recovery depends on the regrowth of axons down appropriate basal laminar tubes so that axons can eventually reach the original target. If the initial nerve injury results in axonal interruption along with injury to the basal laminar structure, regenerating axons can and often do regrow down inappropriate basal laminar tubes, resulting in aberrant regeneration. This reduces functional recovery. In the case of interruption of not only axons and basal laminar structures but the entire nerve trunk as well, sprouting axons are capable of crossing gaps of several millimeters to reach Schwann cell–basal laminar tubes in the distal stump. However, if the gap is too large or if the distal stump is removed, the regenerating axons form a neuroma.

Pathologic changes also occur in the nerve cell body and proximal axonal segment after an axonal transection. These include retrograde axonal atrophy, histologic changes within the cell body known as chromatolysis, retraction of synaptic terminals from the cell body, and even cell death. The changes that occur in the cell body are particularly likely to develop if the transection occurs close to the cell body.

## Axonal Degeneration

In this common pathologic process, the distal portions of the axon begin to degenerate. At times this begins with axonal atrophy and is followed by wallerian-like degeneration. Because the integrity of the myelin sheath depends on the axon as well as the Schwann cell, secondary demyelination occurs. The entire process progresses proximally; hence, the term dying back. If the insult to nerve is temporally limited, regeneration can occur. This pathologic process is frequently referred to as axonopathy.

Distal axonal degenerations can arise from a process that directly affects the distal axonal segments. In addition, because the distal axonal segment depends on axonal transport from the cell body, processes that primarily affect the neuronal cell body

may lead to degeneration of the most vulnerable distal segment. Axonal degeneration is the process that most frequently accompanies a large number of toxic and/or metabolic insults to neurons or their axons.

## Neuronal Degeneration

This pathologic process, frequently referred to as a neuronopathy, results in loss of axons and secondary loss of the myelin sheath similar to that which occurs in axonal degeneration. As noted earlier, this can result in a distal axonal degeneration that proceeds proximally. It may at times be difficult to distinguish the two processes clinically.

## Demyelination

A lesion that affects the myelin sheath and/or Schwann cell with relative sparing of the axon is termed a primary demyelinating process or myelinopathy. This is distinct from the secondary demyelinating process that results from a primary axonal or neuronal process. Resulting from toxic, immunologic, as well as hereditary processes, it may develop in multiple ways but most frequently results in demyelination of one or more segments of axons (segmental demyelination). Conduction velocity is substantially slowed along a demyelinated segment. If the demyelinated segment is long enough (three or more internodes), conduction cannot proceed past it (conduction block). Recovery occurs by remyelination of the demyelinated segment with resultant recovery of conduction. The resulting internodal segments are shorter than the original ones (Fig. 16–5).

## CLAISSIFICATION OF PHYSICAL NERVE INJURY

Physical injury of a peripheral nerve is generally classified along a continuum of three types:

- **Class 1 (neurapraxia)**: A physical nerve injury that results only in segmental demyelination with resultant conduction failure and a secondary sensory and/or motor neurologic deficit. Prognosis for recovery related to remyelination is excellent.
- **Class 2 (axonotmesis)**: A physical injury of nerve that results in focal axonal disruption and distal wallerian degeneration. As a result, nerve conduction fails and a motor and/or sensory deficit ensues. The nerve trunk is in-

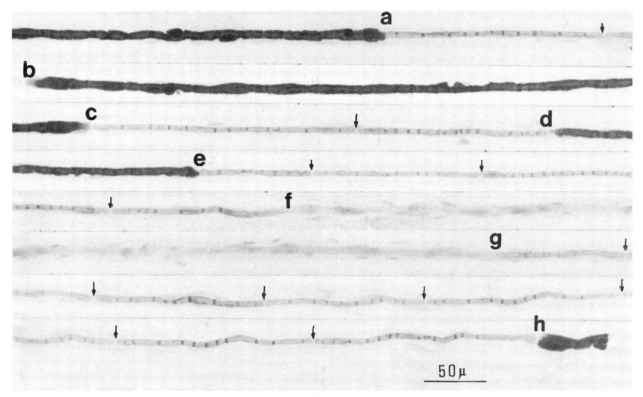

**Figure 16–5** Demyelination and remyelination in the Guillain-Barré syndrome. Consecutive segments of a nerve fiber from a sural nerve biopsy from a patient with demyelinative polyradiculoneuropathy of acute onset. From top left to a, b-c, d-e, and distal to h, the original myelin sheath is still present. Segments a-b, c-d, e-f, and g-h are remyelinated. The newly formed nodes of Ranvier are shown by arrows. Note that new internodes are much shorter than the original ones. The segment f-g is still demyelinated. (From Said G, Thomas PK: Pathophysiology of nerve and root disorders. *In* Asbury AK, McKhann GM, McDonald WI (eds): Diseases of the Nervous System: Clinical Neurobiology, 2nd ed. page 245, 1992, WB Saunders 1992, p 245.)

tact. Assuming the continued integrity of the basal lamina–Schwann cell tubes within the fascicles, recovery occurs by sprouting of the distal stump, regrowth of axons to their original targets, and re-establishment of nerve conduction.

- **Class 3 (neurotmesis)**: A physical nerve injury that results in focal severance of the nerve trunk and all of its axons and connective tissue stucture. Spontaneous recovery is unlikely. Neuroma formation occurs.

## HISTORY IN POLYNEUROPATHY

As with any neurologic process, obtaining a good history is an essential first step in arriving at an etiologic diagnosis in patients with polyneuropathy. It also begins the process by which other central or peripheral disorders that mimic polyneuropathy can be considered.

The most common early symptom in prototypic polyneuropathy is usually sensory disturbance. This can take the form of negative or positive sensory symptoms. Most commonly, it involves the toes, distal foot, and sole. It is largely symmetric, al-

though some minimal side-to-side asymmetry is not uncommon. The sensory change should begin in all distal cutaneous distributions simultaneously or at least with a minimal temporal lag. For example, the large toe dorsum (superficial peroneal), first dorsal web space (deep peroneal), second through fourth toe dorsum (superficial peroneal), fifth toe dorsum (sural), and plantar surface of sole as well as toes (medial and lateral plantar) should all be noted by the patient to have a sensory change. A similar onset should be noted in the digits of the hand and then the palm and hand dorsum. Any substantial asymmetry, focal cutaneous territory involvement, or temporal delay should suggest the possibility of multiple mononeuropathies (mononeuropathy multiplex).

Negative sensory symptoms are common. A loss of sensation is not infrequently described by the patient as a feeling that the foot is wrapped in something, that when walking it feels as if something is between the feet and the floor, or that the feet are wooden. When marked, sensory loss can result in a perversion of sensation such that the toes or feet are perceived as grossly enlarged or the toes are perceived as being in unusual positions. When large-fiber sensory loss (proprioception, discriminative touch) is marked, the patient begins to feel unsteady, particularly when the use of other sensory clues is difficult (e.g., in the dark). When small-fiber sensory loss (pain and temperature) is marked, the patient is unable to perceive temperature with the involved feet on toes or may note the occurrence of injury without pain.

Positive sensory symptoms such as paresthesias and pain can occur. Paresthesias can take the form of pins and needles, tingling, and buzzing. At times, significant paresthesias can be perceived as painful (dysesthesias). Spontaneous pain is often burning, although it can be described as stabbing, aching, searing, or a painful coldness. If hypersensitivity or hyperpathia is present, pain can at times be caused or exacerbated by minimal mechanical or thermal stimulation. This may make walking or wearing shoes difficult.

With progression, the sensory disturbance ascends to produce a graded loss of sensation that is noted by the patient to be worse distally and improved proximally (stocking distribution). With leg involvement in polyneuropathy, the sensory disturbance should be circumferential. Involvement of the distal upper extremities begins when the sensory change ascends to the level of the proximal leg or knee. This too ascends in a graded fashion (glove distribution) and should be circumferential. As the sensory change ascends to the level of the middle to upper thigh, loss of sensation can be perceived in the midabdomen. With progression, this enlarges laterally and rostrally. Sensory loss involves the top of the head and the trigeminal distribution last. This stocking-glove progressive pattern of sensory change is often referred to as length dependent.

Motor symptoms can also take a positive form. The most common positive motor symptom in polyneuropathy is cramping. Less common are fasciculations, myokymia, and muscular enlargement.

Negative motor symptoms take the form of weakness and atrophy. In early polyneuropathy it is common for the patient not to notice distal weakness because weakness of large and small toe extensors as well as intrinsic foot muscles does not result in significant functional disturbance. It is often not until weakness involves the anterior compartment muscles of the legs with resulting footdrop or the intrinsic muscles of the hands with resultant loss of manipulative ability that patients begin to complain. Atrophy is a rare complaint. As with the sensory disturbance, muscle weakness progresses in a graded and length-dependent fashion. In extreme cases, diaphragmatic weakness can result.

Autonomic symptoms can arise in polyneuropathies in which there is mixed-fiber loss that includes small fibers. In the case of polyneuropathies in which small-fiber loss predominates, pain and autonomic symptoms predominate. The presence of dry mouth, constipation, diarrhea, early satiety, postprandial vomiting, increased or decreased sweating, orthostatic symptoms, bladder dysfunction, and erectile dysfunction should be discussed.

The pace of the process should be determined. Polyneuropathies can vary from acute in onset over a few days to evolution over a decade. Toxic- and metabolic-related polyneuropathies with few exceptions usually progress over many weeks to over a few years. Polyneuropathies that progress over many years are often genetically related, although diabetic polyneuropathy and paraproteinemic polyneuropathy can also develop over this time span. Significant fluctuations in polyneuropathic symptoms occur only with repeated exposure to drugs and toxins or in inflammatory demyelinating neuropathies.

The history should also include a thorough exploration of the past medical history and review of symptoms. The presence of medical problems, such as diabetes, known to be associated with the development of polyneuropathy should be determined. However, it should not be assumed that the presence of such problems is in fact the cause of the development of polyneuropathy. Recent illnesses, systemic symptoms, medications, and toxic exposures should be determined. A review of medications should include not only prescription medications but also over-the-counter medications, vitamins, and herbal preparations. The review of toxic exposures should include occupational, home, and avocational chemical use as well as alcohol ingestion. When appropriate, it should be determined whether the patient uses city water, well water, or bottled water. It should be determined whether there is a family history of neuropathy.

## EXAMINATION IN POLYNEUROPATHY

The examination of polyneuropathic patients should be expected to demonstrate symmetric sensory, motor, and reflex findings. As with historical features, any significant asymmetry on the clinical examination raises concern about a multifocal neuropathic process. In addition, with few exceptions, sensory signs predominate and the sensory, motor, and reflex findings should demonstrate length dependence. Weakness and atrophy should be maximal distally with graded improvement proximally. Distal upper extremity motor findings should not be present until there is weakness demonstrable in upper calf and even to some extent in thigh muscles. Sensory loss should also be maximal distally and, as with motor findings, upper extremity sensory loss should not be present until there is sensory loss demonstrable in the upper calf or distal thigh. Reflex loss should coincide with the sensory loss, with the ankle jerks lost first followed by the knee jerks and finger flexor reflexes. The biceps and triceps jerks are lost last. Autonomic signs may include resting supine hypertension, significant orthostatic hypotension with an inappropriate increase in heart rate, lack of sweating, loss of hair growth, and dystrophic skin and/or nail changes.

The sensory examination provides a window into the pathologic involvement of specific fiber sizes. Loss of position sense, discriminative touch, and two-point discrimination and sensory ataxia occur with involvement of large fibers. Reflex loss is also a manifestation of large-fiber loss. Loss of pain and temperature sense and autonomic dysfunction are manifestations of small-fiber involvement. When severe, loss of small fibers and the attendant loss of pain sense may also result in cutaneous ulcers, bone and joint deformity, as well as skin and bone infections. In polyneuropathy, the sensory, motor, and reflex examinations are poor discriminators of a primary axonal versus primary demyelinating process.

## LABORATORY EVALUATION OF POLYNEUROPATHY

The most useful initial step in the laboratory evaluation of polyneuropathy is obtaining an electromyographic and nerve conduction study (EMG-NCS). This procedure confirms the presence and severity of a neuropathy and allows determination of whether the primary pathologic process is an axonopathy or a myelinopathy. This study also provides a sensitive determination of symmetry, which is essential for the diagnosis of polyneuropathy. Conversely, a confluent mononeuropathy multiplex masquerading as a polyneuropathy can be detected. In addition, EMG-NCS can detect the presence of multiple entrapment neuropathies, multiple radiculopathies, plexopathies, and myopathies, that may be confused with polyneuropathy. In the case of a myelinopathy, various electrophysiologic features allow a distinction to be drawn between acquired and hereditary demyelinating neuropathies.

If the electrodiagnostic study is consistent with an axonal polyneuropathy, the differential diagnosis includes a large list of metabolic and toxic factors. Systemic disorders such as diabetes, uremia, hypothyroidism, collagen vascular disease, human immunodeficiency virus infection, vitamin deficiency ($B_{12}$, thiamine), malignancy, amyloidosis, monoclonal gammopathy, and porphyria can be associated with an axonal polyneuropathy. Exposure to toxins such as alcohol, arsenic, lead, organophosphates, thallium, and excessive pyridoxine (vitamin $B_6$) as well as drugs such as isoniazid, amiodarone, metronidazole, disulfiram, various chemotherapeutic medications, antiretroviral medications, nitrofurantoin, and gold can also lead to the development of neuropathy. Hereditary neuropathy (e.g., hereditary motor and sensory neuropathy type II) can also result in a chronic axonal polyneuropathy.

If the electrodiagnostic study is consistent with a demyelinating polyneuropathy, the differential diagnosis is much more restricted. Acute demyelinating neuropathy is with rare exceptions related to Guillain-Barré syndrome. Causes of chronic acquired demyelinating polyneuropathies include inflammatory or autoimmune, dysproteinemic, and various systemic metabolic disorders (e.g., adrenoleukodystrophy, metachromatic leukodystrophy, Refsum's disease). Electrodiagnostic findings in diabetes also frequently demonstrate significant demyelinating features. The cause of chronic demyelinating polyneuropathies also includes hereditary disorders (e.g., hereditary motor and sensory neuropathy type I).

After a thorough evaluation of polyneuropathy, which may include electrodiagnostic studies, laboratory studies, examination of family members, and potentially nerve and/or other tissue biopsy, an etiologic diagnosis is arrived at in roughly 60% to 70% of patients. Thus, 30% to 40% of patients defy a definitive diagnosis and have what is frequently called a cryptogenic neuropathy. Because the development of polyneuropathy can precede the clinical detection of malignancy or other systemic disorders by as many as 2 years or the progression of the process over time can provide clues to the etiology of the disorder, these patients should be followed closely with serial examinations and repetition of selective laboratory studies (Fig. 16–6).

## TREATMENT OF POLYNEUROPATHY

If an etiology for a patient's polyneuropathy can be determined, treatment is, of course, directed at treating the underlying medical problem, stopping an offending drug, or removing a toxin. In many circumstances, effective treatment stops or at least reduces the pace of progression. Less frequently, therapeutic intervention may lead to improvement in neuropathic symptoms or even complete resolution of neuropathy.

The all too frequent symptom of neuropathic pain is unfortunately difficulty to treat. Although particularly common in small fiber–predominant neuropathies, it is also seen in neuropathic disorders involving mixed-fiber populations. Amelioration and at times significant improvement in symptoms can be achieved through both treatment of the underlying cause and use of various medications.

Capsaicin cream, having the advantage of lack of systemic side effects, is perhaps the most reasonable first step in the management of neuropathic pain. Applied to the involved painful areas three or

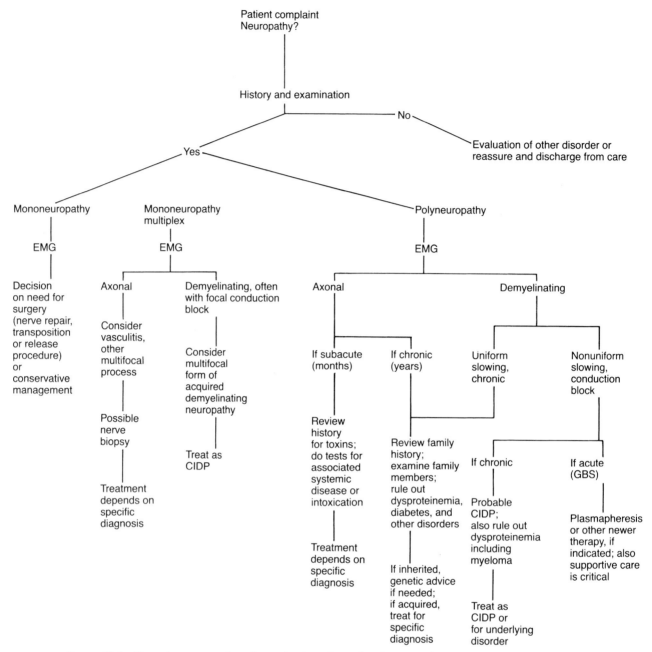

**Figure 16–6** Flow chart approach to the evaluation of peripheral neuropathies. CIDP, chronic inflammatory demyelinating polyradiculoneuropathy: EMG, electromyography; GBS, Guillan-Barré syndrome. (Data from Asbury AK: New aspects of disease of the peripheral nervous sytem. *In* Isselbacher KT, Adams RD (eds): Harrison's Principles of Internal Medicine. Update 4. New York, McGraw-Hill, 1983, p 253.)

four times a day, it can reduce neuropathic pain in perhaps 30% of patients. However, it is most often the case that this agent does not afford complete relief of the pain. Also, the burning that the cutaneous application of capsaicin induces is at times difficult for patients to tolerate. If this agent fails, a systematic trial of monotherapy should be pursued. The drug should be started at a low dose and gradually increased, if tolerated, to the point of an established maximal dose or until side effects occur. Drugs that may be of help in the management of neuropathic pain include tricyclic antidepressants, carbamazepine, diphenylhydantoin, gabapentin, mexiletine, and clonazepam. Selective serotonin uptake inhibitors may also be of some use in polyneuropathic pain. Accurate records of maximal doses taken, blood levels achieved (if available), side effects, and results should be kept for each agent. Polytherapy should be pursued only after the patient fails to respond to monotherapy with multiple agents. Pain medications including narcotics may be necessary as adjunctive or as primary therapy if the preceding medications fail to control discomfort adequately.

# Entrapment Neuropathy

# 17

*Harold Schoenhaus*

Neuropathy secondary to entrapment generally denotes a more chronic malady than that associated with impingement on a nerve. This chronic response can be the result of a small number of etiologies, including biomechanical and iatrogenic causes. The biomechanical causes of an entrapment neuropathy are largely a secondary response to a flatfoot deformity but may also be a response to an antalgic gait. Iatrogenic causes of entrapment neuropathy include the postsurgical state, with concomitant fibrosis and trapping of the nerve. Whatever the etiology, the symptoms correspond to any neuropraxia: paresthesias or paroxysmal losses of sensation or abnormal sensations. If allowed to continue without relief, the entrapment can progress to axonotmesis and, rarely, neurotmesis.

A small number of nerves are commonly involved in the entrapment neuropathies, which comprise tarsal tunnel syndrome, sural nerve entrapment, calcaneal nerve entrapments, peroneal and saphenous nerve entrapment, and common neuroma formation, including Morton's and Joplin's neuromas.

## TARSAL TUNNEL SYNDROME

Many authors have described the clinical existence of posterior tibial nerve injury, but it was not until the 1960s that a description of this syndrome was published, accredited to Kopell and Thompson. In 1962, the syndrome now known as tarsal tunnel syndrome was first named by Keck and Lam in two separate reports. They referred to tarsal tunnel syndrome as the entrapment primarily of the posterior tibial nerve under the flexor retinaculum posterior to the medial malleolus.[1, 2] We now know that the entrapment may occur anywhere proximal to, within, or distal to the flexor retinaculum, as well as within the abductor hiatus (porta pedis). Previously, its presentation was that of a diffuse entity with pain, throbbing, and paresthesias and with multifactorial causes that nobody could pinpoint. Now, with the use of computed tomography and magnetic resonance imaging (MRI), we are able to isolate the cause(s) of this syndrome.

The anatomy of the tarsal tunnel, in addition to the course of the tibial nerve, has been well documented. The tarsal tunnel was described by Sarrafian[3] as a fibro-osseous tunnel, with its floor the medial wall of the calcaneus, its posterior wall the process of the talus, its anterior wall the tibia and the medial malleolus, and its roof the flexor retinaculum.

The flexor retinaculum is a fan-shaped structure of variable thickness. It is attached proximally to the posterior distal portion of the medial malleolus. As it spreads out approximately 10 cm to the distal portion of the sustentaculum tali, it has attachments to the sheaths of its four compartments. From an anterior to posterior perspective, the contents of the tarsal canal include the posterior tibial tendon, flexor digitorum longus tendon, posterior tibial neurovascular bundle, and flexor hallucis longus tendon.[3]

## Etiology

### Intrinsic Factors

Tibial nerve compression can be caused within the tarsal tunnel by many soft tissue masses. Ganglioneuromas, lipomas, neurilemomas, neurofibromas, and synovial sarcomas are the neoplasms most commonly associated with tarsal tunnel syndrome. Takakura and colleagues[4] reported that 36% of 50 cases were due to ganglioneuromas. These space-occupying masses can compress the vasa vasorum surrounding the tibial nerve, causing ischemia of the nerve itself. Other intrinsic causes include venous insufficiency leading to varicosities of the posterior tibial venae comitantes as well as posterior tibial artery aneurysm.

### Extrinsic Factors

Tarsal tunnel syndrome can be secondary to the biomechanics of excessive subtalar joint pronation. Hindfoot valgus or forefoot varus causes pronation at the subtalar and midtarsal joints, which can overstretch the tibial nerve. In addition, the stretching of the flexor retinaculum and the abductor hallucis muscle further compresses the tibial nerve and its branches within the tarsal tunnel and at the porta pedis. Furthermore, excessive pronation can cause posterior tibial tendinitis and tenosynovitis, which can also cause tarsal tunnel syndrome.

Tarsal tunnel syndrome caused by tenosynovitis of the posterior tibial tendon is often a marker for systemic disease, especially when it presents bilaterally. Yamaguchi[5] found a 26% association between tarsal tunnel syndrome and such diseases as rheumatoid arthritis, diabetes mellitus, and myxedema. McGuigan[6] reported that 13% of patients with rheumatoid arthritis had symptoms consistent with tarsal tunnel syndrome. Also, tarsal tunnel syndrome has been described in association with many seronegative spondyloarthropathies such as Reiter's syndrome and ankylosing spondylitis.[7]

Blunt trauma can lead to tibial nerve compression when there is hemorrhage within the tarsal tunnel resulting in scarring and fibrotic adhesions to the nerve. This mechanism is also associated with fractures of the calcaneus, talus, and ankle mortise. Entrapment of the tibial nerve and its branches can also be caused iatrogenically during triple arthrodesis, ankle fusion, or fixation of fractures.

Extrinsic compression of the tarsal tunnel can also be due to accessory musculature.[8] The peroneocalcaneus internus, tibiocalcaneus internus, flexor digitorum accessorius longus, and accessory soleus are accessory muscles that have been found to cause compression of the tarsal tunnel.

## Clinical Symptoms

The symptoms of tarsal tunnel syndrome tend to vary from person to person depending on the etiology and location of the entrapment. Most patients describe a burning or sharp pain in the area of the tarsal tunnel that shoots distally into the plantar foot. Paresthesias, commonly described as pins-and-needles sensations, tend to radiate distally or proximally and can be accompanied by numbness. Patients often describe a feeling of cramping in the arch of the foot that awakens them from sleep. The pain and paresthesias tend to be aggravated by weight bearing and ambulation and worsen as the day progresses. Patients relate temporary relief after removal of shoegear, massage, and cessation of weight bearing.

Physical examination may show localized erythema and edema over the area of the tarsal tunnel. Palpation along the tibial nerve and its branches elicits tenderness proximal and distal to the area of entrapment. This aids in differentiating between proximal tarsal tunnel syndrome and the distal porta pedis syndrome. Percussion over the tarsal tunnel often reproduces the pain and paresthesias

radiating distally or proximally (Tinel's sign). Valleix's points are direct areas of point tenderness that may also be elicited. The symptoms tend to worsen with forced pronation of the foot as the tarsal tunnel is further compressed. If the condition is long standing, loss of sensation can become constant along the distribution of the medial and/or lateral plantar nerves. Other late findings include atrophy of the intrinsic musculature leading to hammer toe deformities.

## Diagnosis

In addition to a complete history and physical examination, diagnostic testing, such as with electromyography and nerve conduction studies, may be useful in confirming the diagnosis. However, variable results have been reported with both these techniques. The sensitivities of these tests have been between 65% and 90.5% for the nerve conduction studies and 54.4% for motor abnormalities. A normal nerve conduction study, therefore, does not exclude the diagnosis of tarsal tunnel syndrome, leaving 9.5% of the population with normal studies. This is a diagnostic problem.[9, 10]

Positive electroconduction nerve findings include sensory latency greater than 3.5 ms over the medial plantar and lateral plantar nerves. A motor latency greater than 6.7 ms in the lateral plantar nerve was more sensitive than a latency of 6.1 ms in the medial plantar nerve.[10] Other positive findings demonstrated that both nerves had motor fibrillations in the abductor hallucis muscle (porta pedis).[1] According to Kaplan and Kernahan,[11] decreased amplitude and increased duration of motor evoked potentials are more sensitive diagnostic indicators of tarsal tunnel syndrome that are distal motor latencies. Wieman and Patel[12] confirmed that standing electrodiagnostic studies are not helpful in deciding which patients with compression neuropathy may be surgical candidates.

Limited electrodiagnostic confirmation of tarsal tunnel syndrome has multiple causes. The nerves curving behind the medial malleolus and under the flexor retinaculum are difficult to pinpoint. There is difficulty in reading the onset of the evoked muscle action potential in muscle-nerve conduction studies.[13] The onset is often sloped, making a precise measurement of the onset tenuous. Moreover, the motor, sensory, and mixed-nerve techniques all fail to distinguish between proximal tarsal tunnel syndrome (involving the posterior tibial nerve) and distal tarsal tunnel syndrome (involving the medial and/or lateral plantar nerves).[14]

Failure of conventional radiographs to show a mass in association with tarsal tunnel syndrome should lead to further diagnostic imaging with computed tomography and/or MRI. MRI is a highly precise diagnostic tool that can demonstrate the presence and extent of the lesion(s) causing tarsal tunnel syndrome.[9] These lesions can be imaged by MRI from several centimeters proximal to the ankle joint to the plantar soft tissue of the midfoot. With the use of MRI, the tarsal canal can be clearly illustrated, including the musculotendinous and neurovascular structures.[9, 15]

In a study by Frey and Kerr,[15] 88% of the positive findings were obtained with MRI. Eighty-five percent of positive electrodiagnostic tests (electromyography and nerve conduction studies) were associated with highly positive MRI findings. Of the causes reported, 20% were idiopathic and 80% were varied. The predominant findings were flexor hallucis longus tenosynovitis, venous variocosities, fibrous scar tissue, and posterior tibial tendon tenosynovitis, from most to least frequent. Other common causes noted on MRI were ganglion cysts, neoplasms (synovial cell sarcoma, most commonly soft tissue sarcoma of the foot),[10, 14] neurilemoma, hemangioma, posttraumatic fracture deformity, abductor hallucis muscle hypertrophy, fluid collection, and valgus hindfoot.[9, 15]

## Differential Diagnosis

A thorough list of differential diagnoses should include any pathology of the medial foot and ankle such as plantar fasciitis, heel pain syndrome, calcaneal bursitis, posterior tibial tendon rupture, tendinitis, prolapsed metatarsal heads with metatarsalgia, tenosynovitis, ligamentous rupture or sprain, frank fractures, stress fractures, neoplasms, bone metastatic carcinoma, peripheral vascular disease, peripheral neuritis, lumbosacral radiculopathy, any peripheral neuropathy, reflex sympathetic dystrophy, plantar nerve entrapment, seronegative arthridities, rheumatoid arthritides, Morton's neuroma, and a mass in the popiliteal fossa.[1, 6]

## Treatment

Depending on the etiology, conservative therapy may or may not be effective. It is extremely important to identify the underlying pathology in each patient as it dictates the therapy. A course of monsteroidal anti-inflammatory drugs (NSAIDs) combined with immobilization to prevent pronation, such as with strappings, braces, or casting, can aid in relief of mild cases of tarsal tunnel syndrome. For patients with more severe symptoms, a local injection of steroid and anesthetic into the tarsal

tunnel combined with orthotic support can be effective. If the condition is long standing, some patients also benefit from physical therapy consisting of whirlpool massage, range-of-motion exercises, and iontophoresis.

In cases of severe entrapment secondary to adhesions or space-occupying masses, surgical exploration of the tibial nerve and decompression of the tarsal tunnel with removal of any masses are often required. Dissection involves opening the tarsal tunnel and the third canal, which contains the neurovascular bundle. The tibial nerve and its branches should be explored both proximally and distally into the porta pedis for any connective tissue adhesions. External neurolysis is performed by releasing any constricting muscle or fascia along the tibial nerve as it divides into the medial and lateral plantar branches. If soft tissue masses are present, great care must be taken to remove them without further damaging the nerve itself. Other surgical options include using silicone elastomer to prevent further adhesions and neurectomy of nerve branches still entrapped after neurolysis.

The newest approach to tarsal tunnel surgery involves an endoscopic approach using the instrumentation designed for carpal tunnel releases. This new technique reduces trauma to the patient and postoperative scarring over the tarsal tunnel. A retrospective study of 16 patients by Day and Naples revealed a success rate of 89%.[16] However, there are limitations of this technique related to indication, surgical skill, and anatomic restrictions.

Postoperatively, patients are kept without weight bearing with crutches for 2 to 3 weeks, with range-of-motion exercises and physical therapy to tolerance initiated during the second week. Time for full recovery can vary from 3 weeks to 3 months.

## Prognosis

The success of therapy often depends on identifying the underlying etiology of tarsal tunnel syndrome. When the condition is properly diagnosed, a treatment plan can be formulated and the need for surgical intervention can be assessed much more quickly. Most studies have had an 80% to 90% success rate after surgical decompression of the tarsal tunnel when the pathology was correctly diagnosed preoperatively.[17] However, the success rate drops to 70% when the etiology is unknown before surgical exploration.[18] Also, Takakura and associates reported that the longer the surgery was delayed after the onset of symptoms, the poorer the results of external neurolysis.[4] Furthermore, recurrence after successful surgical correction seems to be related to control of the biomechanical forces that caused or aggravated the tarsal tunnel syndrome. Finally, it is important to use modalities such as MRI to determine the cause of tarsal tunnel syndrome in order to direct the treatment plan and facilitate quick recovery.

## SURAL NERVE ENTRAPMENT

Entrapment neuropathy of the sural nerve may have several mechanisms, including trauma associated with surgery and musculoskeletal injuries of the distal leg and foot causing fibrosis and scarring around the nerve. Compression neuropathy of the sural nerve has also been described. Intrinsic compression can result from peroneal sheath degeneration or an inflamed and edematous Achilles tendon. Extrinsic sources of compression might include tight stockings and pneumatic ankle or midcalf tourniquets. Nerve overuse injury associated with recurrent microtrauma, caused by the cumulative effects of either tension or compression, occurs more frequently in patients who are anatomically predisposed by the presence of a prominent band of muscle or connective tissue or bony ridge that tethers the nerve.[5]

It is important to understand the course and distribution of the sural nerve in order to appreciate traumatic afflictions and prevent iatrogenic harm. Anatomic variations in the course of the sural nerve are considerable. Surgical incision placement and evaluation and diagnosis of sensory loss of the posterolateral leg, lateral ankle, and lateral foot are aided by a thorough understanding of the diverse branching patterns of the sural nerve.[19, 20]

The sural nerve exits the deep fascia at the junction of the distal and middle thirds of the leg. It has been hypothesized that this may be a site of entrapment.[21] At the ankle, it lies posterior to the peroneal tendons and gives off cutaneous branches to the distal quarter of the leg, lateral cutaneous branches to the heel, and branches to the dorsum of the foot. On the dorsolateral aspect of the foot it communicates with the intermediate branch of the superficial peroneal nerve (Lemont's nerve).[22] Generally, the sural nerve supplies the skin of the lateral surface of the lower third of the leg and the lateral and dorsolateral aspect of the foot.[23]

Clinically, patients usually report pain and numbness along the lateral border of the foot, although the nerve may be entrapped anywhere along its course.[5, 22] The patient may or may not relate a history of trauma to the area. Pain is often described as a burning type aggravated by walking and effort and reproduced with digital pressure (a positive Valleix point). A positive Tinel sign may be elicited on percussion at the point of entrapment.[24] Diffuse swelling and tenderness may also be present behind and below the lateral malleolus. Symptoms are generally unilateral but may be bilateral.[25]

Sural nerve entrapment is often the result of musculoskeletal injuries. Fractures of the fifth metatarsal, cuboid, calcaneus, and fibula may cause fibrosis and entrapment of the sural nerve and its branches. Also, lateral ankle sprains and rupture of the peroneal or Achilles tendon may result in scarring and cause nerve entrapment.[26–28]

The most common cause of sural nerve entrapment is iatrogenic.[5] The sural nerve is placed at considerable risk by incisions commonly utilized in lateral ankle reconstruction using the peroneal tendon (i.e., Elmslie, Watson-Jones).[5, 19, 24] The dissection and manipulation of soft tissue required for isolated subtalar, triple, and ankle arthrodeses and for open reduction with internal fixation of fibular, calcaneal, cuboid, or lateral metatarsal fractures often result in fibrosis and entrapment of the sural nerve. Also, the scarring associated with Achilles' tendon and peroneal tendon repair or tenolysis may result in nerve entrapment.[19, 27] Entrapment of the sural nerve also occurs with flatfoot reconstructions utilizing a lateral incisional approach and ankle athroscopy through a posterolateral portal.[29] Meticulous operative technique with identification and isolation of the sural nerve and its branches is therefore required during these procedures to minimize fibrosis and entrapment of the nerve.[19, 28–30]

Sural nerve compression neuropathy has many pathophysiologies, including mechanical and vascular compromise. Many believe that the primary lesion of compression neuropathies is the vascular compromise of an axonal segment resulting from a change in nerve position, local anatomy, and/or internal or external pressures.[31] Peripheral nerves have both an extrinsic and an intrinsic blood supply.

Intrinsic sources of sural neuropathy caused by compression include but are not limited to an engorged lesser saphenous vein caused by chronic venous insufficiency, ganglions of the peroneal tendons, inflammation and edema from chronic Achilles' or peroneal tendinitis, and enlargement of the peroneal tubercle on the lateral aspect of the calcaneus.[24]

Extrinsic compression of the sural nerve with resulting neuropathy has been less frequently reported. Most cases involve an individual's distal leg, ankle, or foot resting against a hard surface such as a table or stool for a prolonged period of time. Other causes include a tight ankle bracelet, compression stockings, and an ill-fitting ski boot.[32, 33] Ankle and midcalf tourniquets induce a state in which the nerve segment distal to the cuff becomes ischemic while the nerve segment under the cuff is subjected to mechanical compression and ischemia. The prognosis for recovery in cases of extrinsic compression is directly related to the time the ischemic state is maintained and the resulting neuropraxia, axonotmesis, or neurotmesis.[54]

The diagnosis and treatment of lateral foot pain are often difficult. The differential diagnoses are numerous, including osseous abnormalities, sprains, peripheral mononeuropathies, and radiculopathy.[35] The diagnosis of sural nerve entrapment neuropathy as the cause of the pain requires a thorough history and physical examination. Radiographic and MRI studies may prove extremely useful in determining osseous and soft tissue pathology resulting in direct compression or fibrosis along the course of the sural nerve or neuralgia caused by root compression at the level of the fifth lumbar and first and second sacral vertebrae.[25] Electrodiagnostic tests including electromyography and nerve conduction studies may be helpful in determining the exact level of entrapment.[35] One must also include the possibility of underlying vascular pathology as a potential cause of sural neuropathy. In chronic venous insufficiency, an engorged lesser saphenous vein may compress the sural nerve, and therefore a thorough vascular examination may be necessary. Scleroderma and other mixed connective tissue disorders may cause fibrosis and entrapment of the sural nerve as well as microangiopathic changes in the endoneural, perineural, and epineural vessels resulting in ischemia and neuropathy. Suspicion that this is the underlying cause may necessitate appropriate hematologic studies including the erythrocyte sedimentation rate, antinuclear antibody, and rheumatoid factor or possibly biopsy of the sural nerve.[36, 37]

Conservative treatment of sural nerve entrapment includes avoidance of activities or positions that cause obvious irritation or compression of the nerve. Stockings of appropriate size or properly fitting boots may be enough to relieve the painful symptoms. Anti-inflammatory medications, rest, and braces to stabilize the ankle may be of some further benefit. Various physical therapy modalities including whirlpool, moist heat, ultrasonic radiation, and iontophoresis may be useful for entrapment caused by postsurgical scarring. Relief with conservative measures, however, is uncommon.[24]

Surgical intervention is frequently necessary when dense subcutaneous scarring incarcerates the sural nerve or its branches or when a bony prominence is responsible for direct compression and a positive Valleix point test. External neurolysis is performed through an incision over the suspected entrapment site. The nerve is mobilized from surrounding fibrotic or scar tissue. Success of neurolysis is directly related to the soft tissue bed in the postoperative nerve environment. If the surrounding soft tissue bed is of poor quality for transposition of the nerve, progression to immediate neurectomy is often the best surgical option. If neurectomy is performed, the nerve should be resected proximal to the site of entrapment and placed in a good soft tissue environment away from future mechanical irritation, as in fat, or buried in bone. A small amount of soluble steroid may be dispersed over the nerve before closure.[24, 38]

Reflex sympathetic dystrophy after severe sural nerve trauma is not uncommon. It is important to avoid surgical intervention in these cases unless an offending fracture remnant is disturbing the course of the nerve, causing persistent symptoms.[39]

## CALCANEAL NERVE ENTRAPMENT

Entrapment is a condition of regionally localized injury and inflammation in a peripheral nerve that is caused by a mechanical irritation by some impinging anatomic neighbor.[24] Three anatomic landmarks divide the calcaneal nerves. Geographically, the calcaneus and immediately adjacent soft tissue structures are innervated by (1) the medial calcaneal nerve, a branch of the posterior tibial nerve; (2) the inferior calcaneal nerve, the first branch of the lateral plantar nerve, which gives both sensory and muscular innervation; and (3) the lateral calcaneal nerve, a branch of the sural nerve. There is sparse literature describing isolated nerve injuries involving the calcaneal nerves. Foremost, descriptions of these injuries involve etiologies of heel pain similar to those of heel spur syndrome. The clinical descriptions of symptoms vary, including pains classically described as burning, sharp, lancinating, tingling, itching, or stabbing and localized to an isolated area unless multiple nerves are involved in the region of the heel. The courses of these symptoms are similar in that they typically worsen when they are untreated. Diagnosis can most often be made on the basis of a complete history and physical examination. In cases in which the history and physical examination are not definitive, electrodiagnosis can be utilized, including electromyography and nerve conduction velocity tests. Sensory evoked potentials may reveal a decreased conduction velocity through the injured nerve, and electromyography may aid in the evaluation of motor deficits. Electromyographic nerve conduction studies are the only objective method for confirming a diagnosis of peripheral entrapment-compression syndromes.[40]

Etiologies of the entrapment of the calcaneal nerves may be classified as traumatic and nontraumatic. The traumatic factors include direct injury with subsequent hematoma formation, tenosynovitis of adjacent tendons, and several predisposing biomechanical factors.[40] Direct injuries include traction, laceration, compression, and incarceration in scar tissue. Injection injuries as discussed by Clark may also be included.[41] The nontraumatic factors include congenital abnormalities (such as an accessory abductor hallucis muscle) and neoplastic formation, which causes external pressure on the nerve through a mass effect. Also commonly encountered in this classification are fibrolipomas, ganglioneuromas, rheumatoid nodules, and severe varicosities.[40]

To differentiate and isolate pathology of the calcaneal nerves, an understanding of the anatomy is necessary. This includes the dermatome, the pathway of the specific nerve, and the various fascial layers where these nerves may be found. Any approved dermatome map is useful. The medial calcaneal nerve is the first of three branches from the posterior tibial nerve. The calcaneal nerve consists (usually) of two major branches that supply the cutaneous innervation of the medial plantar aspect of the heel. The anterior major branch is interposed between the deep fascia of the proximal part of the abductor hallucis muscle and the medial anterior corner of the tuber calcanei. At this point the deep fascia is tense, thick, and inelastic, causing the nerve to be vulnerable. The posterior calcaneal branch is small and passes the medial edge of the os calcis dorsal to the origin of the abductor hallucis muscle.[42] Tanz indicated that tightening the abductor hallucis, the short toe flexors, and the medial portion of the plantar aponeurosis caused heel pain and that relaxing these structures relieved the pain.[43]

In a series of anatomic dissections of the human foot by Arenson, Cosentino, and Suran, a branch of the lateral plantar nerve was studied. This nerve branch was found to course laterally and deep to the abductor hallucis muscle. It then passes between the most proximal portions of the flexor digitorum brevis muscle and the long plantar ligament. It usually terminates within the most proximal portion of the abductor digiti minimi muscle.[44] It has been reported in the literature that this inferior calcaneal nerve may be responsible for a portion of cases involving the diagnosis of heel spur syndrome, called Baxter's nerve.[45]

The lateral calcaneal nerve is a branch of the sural nerve. The sural nerve travels with the small saphenous vein superficially along the anterior lateral border of the Achilles tendon. The lateral calcaneal nerve branches off as the sural nerve enters the foot and passes inferior to the lateral malleolus. The lateral calcaneal nerve supplies cutaneous innervation to the proximal-lateral and inferolateral heel. Carrel and Davidson suggested that the sural nerve and branches may be subject to internal and external pressures when problems involving the peroneal tendons arise.[40]

Utilizing the information from the history and physical examination, the results of any electrodiagnostic studies, and appropriate anatomic correlation, a secure diagnosis may be rendered. Differential diagnoses may include any metabolic abnormalities (e.g., rheumatoid arthritis, Reiter's disease, psoriatic arthritis), infection, neoplasms (neurilemoma),[46] trauma involving adjacent soft tissue elements, and congenital abnormalities involving the hindfoot, particularly the calcaneal nerves.

Specific methods of treatment must be utilized for each isolated calcaneal nerve injury; invasive therapies such as injectable steroids or surgical intervention are considered in terms of the patients' needs and desired outcome of therapy. Treatment is by conservative measures first, followed by surgical methods when conservative ones fail. Conservative methods of treatment include (1) controlling abnormal pronation by the use of biomechanical orthoses, strapping, or padding; (2) local steroid injections; (3) oral anti-inflammatory medications; and (4) physiotherapy (e.g., whirlpool, ultrasonic radiation).[47] Tanz discussed the use and efficacy of therapeutic strapping and padding in an effort to support and relax the aponeurotic tension on the medial calcaneal nerve branch.[43] The efficacy of first-time steroid injection for painful heel syndrome was discussed by Miller, Torres, and McGuire. They suggested that a steroid injection is a reasonable adjunct to therapy but that it is unlikely to provide permanent pain relief.[48]

Surgical intervention is the final and potentially most permanent correction of the nerve pathology but has associated morbidities. Surgical decompression, release, adhesiotomy (external neurolysis), possibly repair, and neurectomy are the available options. According to Malay and McGlamry, surgical management of localized acquired peripheral neuropathy evolves primarily around external neurolysis.[24] This entails freeing the entrapped nerve from any impinging local structures, incising any adjacent fibrous bands, and dissecting and mobilizing the nerve truck from surrounding scar tissue, when present. When all attempts at salvage or repair have been exhausted, surgical neurectomy is often a preferable treatment option but leads to sensory loss. The prognosis is based on the individual case and depends on the patient's overall mental status and the response of the physical impairment to treatment.

## MISCELLANEOUS ENTRAPMENT SYNDROMES: MORTON'S AND JOPLIN'S NEUROMAS, ANTERIOR TARSAL TUNNEL SYNDROME, AND PERONEAL NERVE ENTRAPMENT

Morton's neuroma is described as an interdigital neuritis of the foot. Many etiologies have been described, including mechanical imbalance of the foot, soft tissue trauma, inflammation, and transient ischemia.[49, 50] This neuroma is most likely a mechanically induced degenerative neuropathy that has a strong predisposition for the second and third interspaces of the foot and a tendency to occur in middle-aged women. The third common digital nerve is most commonly affected. Excessive motion between the third and fourth metatarsals, hypertrophied third and fourth metatarsal heads, digital contractures, irregularly shaped metatarsal heads, entrapment within the deep transverse metatarsal ligament overlying the common digital nerve, and excessive forefoot weight bearing exacerbated by improper shoegear can collectively result in microdegeneration of the common digital nerve.[51] If these conditions persist over a period of time, the common digital nerve can become damaged, hypertrophied, and extremely painful. As the nerve becomes larger, further weight bearing–induced trauma can result, increasing the pain experienced by the patient.[52]

In the early stages of Morton's neuroma, before the classic perineural fibrosis, demyelination, and endoneural fibrosis, patients may experience transient signs and symptoms associated with dorsiflexing the metatarsal phalangeal joints. This biomechanical force on the forefoot causes stretching of the common digital nerve over the distal aspect of the deep transverse metatarsal ligament. Biomechanically, during excessive pronation, third and fourth metatarsal dorsiflexion is increased compared with the more medial metatarsals, also causing nerve irritation.[53] The clinical history includes parethesias and cramping pain in the toes of the affected area. The patient experiences pain on palpation of the affected interdigital space (Molder's sign), and pain can be reproduced by the examiner by compressing the metatarsal heads while dorsiflexing the metatarsal phalangeal joints and then palpating the affected web space. Occasionally, a classical "click" may be elicited while performing this clinical test. Commonly, the neuroma is present in the third or fourth interspace, less commonly in the other interspaces, and rarely in more than one interspace of the same foot.[54] As always, it is important to rule out more proximal nerve pathology before diagnosing intermetatarsal neuroma.

Conservative treatment can include modifying shoegear. A shoe with a wider toe box or a better padded shoe helps to prevent painful discomfort and also aids in slowing the progression of nerve degeneration if no underlying anatomic pathology is present. The NSAIDs have been used successfully to control pain associated with intermetatarsal neuroma. Pain related to an inflammatory process causing neuritis responds best to NSAID therapy.[51]

Unfortunately, a large percentage of patients do not respond to these conservative treatments and need more invasive treatment. Injection therapy is widely accepted and good results have been reported.[55] Injections consist of 1 to 3 mL of local anesthetic, short and long acting, and steroid of phosphate or mixed phosphate and acetate suspensions. Three injections may be given in 1 year. The injection is directed dorsal to plantar and is targeted at the nerve. Side effects of local injection include but are not limited to local hyperpigmentation, local irritation, infection, and, most important, weakening of capsular and tendinous structures. The limit of three injections over a period of 1 year helps to decrease the risks.

Surgical intervention is the final step in treatment, with MRI used to guide localization of the lesion. Regardless of the approach used in isolating the neuroma, recommendations have ranged from resection as far proximally as possible to resection 1 to 2 cm proximal to the bifurcation of the proper digital branches.[50, 56] Retraction of the nerve bifurcation has been consistently regarded as an essential feature in the long-term success of excision of Morton's neuroma.[57, 58] A dorsal incisional approach is favored for the first excision of neuroma. Recurrent neuroma excision warrants a plantar incisional approach.[59] Good surgical dissection technique and proper excision are essential in limiting the recurrence of Morton's neuroma. Endoscopic surgical techniques have also been utilized to cut the transverse metatarsal ligament, thus alleviating compression of the nerve against the ligament.

Joplin's neuroma is described as a neuroma of the medial plantar proper digital nerve. The medial plantar proper digital nerve is a terminal sensory branch arising from the medial plantar nerve and supplies sensation to the medial aspect of the hallux. Entrapment neuropathy of this nerve can result from trauma, tight shoegear, or adhesion secondary to bunion surgery. This nerve lies superficially as it courses along the medial aspect of the hallux, which increases the susceptibility of the nerve to trauma as well as chronic compression.

Patients may present with pain and paresthesias at the medial aspect of the hallux. An incision noted on the medial aspect of the hallux correlated with a proper history and clinical findings can signify Joplin's neuroma.[60] This is a sensory nerve, so full motor function is present to the hallux while sensory loss is noted.

Electrophysiologic studies of the medial plantar proper digital nerve have been attempted to confirm the diagnosis of Joplin's neuroma. In a case report, electrophysiologic studies did not indicate that demyelination is a significant component of Joplin's neuroma. Minimal nerve conduction velocity slowing suggested that axonal degeneration may be a prominent feature of this condition, which was reported previously with Morton's neuroma.[61, 62] Again, MRI is useful for delineation of this lesion from any other mass-occupying lesion.

Conservative treatment includes reducing compression of this nerve by first changing shoegear. Because of the superficial anatomy of the nerve, if epineural inflammation is present, the pain can be easily elicited by palpation of the enlarged area. Care must be taken by the foot surgeon to avoid the area while planning a surgical incision. Adhesions in this area have been reported to entrap the medial plantar proper digital nerve. NSAIDS and shoe modification constitute a combined form of conservative treatment. Once again, surgical excision of the nerve or surgical excision of scar tissue causing entrapment is the final step in treatment. Degenerative joint disease at the first metatarsal phalangeal joint (bunion formation) with osteophytic spurring has been associated with neuritis, and surgical correction of the bone deformity may be needed for relief of symptoms.[52] Injections may be used before surgical intervention when appropriate. These include local anesthetic, both long and short acting, with a mixture of steroid of phosphate or mixed phosphate and acetate suspensions.

Anterior tarsal tunnel syndrome is caused by entrapment of the deep peroneal nerve by the inferior extensor retinaculum. The deep peroneal nerve (also known as the anterior tibial nerve) begins at the bifurcation of the common peroneal nerve at the neck of the fibula, deep to the origin of the peroneus longus. As it travels distally in the anterior compartment of the leg with the anterior tibial artery, it innervates the muscles of the anterior compartment. At the level of the ankle joint, the nerve lies lateral to the artery. Here it divides into two branches as it continues to the dorsum of the foot. The two branches are the lateral and medial terminal branches of the deep peroneal nerve. The lateral terminal branch travels along the dorsum of the foot, deep to the extensor digitorum brevis, which it innervates. Because this branch lies deep to the muscle, entrapment can occur in this area. This area is considered to be in the space of the anterior tarsal tunnel.

The anterior tarsal tunnel is a narrow space between the fascia overlying the talus and navicular and the Y-shaped band of the inferior extensor retinaculum. As the deep peroneal nerve passes through this space, it is deep to the tendons of the extensor hallucis longus and extensor digitorum longus. The deep peroneal nerve divides into its medial and lateral branches just proximal to the most prominent part of the articular surface of the head of the talus.

Patients present with burning, numbness, and/or tingling extending distally over the dorsum of the foot and often to the hallux. They experience fatigue while walking and can wake from sleep because of the pain. Pain is decreased with dorsiflexion and increased with plantarflexion. Pain also can be exacerbated if osteophytes or degenerative changes are seen dorsally at the talonavicular joint.[52, 63] Clinical signs include weakness of extension of the hallux, wasting of the extensor hallucis brevis and extensor digitorum brevis muscles, and decrease in sensation in the first interdigital space.

Electrophysiologic studies show denervation of the extensor digitorum brevis, and nerve conduction velocities show normal velocity proximal to the ankle but increased motor latency distal to the ankle.[64, 65]

Conservative treatment includes padding the area of most concern, which can aid in elimination of compression. Medications including NSAIDS and tricyclic antidepressants such as amitriptyline (Elavil) have been used. If a bony prominence or deformity exists, surgical correction is warranted. The area of surgical correction, or nerve release versus resection, is correlated with the area associated with most symptoms.[66]

The superficial peroneal nerve, also referred to as the musculocutaneous nerve, also begins at the bifurcation of the common peroneal nerve at the neck of the fibula. This nerve travels distally in the lateral compartment of the leg. As it passes distally, it provides branches to the two peroneal muscles and sensory nerves to the skin of the lateral leg. In the distal aspect of the leg the nerve divides into two branches, the medial dorsal cutaneous nerve and a lateral branch called the intermediate dorsal cutaneous nerve. The medial branch then branches distally into the medial dorsal digital nerve and the second common digital nerve. The intermediate dorsal cutaneous nerve branches distally into the third and fourth common dorsal digital branches.

Entrapments of the superficial peroneal nerve typically occur where the nerve pierces the deep fascia and divides into the medial and lateral branches. Patients with entrapment here can present with pinpoint pain or fullness at the area where the nerve penetrates the deep fascia. Pain becomes worse with activity and better with rest. As with other entrapments, burning, numbness, and tingling can be felt along the distributions of the nerve and its branches. Testing for compression has been described by Styf: first, the physician palpates the nerve at the compression site while the patient dorsiflexes and everts against resistance; then the physician passively plantarflexes and inverts the foot while percussing the nerve.[67]

Conservative treatment, including local injections, NSAIDs, padding and strapping of the ankle, and rest, has generally provided little relief in this entrapment.[68] Surgery involves decompression of the nerve as it passes through the deep fascia. Patients can obtain immediate relief, and follow-up data support the procedure.[69]

Saphenous nerve entrapment usually occurs at Hunter's canal after knee surgery, as the infrapatellar nerve is a branch of the saphenous nerve. Saphenous nerve entrapments are of importance to the foot and ankle surgeon because branches of the nerve provide sensation to the medial side of the ankle as well as the medial side of the foot. Surgical correction is warranted for this entrapment and usually involves release of the fibrous roof of Hunter's canal.[70]

The preceding entrapments can be frustrating to the patient as well as the physician if not diagnosed properly and in a timely manner. With all entrapments, proximal disease or pathology must be ruled out first. Diagnostic studies including electrophysiologic studies, nerve conduction studies, radiography, and MRI evaluation can all be helpful in assessing these conditions. A good clinical examination including biomechanics is essential for determination of abnormal motion, which may induce the pain and increase trauma to the nerve.

## REFERENCES

1. Cimino WR: Tarsal tunnel syndrome: Review of literature. Foot Ankle 11:47–52, 1990.
2. Keck C: The tarsal tunnel syndrome. J Bone Joint Surg 63A:180–182, 1962.
3. Sarrafian S: Anatomy of the Foot and Ankle: Descriptive. Topographic. Functional. Philadelphia, JB Lippincott, 1983, p 119.
4. Takakura Y, Kitada C, Sagimoto K, et al: Tarsal tunnel syndrome: Causes and results of operative treatment. J Bone Joint Surg 73B:125–128, 1991.
5. Yamaguchi D: Carpal tunnel syndrome. Minn Med 48:22–26, 1965.
6. McGuigan L: Tarsal tunnel syndrome and peripheral neuropathy in rheumatics. Ann Rheum Dis 42:128–131, 1983.
7. Olivieri I: Tarsal tunnel syndrome in seronegative spondyloarthropathy. Br J Rheum 28:537–538, 1989.
8. Sammarco GJ, Stephans MM: Tarsal tunnel syndrome caused by the flexor digitorum longus accesorius. J Bone Joint Surg 72A:453–454, 1990.
9. Deutsch AL, Mink JH, Kerr R: MRI of the Foot and Ankle. New York, Raven, 1992, pp 349–351.
10. Belding RH: Neurilemoma of the lateral plantar nerve producing tarsal tunnel syndrome: A case report. Foot Ankle 14:289–291, 1993.
11. Kaplan PE, Kernahan WT: Tarsal tunnel syndrome: Electrodiagnostic and surgical correlation. J Bone Joint Surg 65A:96–99, 1981.
12. Weiman TJ, Patel VG: Treatment of hyperaesthetic neuropathic pain in the diabetic: Decompression of the tarsal tunnel. Ann Surg 221:660–665, 1995.
13. Johnson EW, Ortiz PR: Electrodiagnosis of the tarsal tunnel syndrome. Arch Phys Med Rehab 47:776–780, 1996.
14. Felsenthal G, Butler DH, Shear MS: Across tarsal tunnel motor nerve conduction technique. Arch Phys Med Rehab 73:64–69, 1992.
15. Frey C, Kerr R: Magnetic resonance imaging and the evaluation of tarsal tunnel syndrome. Foot Ankle 14:159–164, 1993.
16. Day FN, Naples JJ: Tarsal tunnel syndrome: An endoscopic approach with 4–28 month follow-up. J Foot Ankle Surg 33:244–248, 1994.
17. O'Malley GM, Lambdin CS, McCleary GS: Tarsal tunnel syndrome: A case report and review of the literature. Orthopedics 8:758–760, 1985.
18. Stern DS, Joyce MT: Tarsal tunnel syndrome: A review of 15 surgical procedures. J Foot Surg 28:290–294, 1989.
19. Lawrence SJ, Botte MJ: The sural nerve in the foot and ankle: An anatomic study with clinical and surgical implications. Foot Ankle 15:490–493, 1994.
20. Hjuene DB, Bunnell WP: Operative anatomy of nerves encountered in the lateral approach to the distal part of the fibula. J Bone Joint Surg 77A:1021–1024, 1995.
21. Coert JH, Dellon AL: Clinical implications of the surgical anatomy of the sural nerve. Plast Recon Surg 94:850–855, 1994.
22. Pringle RM, Protheroe K, Mukherjee SK: Entrapment neuropathy of the sural nerve. J Bone Joint Surg 56B:465–468, 1974.
23. Ortiguela ME, Wood MB, Cahill OR: Anatomy of the sural nerve complex. J Foot Surg 29:119–121, 1990.
24. Malay DS, McGlamry ED, Nava CA: Acquired neuropathies of the lower extremities. In McGlamry ED (ed): Comprehensive Textbook of Foot Surgery, Vol 2, pp 1110–1114. Baltimore, Williams and Wilkins, 1987.
25. Mozes M, Ouaknine G, Nathan H: Saphenous nerve entrapment simulating vascular disorder. Surgery 77:299–303, 1975.
26. Mitsumoto H, Wilbourn AJ: Causes and diagnosis of sensory neuropathies: A review. J Clin Neurophysiol 11:553–567, 1994.
27. Myerson M, Quill GE: Late complications of fractures of the calcaneus. J Bone Joint Surg 75A:331–339, 1993.
28. Gould N, Trevino S: Sural nerve entrapment by avulsion fracture of the base of the fifth metatarsal bone. Foot Ankle 2:153–155, 1981.
29. Ferkel RD, Dalton HD, Guhl JF: Neurological Complication of Ankle Arthroscopy. Arthroscopy 12:200–208, 1996.
30. Hjuene DB, Bunnell WP: Operative anatomy of nerves encountered in the lateral approach to the distal part of the fibula. J Bone Joint Surg 77A:1021–1024, 1995.
31. Shaffrey ME, Shaffrey CL, Persing JA, et al: Diagnosis and treatment of entrapment neuropathies. In Kassell (ed): Contemporary Topics in Neurosurgery. Contemporary Neurology Series. Philadelphia, FA Davis, 1994.
32. Reisin R, Pardal A, Ruggieri V, Gold L: Sural neuropathy due to external pressure: Report of three cases. Neurology 44:2408–2409, 1994.
33. Lindenbaum BL: Ski boot compression syndrome. Clin Orthop 109–110, 1979.
34. Lundborg G: Structure and formation of the intraneural microvessels as related to trauma, edema formation, and nerve function. J Bone Joint Surg 57A:938–948, 1975.
35. Shear MS, Baitch SP, Shear DB: Sinus tarsi syndrome: The importance of biomechanically based evaluation and treatment. Arch Phys Med Rehab 74:777–781, 1993.
36. Gillilaud BC: Progressive systemic sclerosis. In Braunwald E et al (eds): Harrison's Principles of Internal Medicine, Vol 2. New York, McGraw Hill, 1987, pp 1428–1432.
37. Corbo M, Nemi S, Iannaccone S, et al: Peripheral neuropathy in scleroderma. Clin Neuropathol 12:63–67, 1993.
38. Downey MS: Surgical treatment of peripheral nerve entrapment syndrome. In Oloff LM (ed): Musculoskeletal Disorders of the Lower Extremities. Philadelphia, WB Saunders, 1994, pp 702–703.
39. Schon LC: Nerve entrapment, neuropathy, and nerve dysfunction in athletes. Orthop Clin North Am 25:47–59, 1994.
40. Carrel JM, Davidson DM: Nerve compression of the foot and ankle: A comprehensive review of symptoms, etiology, and diagnosis using nerve conduction testing. J Am Podiatr Med Assoc 65:322–341, 1975.
41. Clark WK: Surgery for injection injury of peripheral nerves. Surg Clin North Am 52:1325–1328, 1972.
42. Hennicson AS, Westtin NE: Chronic calcaneal pain in ath-

letes: Entrapment of the calcaneal nerve. Am J Sports Med 12:52–54, 1984.

43. Tanz SS: Heel pain. Clin Orthop 28:169–178, 1963.

44. Arenson DJ, Cosentino GL, Suran SM: The inferior calcaneal nerve: An anatomical study. J Am Podiatr Med Assoc 70:552–560, 1980.

45. Baxter DE, Pfeffer GB: Treatment of chronic heel pain by surgical release of the first branch of the lateral plantar nerve. Clin Orthop 279:229–236, 1992.

46. Brieststein RJ: Compression neuropathy secondary to neurilemoma. J Am Podiatr Med Assoc 75:160–161, 1985.

47. Altman MI, Hinkes MP: Heel neuroma: A case history. J Am Podiatr Med Assoc 72:517–519, 1982.

48. Miller RA, Torres J, McGuire M: Efficacy of First-Time Steroid Injection for Painful Heel Syndrome. Foot Ankle Int 16:610–612, 1995.

49. Haeri GB, Fornasier VL, Schatzker J: Morton's neuroma: Pathogenesis and ultrastructure. Clin Orthop 141:257, 1979.

50. May VR: The enigma of Morton's neuroma. In Bateman JE (ed): Foot Science. Philadelphia, WB Saunders, 1976, p 222.

51. Wu KK: Morton's interdigital neuroma: A clinical review of its etiology, treatment, and results. Forefoot Ankle Surg 35:112–119, 1996.

52. Scon LC: Nerve entrapment, neuropathy, and nerve dysfunction in athletes. Orthop Clin North Am 25:47, 1994.

53. Murphy PC, Baxter DE: Nerve entrapment of the foot and ankle in runners. Clin Sports Med 4:753, 1985.

54. Youngswick FD: Intermetatarsal neuroma. Clin Podiatr Med Surg 11:579–592, 1994.

55. Dellon AL: Treatment of Morton's neuroma as a nerve compression. The role for neurolysis. J Am Podiatr Med Assoc 82:399–402, 1992.

56. Amis JA, Swirhus SW, Liwnicz BH: An anatomic basis for

57. Bradley N, Miller WA, Evans JP: Plantar neuroma: Analysis of results following surgical excision in 145 patients. South Med J 69:853–854, 1976.

58. Bickel WH, Dockerty MD: Plantar neuromas, Morton's toe. Surg Gynecol Obstet 84:111–116, 1947.

59. Kuwada GT: Plantar incisional approaches: Current perspectives. J Am Podiatr Med Assoc 85:15–21, 1995.

60. Ames PA, Lenet MD, Sherman M: Joplin's neuroma. J Am Podiatr Med Assoc 70:99–101, 1980.

61. Cichy SW, Claussen GC, Oh SJ: Electrophysiological studies in Joplin's neuroma. Muscle Nerve 18:671–672, 1995.

62. Oh SJ, Kim HS, Ahmad BK: Electrophysiological diagnosis of interdigital neuropathy of the foot. Muscle Nerve 7:218–225, 1984.

63. Zongzhao I, Jiansheng Z, Zhao I: Anterior tarsal tunnel syndrome. Foot Ankle 73:471–473, 1991.

64. Anderson BL, Wertsch JJ, Stewart WA: Anterior tarsal tunnel syndrome. Arch Phys Med Rehab 73:1112–1117, 1992.

65. Kanbe K, Hitoshi K, Shirakura K: Entrapment neuropathy of the deep peroneal nerve associated with the extensor hallucis brevis. J Foot Ankle Surg 34:560–562, 1995.

66. Dellon AL: Deep peroneal nerve release. Entrapment on the dorsum of the foot. Foot Ankle 11:73, 1990.

67. Styf J: Entrapment of the superficial peroneal nerve: Diagnosis and results of decompression. J Bone Joint Surg 71:131, 1989.

68. Kernohan J, Levack B, Wilson JN: Entrapment of the superficial peroneal nerve. J Bone Joint Surg 67B:Jan, 1985.

69. Kopell HP, Thompson WL: Peripheral Entrapment Neuropathies. Baltimore, Williams and Wilkins, 1963, p 171.

70. Worth RM, Kettelkamp DB, Defalque RJ, et al: Saphenous nerve entrapment. Am J Sports Med 12:80–81, 1984.

# Myopathies

**18**

*Richard H. Bennett*

The number and diversity of neuromuscular diseases are ever increasing. Our understanding has paralleled the rapid advances of the basic as well as clinical sciences. Most myopathic disorders affect the lower extremities at some point in their evolution. Myopathic diseases typically present with a distinct set of symptoms and physical findings; symptoms are often subtle and difficult to distinguish from complaints of anxiety, depression, and chronic disease rather than neuromuscular elements. Weakness and fatigability are key features, and inquiring about an individual's ability to walk, run, climb stairs, and arise from a seated position is extremely important. Proximal arm strength should be assessed by recording weakness with the arms placed above the shoulder level. Drooping of the eyelids, a change in facial expression, and difficulty with swallowing or speaking are commonly seen.

Muscle weakness is most commonly observed in proximal shoulder or pelvic muscles. Certain muscle diseases may be distinguished by a predilection for particular areas of the body (e.g., myotonic dystrophy affecting the distal muscles of the forearm and fascioscapulohumeral muscular dystrophy affecting the proximal neck, face, and shoulder muscles). Pain or tenderness is often prominent in inflammatory disease, whereas in more indolent muscular dystrophies the course is painless. Weakness is frequently accompanied by muscle wasting or atrophy, but early in certain diseases, such as Duchenne's muscular dystrophy, weakness is present with hypertrophy reflecting fat replacement.

Muscle strength has typically been graded using the rating system of the Medical Research Council of Great Britain: 0, complete paresis; 1, minimal contraction with gravity eliminated; 2, weak contraction against gravity; 3, moderate weakness; 4, minimal detectable weakness; and 5, normal strength. Further gradations with + and − may also define strength.

Whereas in primary neuropathies, deep tendon reflexes are frequently lost when minimal clinical symptoms are present, deep tendon reflexes are frequently maintained until muscle diseases become far advanced.

Involuntary muscle movements may be present. Fasciculations, twitches, spasms, cramps, contractures, and myotonia are commonly seen. In advanced muscle diseases, scoliosis of the spine and tendon contractures of the hips and calves develop.

Laboratory studies highlight myopathic disorders. Elevations of creatine kinase, serum glutamic-oxaloacetic transaminase, and serum glutamic-pyruvic transaminase are frequently noted. An elevated sedimentation rate is a nonspecific finding that may also reflect the presence of an underlying inflammatory condition.

In certain myopathies, analysis of DNA from blood and tissue and genetic linkage analysis are extremely important in defining genetic disorders.

An electromyogram characteristically reveals myopathic findings that are present in all muscle disorders. Small-amplitude, polyphasic motor unit potentials that are recruited rapidly with minimal effort in weakened muscles may be accompanied by signs of active denervation such as fibrillations and positive sharp waves with increased insertional activity. Complex repetitive discharges may also be seen, reflecting the destruction of distal nerve terminals that are located intramuscularly. Histologic analysis with muscle biopsy typically reveals variations in fiber size with necrosis, fat replacement, and endomysial inflammation.

## MUSCULAR DYSTROPHY

The most common of the genetically acquired muscular dystrophies is Duchenne's muscular dystrophy. This is one of the most common of the lethal diseases involving progressive dystrophy of skeletal muscles. There are three main presentations: proximal muscle weakness, elevated levels of creatine kinase, and malignant hyperthermia after exposure to halothane anesthesia. Proximal muscle weakness and muscle hypertrophy with tendon contractures develop in early childhood. Motor milestones are delayed. Most affected individuals walk 3 to 6 months later than their peers. Proximal leg weakness is characteristically detected, with inability to rise from a squatting or seated position without use of the hands (Gowers' sign). Calf pseudohypertrophy is commonly seen. Contractures of the tendons leading to toe walking and scoliosis also develop.

The disease progresses and leads to wheelchair dependence by age 7 to 14, and death caused by respiratory failure usually occurs by age 20. The disease primarily affects boys, and females are carriers (X linked). The disease is caused by a mutation of the X chromosome (Xp21). The protein product of the gene, dystrophin, is absent or markedly deficient. Dystrophin is a component of the muscle membrane cytoskeleton. The disease affects approximately 1 in 3500 male births. Although the disease is X linked, there is a high spontaneous mutation rate of 1 in 10,000 gametes. Sporadic cases of myopathy with elevated creatine kinase levels and with dystrophin deletion can be seen in females. A heterozygous defect in dystrophin can lead to a benign, more indolent disease (Becker's muscular dystrophy).

As the disease is inherited, affected individuals can be identified by genetic procedures. Genetic linkage analysis with direct assessment of dystrophin in fetal muscle tissue or in DNA blood samples has shown considerable promise. Although molecular diagnostic tests are still in various stages of development, refinement is rapid, and these techniques are particularly sensitive for diagnosis of Duchenne's muscular dystrophy.

Treatment is primarily symptomatic. Contractures of tendons lead to toe walking. Physical therapy with frequent stretching and surgical tendon lengthening are frequently applied. Tendon releases at the hip girdle may also be helpful. Braces (knee-foot orthosis) may prolong mobility and provide stability. Lordosis or scoliosis eventually develops, requiring careful wheelchair design. Respiratory and cardiac involvement often occurs and requires monitoring and treatment.

No medical therapies are effective. Corticosteroids can slow progression to some extent but are associated with serious side effects when taken over long periods of time.

Other important hereditary myopathies include limb-girdle muscular dystrophy and facioscapulohumeral muscular dystrophy. These autosomal dominant or recessive conditions are characterized by their pattern of presentation and, unlike Duchenne's muscular dystrophy, are not considered fatal disorders.

## INCLUSION BODY MYOSITIS

Inclusion body myositis has emerged as a distinct entity. First recognized in 1967, it accounts for the vast majority of steroid-nonresponsive inflammatory myopathies in patients older than 50 years. The diagnosis is established by the presence of microtubular filamentous inclusions in muscle biopsy specimens. A typical patient exhibits proximal distal weakness of the quadriceps muscles and foot extensors. In other individuals, the disease may begin with weakness in the distal muscles of the hand that interferes with fine motor movements such as pinching, grasping, and buttoning. Forty percent of the individuals develop dysphagia at some point. The disease progresses slowly to the arms and hands. The quadriceps muscles are almost always involved early in the disease, which accounts for the high frequency of falling. Selective weakness of the flexors of the third, fourth, and fifth fingers is considered characteristic of this disorder. Putative or definite autoimmune diseases may be present in 15% of patients with inclusion body myositis. This incidence parallels the incidence of such diseases in polymyositis. The biologic basis of this condition remains unknown. Infiltration of CD8+ cytotoxic T cells with macrophages has been noted. A role of viruses or prions as precursors of the development of microtubular filaments has been hypothesized.

Unlike other inflammatory neuropathies, inclusion body myositis is unresponsive to steroids. Thus, the treatment is entirely symptomatic. Inclusion body myositis is a slow but relentless progressive myopathy that, at worst, confines the patient to a wheelchair. Physical therapy and occupational therapy are particularly helpful in maintaining functional capabilities, especially in relation to ambulation and hand use.

## ENDOCRINE MYOPATHIES

Various endocrine disorders have been associated with a myopathic presentation. Chronic exogenous corticosteroid administration may result in profound weakness, especially with the use of synthetic fluorinated corticosteroids (e.g., triamcinolone). A severe acute myopathy that prolongs ventilator dependence has been described in patients treated concurrently with high-dose corticosteroids and nondepolarizing neuromuscular blocking agents. Individuals who are experiencing status asthmaticus are particularly sensitive to this condition. Primary pituitary and adrenal syndromes may also present with myalgias and weakness. Serum creatine kinase levels are typically normal in chronic corticosteroid myopathy. Electromyographic findings are variable with myopathic findings frequently noted. Chronic corticosteroid myopathy is reversible when medication is stopped.

Hyperthyroidism and hypothyroidism are also associated with myopathic findings. Thyroid toxic myopathy, commonly seen in Graves' disease, may be associated with other neuromuscular disorders such as myasthenia gravis, periodic paralysis, and thyroid ophthalmopathy.

Hypothyroidism in adults is characterized by lethargy and nonspecific weakness. In severe thyroid disorders that develop in utero or in early life, atypical enlargement of muscles as an expression of myxedema may be seen.

## METABOLIC MYOPATHIES

Disturbances of glycogen and lipid metabolism may present with myopathic symptoms and findings. In addition to muscle weakness, muscle contractures, myoglobinuria, and rhabdomyolysis may occur. Disorders of glycogen and metabolism present with painless muscle cramps (i.e., contractures) that occur during intense or ischemic exercise. Lipid storage myopathies are associated in some cases with decreased muscle carnitine. Cramps and myoglobinuria are frequently seen with carnitine palmityltransference deficiency.

## DRUGS AND TOXINS

Numerous drugs have been associated with myopathic conditions. Emetine, chloroquine, steroids, cimetidine, ipecac, lovastatin, zidovudine, and D-penicillamine are a few such drugs. Alcoholic myopathy can occur either acutely or chronically and may likewise present with fulminant myoglobinuria.

## INFECTION

Infections may be primary or secondary causes of myopathy. Trichinosis, viral and bacterial infections, eosinophilic inclusions, sarcoidosis, and infection with human immunodeficiency virus type 1 are examples.

## CONGENITAL

Examples of congenital myopathy include central core disease, nemaline rod myopathy, and various mitochondrial diseases. Muscle biopsy in patients with mitochondrial diseases characteristically reveals ragged red fibers and lactic acidosis.

## MYOTONIC DYSTROPHY

Myotonic dystrophy is characterized by distal muscle weakness associated with myotonic muscle activity. It is characterized by spontaneous repetitive high-frequency discharges of muscle fibers. A complex multisystem disease, it is associated with premature frontal balding, cataract development, endocrinopathies, mental retardation, gonadal atrophy, and a primarily distal myopathy. There is a defect on the proximal long arm of chromosome 19 in the majority of cases. Treatment is symptomatic. Phenytoin (Dilantin) can diminish spontaneous myotonia, but the disease itself has no specific cure.

### BIBLIOGRAPHY

Barohn RJ, Jackson CE, Rogers SJ, et al: Prolonged paralysis due to nondepolarizing neuromuscular blocking agents and corticosteroids. Muscle Nerve 17:647–654, 1994.
Dalakas MC: Polymyositis, dermatomyositis, and inclusion-body myositis. N Engl J Med 325:1487–1498, 1991.
Dalakas MC: Polymyositis. *In* Gilman S, Goldstein GW, Waxman SG (eds): Neurobase, 3rd ed. San Diego, Arbor Publishing, 1995.
Engel AG, Yamamoto M, Fischbeck KH: Dystrophinopathies. *In* Engel AG, Franzini-Armstrong C (eds): Myology, 2nd ed. New York, McGraw-Hill, 1994, pp 1130–1187.
Moser H: Duchenne muscular dystrophy: Pathogenetic aspects and genetic prevention. Hum Genet 66:17–40, 1984.
Rowland LP (ed): Merritt's Textbook of Neurology. Philadelphia, Lea & Febiger, 1995.

# Reflex Sympathetic Dystrophy: Complex Regional Pain Syndrome, Type I

# 19

*Robert L. Knobler*

"My left foot is so swollen that I can't even get a shoe on it." "My foot stays so cold, there is nothing that I can do to warm it up. I'm wearing two socks on it already, but it is ice cold and feels like it is on fire at the same time." "I walk a few feet and my foot starts turning purple, swelling, and cramping up." "I have not done anything, and my foot started turning in. No matter how hard I try to straighten it out, I can't." "I don't understand this, I never even hurt my right foot, but I have pain there, at exactly the same spot that hurts so badly on my injured left foot." "My doctor told me there was no explanation for this pain and that he thought it was all in my head." "Why does my foot bother me so much when it is my knee that was injured?" These are some of the common complaints (Table 19–1) of people who have the painful condition of reflex sympathetic dystrophy (RSD) affecting the lower extremity.

Whether it follows an arthroscopic procedure of the knee, a broken tibia supported with a cast, or a sprained ankle, RSD becomes a nightmare of pain that preoccupies people's every waking moment and limits their sleep. At the start, the only relief (Table 19–2) seems to come from holding the affected limb motionless without anything touching it. Ironically, although this "guarding" of the limb seems to provide relief for the moment, it allows the condition to progress, which is a process that can occur rap-

idly and with permanent sequelae. Therefore, delay in treatment can have serious consequences. Even more ironically, treatment—movement therapy—is extremely simple to carry out, but the pain is so severe that it is not often followed as rigorously as it should be.

From the perspective of both diagnosis and treatment, RSD is one of the more difficult disorders that can affect any part of the body. In this chapter, the focus is on the diagnosis and management of RSD affecting the lower extremity.

It is exceptional to find RSD as a primary disorder without an obvious cause. Instead, RSD is almost always secondary, most often associated with a physical trauma of some sort, typically to an extremity. Simply stated, RSD is characterized by a collection of symptoms (Table 19–3), of which pain is almost always the signal complaint, with varying degrees of swelling; sweating; color and temperature changes; altered growth of the skin, hair, and nails; and finally alterations of control of movement of the affected extremity also found. Fluctuation of these symptoms with a dependent posture, activity, and low ambient temperatures, as well as spread of the pain to previously unaffected parts of the body, further adds to the difficulties in recognition and acceptance of this condition as well as to difficulties in motivating and evaluating the success of treatment strategies.

With this diverse collection of complaints, it is not unusual for the average qualified clinician encountering such a presentation for the first time to be incredulous, even if previously aware of the existence of RSD as a clinical entity.

Disbelief is further supported by the nature of the principal pain complaint of RSD, which is best characterized as a burning and/or aching pain, although other adjectives also apply to the multiplicity of pain forms emerging (e.g., shooting, stabbing, squeezing, throbbing). It is typical to find that as the RSD pain evolves, sometimes rapidly, its legitimacy

Table 19–1  **Common Complaints**

Pain out of proportion to injury
Swelling
Coldness
Color change
Cramping
Altered posture of limb
Decreased movement
Mirror image spread of pain
Worse at the end of the limb (distally)
Impaired sleep
Altered pattern of urination
Blurred vision

**Table 19–2  Maneuvers of Relief**

Holding limb motionless (guarding)
Restricting contact of limb
Keeping affected area warm

is further questioned because it is often character-ized as being painful out of proportion to the precip-itating trauma by both the patient and the clinician. However, it should be made clear that there are two separate pains, that of the precipitating injury and the secondary pains of the RSD.

It is not yet established whether it is the trauma or the secondary issue of immobilization, either in an attempt to compensate for worsening pain and spasm upon movement or because of the need for casting or splinting, that can lead to progressive worsening of this condition over time.

Whatever the cause, certain features of RSD, such as its regional (limb-based) rather than neuro-anatomic distribution (nerve root or peripheral nerve based), its maximal severity distally even if initiated by trauma to a more proximal location, its mirror-image spread to a previously unaffected limb, and its progressive worsening in the presence of presumptively effective treatment, have created a mystique of disbelief regarding the validity of this painful condition.

These problems are compounded by the addi-tion of reactive depression in response to the grow-ing number of unanticipated problems that limit the ability to function normally in activities of daily living and employment because of pain, while man-ifesting little in the way of outwardly visible fea-tures to convince those unfamiliar with RSD of how the patient's life has been changed. It can only be imagined how the admonition and suspicion, "It's all in your head," from treating physicians, family and friends, and worker's compensation personnel, because of inadequate understanding of RSD, can be completely demoralizing at this point. The sense of hopelessness associated with inadequate pain

**Table 19–3  Common Symptoms and Signs**

Pain (burning or aching), regional distribution
Swelling
Sweating
Color change (dusky, purple-red)
Temperature change (cold, warm)
Altered growth: skin, hair, and nails
Movement disorder
 Spasms
 Tremor
 Decreased ability to initiate movements
 Weakness
 Altered posture (focal dystonia)
 Increased tone and reflexes
Sensitivity to posture, activity, and low ambient temperature

management and lack of psychosocial support has even led to suicide in this population of patients with pain.

Movement, however, has been recognized as the key to successful treatment, especially when it is initiated early. Additional therapeutic strategies, such as nerve blocks and medications, are designed to reduce pain and thereby facilitate movement. These steps alone are particularly important when treatment of the precipitating injury, such as a cast for a broken bone, delays the onset of movement therapy. Amazingly, early mobilization and move-ment therapy, particularly in an aquatic environ-ment, which provides buoyancy and support while reducing the negative effects of gravity and fluctua-tions in ambient temperature, is the treatment strat-egy associated with the best clinical outcome.

Perhaps the importance of early mobilization can be best appreciated by recognizing that RSD is less common in professional athletes, such as foot-ball players, who are injured in games. Typically, they undergo a rapid evaluation to determine whether there is a contraindication to physical ther-apy, such as a fracture or torn ligament. The diagno-sis of RSD may never even have been considered in these individuals.

The major focus of treatment is the application of strategies to get the professional player back into action as rapidly as possible. There is early and consistent application of gentle, but regularly ap-plied, physical therapy measures and adjunctive medical therapies, if needed, to accomplish this goal. Because pain is expected to be part of "playing the game," pain out of proportion to the injury and other features that might lead to suspicion of the diagnosis of RSD are rarely a concern. Although there may be profound pain as the treatment regi-men is initiated and continues, the early application of movement therapy typically results in rapid reso-lution of the painful symptoms before there is an opportunity to recognize RSD as a secondary diag-nosis.

In contrast, for the general public, the diagnosis of RSD may not be recognized either but for entirely different reasons (Table 19–4). In general practice, this diagnosis is rarely considered in the earliest stages of RSD. This is due in part to (1) general lack of awareness of the existence of this condition and sometimes frank disbelief; (2) difficulty in differenti-ating between pain, swelling, and color changes as-sociated with the precipitating injury and the early symptoms and signs of RSD; (3) limited understand-ing of the fact that RSD may develop quite early after an injury, with features of pain that are out of proportion the injury sustained; (4) limited accep-tance of the regional rather than nerve root or pe-ripheral nerve distribution of the pain of RSD; (5)

**Table 19–4  Reasons for Failure to Diagnose Reflex Sympathetic Dystrophy**

Lack of awareness of its existence
Difficulty differentiating pain of precipitating injury from the pain of RSD
Limited understanding of RSD time course
  Early onset
  Pain out of proportion to injury
Limited acceptance of regional distribution of pain in RSD
Overstatement of psychologic factors (i.e., reactive depression) as cause of RSD rather than effect of RSD
Sense that patient is noncompliant because of reluctance to continue movement therapy related to persistent pain with movement
Lack of definitive diagnostic test

RSD = reflex sympathetic dystrophy.

overstatement of psychologic factors, such as reactive depression, as a cause of the complaint of pain rather than an effect of RSD; (6) a sense that patients are noncompliant when they fail to continue movement therapy because the pain is worsened with movement; and (7) lack of a definitive diagnostic test for this disorder, so that there must be complete reliance on what may be considered by some to be "vague" clinical criteria to establish the diagnosis of RSD.

For these reasons (see Table 19–4), there has been hesitancy to make the clinical diagnosis of RSD early because of a singular focus on treating the injury at that time and the common but incorrect perception that RSD is an oversubscribed "wastebasket" diagnosis for any form of chronic pain after an injury instead of a disorder having specific diagnostic criteria.

These perceptions must change, because RSD has proved to be most treatable when it first develops. Therefore, it must be properly diagnosed as soon after the injury as possible because of the importance of initiating the relatively simple treatment modality of movement therapy as early and consistently as possible. Therapeutic measures must be a gentle but sustained effort, not unlike the course pursued in the treatment of professional athletes.

It should be noted that in practice, physical therapy measures and adjunctive medical therapies, if applied at all after an injury to the average person, tend to be short lived. This is particularly because pain that is already present is almost certain to intensify with movement. The perception of patients is that they are worse with therapy, because they hurt more despite recommendations to continue physical therapy measures. An important distinction to be made, however, is that no permanent harm results from the transient pain associated with the use of gentle movement therapy. Nevertheless, it is in this clinical setting that the persistent pain

of RSD is usually first recognized, often weeks or months after the injury first occurred.

Although increased pain and spasm on movement are characteristic of RSD, only gradually increased movement can overcome this syndrome. Because it is well recognized that RSD is likely to but does not always progress in the presence of immobilization, it is imperative that physical movement continue. Nerve blocks help to facilitate this course of treatment through reduction of pain and other symptoms, as does the use of aquatic therapy and, if needed, medications, sometimes in combination therapy to address the pain, spasm, and depression.

## DIAGNOSTIC TERMINOLOGY

The International Association for the Study of Pain (IASP) has suggested a new nomenclature, proposing the name complex regional pain syndrome (CRPS), type I, as the designation for RSD. This is to distinguish RSD from complex regional pain syndrome, type II, causalgia (Table 19–5).

Causalgia, or CRPS, type II, is the term applied to painful conditions with a clinical picture identical to that of RSD, with the exception that they are secondary to an incomplete but definitive peripheral nerve lesion, such as a traumatic lesion to the femoral nerve. In contrast, RSD is not associated with a demonstrable partial nerve lesion. RSD (CRPS, type I) most likely reflects local trauma to nerve endings in the skin that are below the level of detection of present testing techniques. However, these pain syndromes are otherwise identical.

In the past, there was even greater confusion regarding terminology, because many different diagnostic names (Table 19–6) were being used clinically to describe essentially the same disorder. The reasons for this confusion (Table 19–7) were that (1) different specialists (orthopedic surgeons, rheumatologists, neurologists, anesthesiologists) used specific terms unique to their specialties to describe the painful conditions they observed in their own unique fashion, (2) different diagnoses were applied to painful conditions because they affected different regions of the body, and (3) different diagnoses were applied to painful conditions after a specific injury. However, the clinical features of RSD are all painted

**Table 19–5  Nomenclature**

Complex regional pain syndrome (CRPS)
  Type I, RSD, no nerve injury demonstrated
  Type II, causalgia, partial (incomplete) nerve injury

RSD = reflex sympathetic dystrophy.

**Table 19–6  Older Names for Reflex Sympathetic Dystrophy or Causalgia**

Algodystrophy
Major causalgia
Minor causalgia
Shoulder-hand syndrome
Sudeck's atrophy
Traumatic arthritis
Posttraumatic pain syndrome
Chronic traumatic edema
Traumatic vasospasm
Posttraumatic angiospasm
Spreading neuralgia
Posttraumatic osteoporosis

from the same palette, irrespective of the name applied to the diagnosis, so there is no difference in the spectrum of complaints and findings in any of these disorders. The unification of these varied conditions under the umbrella term complex regional pain syndrome is therefore quite helpful in terms of both focusing our interest on enhanced understanding of the pathogenesis of this condition and developing and administering more targeted forms of treatment.

The IASP change in nomenclature to emphasize the "complex" and "regional" aspects of the pain is quite useful. The complexity of the CRPS disorders reflects their ability to spread to other limbs (often in a mirror-image fashion), subtle features of autonomic dysfunction (which often go unrecognized until the condition progresses to a more severe form), and dissociation of the numerous symptoms found in CRPS from one another (e.g., pain, swelling, sweating, color change, temperature change), which characterize the disorders.

The regional distribution of the pain in CRPS mirrors the network-like organization of the sympathetic fibers along blood vessels. This pain pattern has often been criticized by physicians as "nonanatomic" and therefore has often been assumed to be "nonphysiologic," in contrast to the traditionally recognized defined distribution of a nerve root or peripheral nerve lesion, which is emphasized throughout anatomically based training.

In this regard, there are some who believe that the best way to establish a clinical diagnosis of RSD,

**Table 19–7  Reasons for Multiple Names of Reflex Sympathetic Dystrophy**

Specialty unique naming
  Orthopedists
  Rheumatologists
  Neurologists
Region-specific diagnoses
  Shoulder-hand syndrome
Injury-specific diagnoses
  Traumatic vasospasm

**Table 19–8  Classification of Pain**

Sympathetically mediated pain (SMP)
  Responsive to sympathetic nerve blocks
Sympathetically independent pain (SIP)
  Unresponsive to sympathetic nerve blocks
  Centralization

which is accepted as a pain syndrome mediated through hyperactivity of the sympathetic nervous system, is through demonstration of a positive response to a placebo-controlled, sympathetic nerve block rather than on clinical features alone. However, this too has its shortcomings.

When a patient responds with pain reduction to a properly performed sympathetic block (which blocks sympathetic activity and warms the limb), the pain may be considered sympathetically mediated pain (SMP). However, failure to respond to a such a nerve block does not preclude the diagnosis of RSD, because the patient may have progressed to a state of sympathetically independent pain (SIP) yet still suffer from RSD (Table 19–8).

The change from SMP to SIP is well recognized clinically. It has no relation to the three stages of RSD (I to III), which have been recognized (Table 19–9) and described as the acute, dystrophic, and atrophic stages. Instead, the progression from SMP to SIP is best conceptualized as "centralization" of the pain, from the point of peripheral origin to within the central nervous system (CNS), and has been considered by some to be a learning phenomenon. However, data for animal models of chronic neuropathic pain have demonstrated that there is a point in time after which there are permanent degenerative changes localized within the spinal cord dorsal root entry zone (DREZ). This is the region of the CNS where afferent sensory fibers, sympathetic fibers, and descending efferents converge and is the first relay station of the CNS where sensory input and painful sensations can be modulated.

The dropout of neurons in the DREZ has been attributed to vigorous and aberrant release of excitatory neurotransmitters into this region as part of the triggered persistent pain response. Excitatory neurotransmitters are toxic when present in abundance. This loss of neurons renders the pain unresponsive to previously viable peripheral measures, such as nerve blocks and movement therapy, hence the change from SMP to SIP. The anatomic and physiologic changes in the DREZ, secondary to per-

**Table 19–9  Stages of Reflex Sympathetic Dystrophy**

| Stage I | Acute |
| Stage II | Dystrophic |
| Stage III | Atrophic |

sistence of the pain syndrome and release of excitatory neurotransmitters, now require an altered treatment strategy to achieve pain relief and restore movement.

It should be noted that there are many links between the sensory and pain pathways and the control of movement. This should not be a surprising association in the context of recognizing that a primary goal of aversive movement is to avoid pain (i.e., withdrawal reflex). The goal of treatment remains relief of pain and restoration of movement, but the changes in the DREZ render further sympathetic blockade ineffective in the relief of pain symptoms. At this point, narcotic medications and possibly invasive procedures, such as use of the dorsal column stimulator and morphine pump, become the only modalities that allow adequate pain relief to facilitate movement.

Stated another way, failure to respond to a properly performed sympathetic block does not rule out RSD when the clinical features of RSD are present. Instead, it provides information indicating that there has been progression to the SIP state. Although the patient no longer responds to a sympathetic block, it should be clear that the clinical diagnosis remains that of an advanced stage of RSD. This should help to guide the clinician with certainty in the need for and justification of the use of pain-relieving medications in the treatment of this disorder.

Therefore, the diagnosis of RSD is best made on the basis of its clinical features. This diagnosis may or may not be supported by laboratory studies, where possible, and then further differentiated as either CRPS type I or type II.

## CLUES TO PATHOGENESIS

Involvement of the sympathetic nervous system, almost selectively, suggests two distinct possibilities that are not mutually exclusive: (1) a sympathotropic factor is released as a result of trauma and (2) a sympathetic ganglionic inflammatory process, with potential systemic effects, is activated as a result of trauma. Experimental studies support both of these possibilities.

Traumatic injury of peripheral nerves has been demonstrated experimentally to lead to the synthesis and release of nerve growth factor (NGF), which is normally present only during developmental stages and declines to low basal levels in the adult. NGF is the most potent sympathotropic factor recognized, with equally dramatic impact on the dorsal root ganglion sensory neurons as well.

The induction and release of NGF are accompanied by induction of the NGF receptor. In addition to its trophic actions on the sympathetic and dorsal

**Table 19–10  Hypothetic Pathogenesis of Reflex Sympathetic Dystrophy**

Trauma
Release of NGF, SP, IL-2
Stimulation of dorsal root ganglia and sympathetic ganglia
Release of excitatory amino acid neurotransmitters
Stimulation of NMDA receptors
Dorsal root entry zone degeneration
Activation of neurogenic inflammation
Reflex sympathetic dystrophy

NGF = nerve growth factor; SP = substance P; IL-2 = interleukin-2; NMDA = N-methyl-D-aspartate.

root ganglion cells, NGF has been recognized to have profound effects in stimulating inflammation. These include activation of the complement system and promoting the expansion of antibody-producing B cells of the immune system. Of further interest, injection of NGF into humans as part of therapeutic clinical trials for the treatment of chemotherapy-induced peripheral neuropathy reproduced the burning pain characteristic of RSD at the site of the injection.

In this way trauma, whether to nerve endings alone, as in a sprain, or through an incomplete nerve injury, as in a gunshot or knife wound, would lead to the induction and release of NGF. The NGF signal would activate both the dorsal root ganglia and sympathetic ganglia. The activation of these neuronal cell populations (Table 19–10) would (1) heighten their sensitivity in all modalities, (2) lead to the release of excitatory neurotransmitters within the DREZ, and (3) produce potentially destructive lesions of these ganglionic or locally (limb) affected structures as a result of activation of inflammatory processes (specifically, the complement system and antibody-producing B cells).

Histopathologic investigation of sympathetic ganglia surgically removed in an effort to treat RSD has been performed (Table 19–11). These ganglia were not previously traumatized by sympathetic nerve blocks at their location, because they were taken from sites remote from those at which sympathetic nerve blocks had been administered to these patients. The ganglia analyzed demonstrated findings such as neuronal vacuolization and atrophy, axonal beading, endothelial cell damage with early thrombus formation, and perivascular lymphocytic

**Table 19–11  Histopathology of the Sympathetic Ganglia in Reflex Sympathetic Dystrophy**

Neuronal vacuolization
Axonal beading
Atrophic neurons
Endothelial damage, early thrombus formation
Perivascular lymphocytic infiltration

infiltration. These findings are consistent with the interpretation of both "activated" neurons and an active inflammatory process. Some investigators, such as Fields and Basbaum, have described similar experimental findings as reflex neurogenic inflammation.

Ultrastructural changes observed in the sympathetic ganglia removed corroborate the histopathologic findings (Table 19–12). These include the presence of intracytoplasmic vacuoles, secondary demyelination, onion bulb–like structures, dilated endoplasmic reticulum, and abnormal mitochondria within the neuronal cells of the sympathetic ganglia. These findings are also consistent with both NGF-activated neurons and an active inflammatory process.

Other candidate sympathotropic and immunogenic molecules are produced in response to local trauma. These include substance P (SP) and the lymphokine interleukin-2 (IL-2). SP is released from nerve terminals as an early posttraumatic event. SP functions as a potent vasoactive molecule that has profound actions during inflammatory events but is a mediator of painful stimuli as well as having properties overlapping those of NGF. SP has also been shown to have direct stimulatory effects on sympathetic neurons and cells of the immune system but may no longer play a role when the disease process is established, because it was not detected locally in skin from patients with long-established RSD.

IL-2 is an immune system signal normally associated with the expansion of reactive lymphocytes important in both cellular and humoral immunity. It may be derived from inflammatory cells specifically recruited and activated by the local release of cytokines in response to trauma. Alternatively, IL-2 may be released from nonspecifically recruited cells trafficking through a traumatic lesion that are activated by the tissue factors present within the lesion. In either case, IL-2 has been shown to stimulate sympathetic neurons selectively, in addition to its known immunologic effects.

Therefore, NGF, SP, and IL-2 are three separate mediators that can selectively stimulate sympathetic neurons in response to an injury. It is easy to see that these molecules can be present in increased quantities after a local injury as part of the local

tissue response. Their impact on the sympathetic neurons associated with the affected region can be dramatic. From the perspective of survival, increased sensitivity to painful stimulation is advantageous because it contributes to a tendency to protect the affected limb from further trauma, as well as enhancing the response of withdrawal from further painful, and perhaps dangerous, stimuli. However, it is essential to move the affected limb in order to overcome the downside of this protective mechanism, progression of the pain syndrome.

Potentially related painful phenomena, independent of the pain resulting from the initial injury and that from the development of RSD, may contribute to further progression of the pain syndrome. This would occur through activation of herpesvirus infections latent within the sympathetic and/or dorsal root ganglion cells as a direct consequence of local trauma. Activation of herpesvirus replication is followed by both direct herpes-associated damage and immune attack related to an antiherpetic response. Experimentally, local trauma in the distribution of a neuron latently infected with herpesvirus has been demonstrated to reactivate the herpesvirus infection, leading to lytic replication in the neuron. In an immunologically intact individual, an antiviral inflammatory response also follows in the distribution of sympathetic and dorsal root ganglion cells in the region of injury.

Further studies are in progress to determine whether herpesvirus antigens are detectable in sympathetic ganglia removed at the time of surgical sympathectomy. A variety of localized skin reactions have been recognized in RSD and reflect the deposition of immune complexes in the skin. At present, these skin lesions are the most compelling observation of the involvement of cytokine, immune, and viral mechanisms in RSD. Thus, at least two separate mechanisms of trauma-induced changes, sympathotropic (NGF, SP, and IL-2) stimulation and herpesvirus reactivation, can contribute to the histopathologic features of RSD. These initiating events could then trigger subsequent events through humoral and inflammatory mechanisms.

In addition to the pain precipitated by trauma, RSD has been observed to occur after lesions of the CNS with associated immobilization. Immobilization may affect multiple levels within the neuraxis, either independently or in concert. One phenomenon is widening of the cortical receptive field, as in denervation supersensitivity, thus increasing the peripheral area of hypersensitivity. Therefore, multiple pathways, whether related to peripheral trauma or to CNS disease, can affect the pathogenesis of RSD. Furthermore, these mechanisms suggest interesting and testable hypotheses for the pathogenesis

**Table 19–12   Ultrastructural Changes of the Sympathetic Ganglia in Reflex Sympathetic Dystrophy**

Intracytoplasmic vacuoles
Secondary demyelination
Onion bulb–like structures
Dilated endoplasmic reticulum
Abnormal mitochondria

of this disorder, which must be better understood in order to provide more effective treatment.

## CLINICAL AND DIFFERENTIAL DIAGNOSIS

RSD can occur in any age group, tends to be more common in women than men for reasons that are not well understood, and usually follows injury to either a limb or another part of the body. The injury precipitating RSD need not be severe. The pain, however, persists beyond the anticipated time of recovery and is described as worse than expected from the scope of the injury. For example, injuries may range from minor traumas such as sprains and traction injuries to more damaging crush injuries or fractures, with which the anticipated recovery time is 6 to 8 weeks. Therefore, clinical suspicion of RSD should arise if traumatic pain persists, although not all sources of persistent pain are associated with RSD. In addition to injury, RSD may occur in the context of a paralyzed limb, stroke, tumor, or other CNS lesions.

The distribution of the pain in RSD is not typically within the territory of peripheral nerves or nerve roots but is regional and primarily distal. This is consistent with the regional distribution of the sympathetic nervous system. During the initial phase of RSD, many of its symptoms and signs are attributable to overactivity of the sympathetic nervous system supplying the affected area(s) of the body, although burning or deep aching pain remains the cardinal feature of RSD.

The sometimes minimally traumatic origins and regional distribution, often with subsequent spread to mirror-image regions of the opposite limb, coupled with limited familiarity with the spectrum of symptoms and signs associated with the earliest stages of this disorder, have resulted in persistent skepticism regarding the validity of this diagnosis. Patients are often labeled as having a "psychogenic" source of their persistent pain rather than a physical disorder. It is not hard to see that reactive depression can develop under these circumstances, yet this is secondary to the persistent pain and consequent impairment of function.

Sympathetic hyperactivity is clinically recognized by its interaction with somatic nerve fibers and the direct involvement of sympathetic nerves that help to regulate blood flow and blood pressure. Interaction with somatic neurons and nerve fibers leads to altered sensation and altered movement.

Altered sensation includes such features as burning and/or deeply aching and throbbing pain, allodynia (altered perception of simple somatic sensations, such as light touch, as painful), hyperesthesia (increased sensitivity and lowered threshold to tactile and painful stimuli), and hyperpathia (increased pain perception, although with an elevated threshold to stimulation). All of these features are experienced as worse with movement, a dependent posture, and low ambient temperature. This leads to resistance of the patient to mobilization of the affected extremity. In addition, there are abnormalities of movement, which include difficulties in initiating movements, dystonic posturing, localized spasms with movement, increased muscle tone, brisk reflexes, and tremors.

Direct involvement of the sympathetic nervous system includes tissue swelling (which is worst in a dependent posture, with increase in physical activity, and with low ambient temperatures), color change (mottling of the skin, purple discoloration related to venous stasis), temperature changes (usually coolness, although increased skin temperature may be present variably in the earliest stages of the disorder), increased sweating, and trophic changes (shiny skin, early hair growth and later hair loss, brittle nails).

It is at this stage that the disorder may be most responsive to sympathetic nerve blocks. Sometimes a positive response with pain relief by virtue of the block is considered "diagnostic" and taken as proof of the presence of RSD. However, as already discussed, there may be loss of responsiveness to sympathetic blocks because of progression of the condition to the SIP phase. Therefore, lack of response to a nerve block does not prove that the individual does not have RSD and does not mean that RSD is ruled out.

Clinical worsening of the disease may involve spread to other extremities and other parts of the body and the appearance of generalized symptoms including fevers and skin reactions suggestive of ongoing inflammation. The most advanced stage of RSD (stage III) is usually readily recognized because of its associated physical manifestations of atrophy and altered posturing of the affected extremity. Unfortunately, in stage III RSD reversal of symptoms is least likely, and commonly only partial pain relief can be achieved. Therefore, efforts to improve the awareness and recognition of RSD at earlier, more treatable stages, coupled with intensively applied treatment strategies, are warranted.

The pain and setting of the clinical presentation of RSD help to differentiate this condition from many other painful disorders (Table 19–13). However, it is imperative to note that there may be confounding underlying or coexistent painful radiculopathies, nerve entrapment conditions, or other painful conditions that must be considered in the differential diagnosis of RSD pain. This list includes lumbar radiculopathy, sciatica, tarsal tunnel syndrome, Morton's neuroma, diabetes, and idiopathic

**Table 19–13  Differential Diagnosis of Reflex Sympathetic Dystrophy**

Diabetes mellitus
Idiopathic painful polyneuropathy
Lumbar radiculopathy
Sciatica
Tarsal tunnel syndrome
Morton's neuroma

**Table 19–15  Diagnostic Sympathetic Nerve Blocks**

Effective in sympathetically maintained pain (SMP)
Ineffective in sympathetically independent pain (SIP)
Provide pain relief, albeit transiently, in SMP
Produce a rise in skin temperature when properly performed technically

painful polyneuropathy. These diagnoses can be excluded through the history and examination, supplemented with specific diagnostic testing where appropriate, such as electromyography or nerve conduction velocity studies, evoked potential testing, nerve and muscle biopsy, serologic studies for Lyme disease and syphilis, metabolic studies to search for an endocrinopathy, and blood work to look for antimyelin or antimembrane antibodies.

## DIAGNOSTIC TESTS

Diagnostic tests of value in corroborating the clinical diagnosis of RSD include thermography, triple-phase bone scan, plain radiographic examination of bone, magnetic resonance imaging (MRI) with gadolinium, diagnostic nerve block, electromyography and nerve conduction velocity studies, and quantitative sensory testing, all of which are listed in Table 19–14.

Thermography can reveal quantitative differences in limb temperatures in affected extremities,

**Table 19–14  Diagnostic Tests in Reflex Sympathetic Dystrophy**

Thermography—quantitates limb temperature differences, reflecting C-fiber dysfunction, but is too nonspecific to be relied on for diagnosis.
Triple-phase bone scan—may show increased uptake in the area affected by RSD. It is of value when positive but cannot be used to rule out RSD if negative.
Plain X-rays of bone—may show demineralization in the affected extremity. As with the triple-phase bone scan, it is of value when positive but cannot be used to rule out RSD if negative.
MRI with gadolinium—shows skin thickening, subcutaneous contrast enhancement, and occasionally soft tissue edema in stage I RSD. Shows muscle atrophy in stage III RSD. It is not definitive for stage II RSD.
Diagnostic nerve block—pain relief when there is sympathetically maintained pain (SMP) but no relief when there is sympathetically independent pain (SIP).
Electromyography and nerve conduction velocity—C-fiber abnormalities characteristic of RSD are below the level of detection of this technique.
Quantitative Sensory Testing—Identifies a raised threshold to sensory stimuli in severely affected extremities (stage III), but further testing of the technique is needed regarding specificity.

RSD = reflex sympathetic dystrophy; MRI = magnetic resonance imaging.

which are a function of C-fiber involvement in this disorder. However, these differences can also frequently be appreciated qualitatively by palpation and are not unique to RSD. Therefore, controversy has arisen regarding this form of evaluation, primarily because of interpretation of the results of the test with regard to a number of other disorders. At present, this technique is claimed to be too imprecise to be relied on in the diagnosis of RSD because of the significant pain relief when the disorder has progressed to the stage of SIP. Failure to recognize the occurrence of a transition from SMP to SIP and the impact of this change on the utility of a sympathetic nerve block in establishing the clinical diagnosis of RSD can undermine the diagnostic process (Table 19–15).

Electromyography and nerve conduction velocity studies cannot demonstrate the small-fiber pathology mediating the effects of RSD, because C-fiber function is below the level of detection of these studies. Quantitative sensory testing is a technique currently under study that appears to identify a raised threshold to sensory stimuli in RSD-affected extremities. It remains to be determined whether these are findings unique to RSD or are nonspecific.

## STAGING OF REFLEX SYMPATHETIC DYSTROPHY

Stage I RSD is described as the acute stage and is characterized by widespread variability in the nature of the symptoms present at any one time (Table 19–16). The pain, however, is best described as being out of proportion to the precipitating insult and is quite intense. Autonomic signs of swelling and discoloration may be masked by traumatically induced inflammatory changes in the tissue. The limb may be warmer or cooler to the touch at any given moment. The pain is described as a burning and/or deep aching pain and is worsened by movement, a dependent posture, and emotional distress. This leads to a tendency to "guard" the limb and limit its movement or any degree of contact causing friction. The pain, swelling, and discoloration often spread to the opposite limb in a mirror distribution and still later become generalized throughout the entire body.

Allodynia (distortion of all sensation as pain-

**Table 19–16  Magnetic Resonance Imaging Findings of Reflex Sympathetic Dystrophy**

Stage I
  Skin thickening
  Skin enhancement with gadolinium
  Subcutaneous edema
Stage II
  Inconsistent findings
Stage III
  Muscle atrophy

ful), hyperalgesia (increased areas of sensitivity to painful stimuli), and hyperpathia (an increased pain threshold with a disproportionate increase in perceived pain when the threshold is crossed) are seen. Edema is usually present in the affected area intermittently, along with increased hair growth (thicker and darker) and enhanced nail growth. The skin is initially hyperhidrotic. Bone changes (periarticular demineralization) are possible. This is the earliest stage of the disease. This stage is most responsive to treatment and generally corresponds to the SMP phase.

In contrast to the opinions that commonly appear in textbooks, there is no preset cadence at which all individuals progress, and it is conceivable for a patient to remain in stage I indefinitely. However, when progression occurs it tends to occur within 3 to 6 months after the onset of symptoms, although this varies from person to person. Therapeutic mobilization of the limb at the patient's own pace, but with regularity, is associated with the best outcome.

Stage II RSD is the dystrophic stage and is marked by constancy of pain and "brawny"-appearing edema. Sleep disruption, anxiety, and depression are associated with this progression. The skin changes from moist (hyperhidrotic) to dry (hypohidrotic), shiny, cyanotic, and hypothermic, with a mottled meshwork pattern of the vessels described as livedo reticularis. Hair loss in the affected region and dulled, ridged, and cracked nails now appear. X-ray films commonly show diffuse osteoporosis, as well as cystic changes and subchondral bone erosion. This stage may correspond to the switch from SMP to SIP as described.

Stage III is the atrophic stage and is not difficult to diagnose because of the often striking atrophy coupled with tight, shiny skin and dramatically altered posture of the affected limb. The skin is thin, shiny, dry, and cold. Proximal migration of the pain occurs, if it has not already done so. This pattern is in contrast to the distal spread of radicular pain. Irreversible skin, cartilage, muscle, and bone damage is evident. These findings include fascial thickening and limb contractures. The tips of the fingers and toes may appear tapered. Dupuytren's con-

tracture is often seen. X-ray films show bone demineralization and ankylosis. There is atrophy of muscle groups in the affected limb. The patient may be wheelchair dependent. The movement disorder of RSD (difficulty initiating movements, tremor, weakness, spasm, increased reflexes, and dystonic posturing) is most dramatic at this stage.

Clinical worsening of the disease may also involve spread to other extremities and the appearance of generalized symptoms such as fevers and skin reactions suggestive of ongoing inflammation, as well as somatic changes such as decreased vision, hearing, and swallowing; broken teeth; and disrupted bladder and bowel functions. The latter are also further compromised by some of the medications used in an effort to provide symptomatic relief.

## SYMPTOM COMPLEX OF REFLEX SYMPATHETIC DYSTROPHY

Sympathetic hyperactivity is clinically recognized as a constellation of variable symptoms that include burning or deep aching limb pain, which is maximal distally. The pain is regional and does not follow a nerve root, plexus, or peripheral nerve pattern, although secondary nerve entrapment (i.e., tarsal tunnel syndrome) may occur as a consequence of local tissue swelling. Additional features include allodynia (mechanical sensation perceived as pain) and hyperesthesia, which leads the patient to guard the affected extremity, preferring to wrap the limb than to risk contact with even a gentle breeze.

Other features are also often present, such as tissue swelling (worst in a dependent posture or with activity), color change (mottling of the skin, purple discoloration related to venous stasis), temperature change (initially variation between warmth and coolness and later only coolness), increased sweating early and decreased sweating later, as well as trophic changes (shiny skin, altered hair growth, brittle nails). Bone demineralization in the affected extremity is commonplace and can be apparent on a plain film.

Abnormalities of movement are frequently present and include difficulty in initiating movements, weakness, dystonic posturing, a variety of tremors, spasms, and increased tone and reflexes. These characteristics probably reflect the varied levels of interplay between the sympathetic nervous system and the somatic motor neurons in the anterior horn.

It has also come to be recognized that more than the initial site of involvement can become affected in RSD. The bladder and the eyes are two of the sites that most commonly reflect problems related to RSD. This may reflect the heavy sympathetic innervation of these structures or represent the effects of the medications used to help control the symptoms. In either event, their involvement can be disconcerting to the affected patient and may mislead the unsuspecting clinician in reaching a proper diagnosis. Symptomatic treatment of involvement of the eyes and the bladder is the best that can be offered at present.

## THERAPEUTIC PRINCIPLES

It must be emphasized that RSD is extremely painful and associated with severe spasms on even minor movements. These factors tend to combine to make the average patient quite reluctant to move an affected extremity, without specific and persistent encouragement, for fear of worsening the situation. In contrast, the professional athlete benefits from sustained therapeutic efforts because of the need for early mobilization. Working through pain is the athlete's motto. Athletes are not in fear of worsening their condition as a result of pain associated with their training regimen because of their level of motivation and the observation that consistent efforts lead to their improvement.

We must apply a similarly enthusiastic and supportive approach to the general public in treating RSD. This is especially important because treatment strategies generally recommended for dealing with trauma to a limb, such as a sprains, traction injuries, or broken bones, often utilize immobilization of the limb, including splinting or casting, further limiting the potential for movement necessary for remediating the painful condition of RSD.

Current treatments of RSD are based on decreasing the sympathetic activity in the affected extremity through the use of medications to limit the degree of pain associated with therapeutic programs of movement and physical therapy (Table 19–17). If mobility is restricted (by guarding or by a cast),

**Table 19–17  Recommended Treatment of Reflex Sympathetic Dystrophy**

First tier
  Identify underlying disease: fracture, sprain, radiculopathies,
    spinal stenosis
  Symptomatic treatments: drugs (antidepressant,
    anticonvulsant, analgesic)
  Physical therapy: regular, repetitive as tolerated, self-
    directed, aquatherapy
  Counseling of patient and family in chronic pain
    management techniques
Second tier
  Blocks: chemical sympathectomy
  Surgical sympathectomy
  Dorsal column stimulator
  Morphine pump
  Counseling of patient and family in chronic pain
    management techniques

there is rapid progression to more advanced stages of RSD, or there is severe edema of the affected limb, sympathetic nerve blocks should be attempted, usually in a series of five on alternate days if initially effective.

Rarely, if RSD is diagnosed early and is not particularly responsive to physical therapy but there is limited yet definite responsiveness to sympathetic blocks, surgical sympathectomy may be considered. Caution should be used in performing surgical sympathectomies on more than one limb because of potential problems with the control of blood pressure, but this has not proved a major problem in practice. However, the use of therapeutic surgical sympathectomy has fallen into some disfavor. It is a challenging procedure and there may be a postsympathectomy pain syndrome at the surgical site as well as recurrence of the original pain. Crossed sympathetic nerve blocks are suggested as one way of handling this recurrent pain.

Many other treatments have been advocated over the years, but their effectiveness has not been established beyond anecdotal reports. Included among this group are systemic steroids, calcitonin, calcium channel blockers, and α-adrenergic blockers. An additional issue related to the use of the latter two groups of agents is the frequent occurrence of hypertension in the context of chronic pain syndromes, for which those and other antihypertensive therapies are appropriate. Similarly, diuretics have been used judiciously in an effort to control local edema, but this requires close monitoring of the patient and should be reserved for the most extreme circumstances, using compression stockings instead.

Greater effectiveness has been achieved empirically through the early use of nonsteroidal anti-inflammatory drugs (NSAIDs); antidepressants (amitriptyline [Elavil], fluoxetine [Prozac], sertraline [Zoloft], and venlafaxine [Effexor]); and anticonvulsants (phenytoin [Dilantin], carbamazepine [Tegretol], gabopentin [Neurontin], and clonazepam [Klonopin]). Narcotic analgesics may frequently be required for adequate pain relief (propoxyphene hapsylate–acetaminophen [Darvocet], acetaminophen [Tylenol] with codeine, oxycodone-acetaminophen [Percocet], hydrocodone-acetaminophen [Lorcet 10/650], hydromorphone [Dilaudid], meperidine [Demerol], and morphine sulfate [MS Contin; MSIR]). Attention to the combination of therapies used and the prospect that medication is provided by more than one source is necessary. A contract with the patient detailing the medications and sources is helpful in this regard.

If diagnosed early and treated with aggressive physical therapy early, RSD can be successfully treated. However, there is often a long lag between onset of symptoms and the initiation of a program of sustained aggressive therapy for reasons that have already been addressed. A consequence of this delay is often progression of the syndrome with a need for more potent medications to help keep the pain at more tolerable levels and allow the individual to perform activities of daily living.

Early involvement of the sympathetic nervous system in RSD, almost selectively, suggests release of a sympathotropic factor as a result of trauma. NGF is rapidly inducible after nerve injury, as is the NGF receptor. In addition to its trophic actions on the sympathetic and dorsal root ganglion cells, NGF has been recognized to have profound effects in mediating pain and stimulating inflammation. Other candidate sympathotropic molecules include SP and the lymphokine IL-2. SP is released from nerve terminals as an early posttraumatic event and is a potent vasoactive molecule that has profound actions during inflammatory events and a mediator of painful stimuli as well as having properties overlapping those of NGF. SP has also been shown to have direct stimulatory effects on sympathetic neurons but may no longer play a role when the disease process is established, because it was not detected locally in skin from patients with established RSD. Capsaicin, derived from red-hot chili peppers, causes depletion of this molecule and has been advocated by some for the treatment of RSD. However, the action of SP in the genesis of the pain of RSD may be an early event, rendering capsaicin ineffective by the time it is used clinically.

## SPECIFIC THERAPY

In determining the specific course of treatment, consideration must be given to the severity of the underlying clinical disorder, duration of illness, past response to treatment regimen, side effects, and likely need for treatment. It is imperative to consider the risk-benefit ratio of the specific treatment chosen. This is especially true of the agents that are used in the treatment of RSD and their associated risks. A generalized approach was provided in Table 19–17.

A limited degree of pain control is first attempted with NSAIDS, tricyclic antidepressants, and anticonvulsants individually or in some combination that works best for the individual patient. A more potent analgesic may be needed to overcome severe pain and to help the patient sleep at night. However, these measures are usually ineffective alone in completely controlling the pain. The patient must be reassured that despite the pain, in the absence of an underlying structural abnormality (such as torn ligaments or a fracture), no harm is done by movement of the painful limb and regular movement is the surest way to combat the pain of early stage I RSD.

Patients are usually reluctant to accept physical therapy as a treatment because of the intensity of the pain, but they must be motivated to move if there is no structural instability, such as in orthopedic injuries with casts. In the event of the latter, a course or more of five nerve blocks is administered to the affected region until movement can be resumed. When patients attempt to reduce pain by guarding the limb, they are actually making the condition worse. Physical therapy is believed to lead to more rapid resolution of the underlying nerve injury. A particularly effective form of physical therapy is aquatic therapy. Patients simply need to move around in a pool, in which the water supports the limb against gravity while simultaneously providing resistance to motion.

I prefer a self-directed physical therapy program, because some patients are inclined to stop treatment if the limb is manipulated too vigorously, and they work better at their own pace. However, some patients need the structure of a therapist-directed program. The addition of an aquatic component is helpful and need not involve anything more complicated than getting into lukewarm water and moving around.

Throughout the self- or therapist-directed physical therapy program, I advocate the continued use of either the antidepressant Elavil (preferred over the generic amitriptyline, titrating up to 150 mg at bedtime in 10-mg intervals initially) or the anticonvulsant Neurontin (gabapentin, titrating up to as much as one or two 300-mg capsules three times daily, but beginning with 100 mg at bedtime, for the relief of the burning pain. Klonopin, 0.5 mg, one or two tablets at bedtime, helps to aid sleep by aiding in the control of spasms, and an NSAID with food reduces acute inflammation and provides some pain relief.

The use of tizanidine (Zanaflex), the antispasticity agent, has also proved helpful for the treatment of activity-induced spasms and stiffness in the legs that interferes with movement of the affected limb during daytime activities and with falling asleep. The 4 mg tizanidine tablet is cross-scored, so that it can easily be broken into quarter tablets, providing four 1 mg doses per tablet. Patients are started on one quarter of a tablet at bedtime and instructed to use as much as one quarter tablet at two-hour intervals during the day or during periods of physical therapy if necessary. This is because when this medication is first started, patients find that they can get quite tired from even this low dosage. Starting at bedtime helps them to get to sleep and allows them the opportunity to gradually escalate the dosage as needed. The maximum dose is eight full tablets per day, but it is unlikely that this amount will be needed. Most find that a dose of one to 12 mg per day is adequate to control their symptoms.

If needed, I frequently prescribe a codeine-containing (Tylenol 3, one to two tablets at 4-hour intervals, limiting these to six tablets per day) or a hydrocodone-containing (Lorcet 10/650, one to two tablets at 4-hour intervals, limiting these to six tablets per day) narcotic analgesic. Narcotic analgesics may be added at any stage of treatment as an adjunct for pain control.

The use of baclofen (Lioresal), titrating slowly up to 10 to 20 mg, using one to two tablets three times daily, helps to overcome both dystonic posturing and falls resulting from sudden weakness and collapse of the lower extremities. Such falls may be particularly problematic in patients with RSD secondary to a brachial plexus traction injury (neurogenic thoracic outlet syndrome), which should also be treated if present to achieve better pain relief of the RSD. Surgery in the context of RSD is always a matter of concern, but it has been performed successfully by arranging for blocks before to the procedure and then again afterward.

These initial steps may be followed by additional chemical sympathetic blockade with local anesthetic (the blocks at our center are performed by anesthesiologists), surgical sympathectomy, dorsal column stimulation, and finally a morphine pump. Some form of counseling is of value if the pain persists to help both the individual and family members adjust to the alteration in lifestyle that often accompanies severe chronic pain.

More severe pain requires the use of a stronger narcotic analgesic. This may include methadone, used in 5- to 10-mg increments, with one or two tablets up to three times a day, or continuous-release morphine in the form of MS Contin twice daily (15-, 30-, 60-, and 100-mg tablets are available), which is supplemented with immediate-release morphine in the form of MSIR at 15 to 30 mg up to four times daily for breakthrough pain. I have found that divalproex sodium (Depakote), in doses ranging from 125 mg at bedtime to 250 mg up to four times per day, has helped to stabilize patients' needs for narcotic medication, perhaps through altering tolerance, but this is not known at present.

Localized limb pain has also been treated successfully with a dorsal column stimulator. This technique can be quite helpful if there is truly isolated limb pain, but the disadvantage is that the patient cannot have an MRI study with this paramagnetic device in place.

With more diffuse pain that becomes resistant to oral narcotics (tolerance) or when the patient cannot tolerate gastrointestinal side effects (antiperistalsis of the stomach—gastroparesis—with reflux and nausea and chronic constipation), effective treatment has been achieved with the intrathecal delivery of much lower doses of morphine directly into the spinal fluid, and bypassing the gastrointestinal system, through the use of a pump delivery system.

Also, a variety of surgical ablative procedures that alter the patient's response to pain in the most severe circumstances are truly last-resort measures for treatment. If these measures fail, the only recourse is medication management and supportive counseling. Suicide has been a choice of some patients who have had difficulties in adjusting to their pain, so ongoing evaluation of how affected patients cope is needed for truly comprehensive management, and a team approach is suggested to avoid "burnout" of both the patient and the caregivers.

## SUMMARY

Current treatments of RSD are based on decreasing the sympathetic activity in the affected extremity through the use of physical therapy, sympathetic nerve blocks, surgical sympathectomy, and related treatments. Therapeutic intervention is evolving along with our understanding of RSD. At present, early mobilization in an aquatic setting appears to be the best modality for treating the new onset of symptoms. Removing as many of the triggers of pain as possible would appear to be the next modality. Finally, medications to address the chronic pain are the last, but essential, resort.

## BIBLIOGRAPHY

Campbell JN, Raja SN: Reflex sympathetic dystrophy. Neurology 45:1235–1236, 1995.
Dubner R, Ruda MA: Activity dependent neuronal plasticity following tissue injury and inflammation. Trends Neurosci 15:96–102, 1992.
Haugen PK, Letourneau PC: Interleukin-2 enhances chick and rat sympathetic, but not sensory, neuritic outgrowth. J Neurosci Res 25:443–452, 1990.
Knobler RL: Reflex sympathetic dystrophy. In Johnson RT, Griffin JW (eds): Current Therapy in Neurologic Disease, 5th ed. St. Louis, CV Mosby, 1996, pp 80–84.
Kozin F: Reflex sympathetic dystrophy syndrome: A review. Clin Exp Rheumatol 10:401–409, 1992.
Morgan EL, McClurg MR, Janda JA: Suppression of human B lymphocyte activation by beta endorphin. J Neuroimmunol 28:209–217, 1990.
Price RW, Katz BJ, Notkins AL: Latent infection of the peripheral ANS with herpes simplex virus. Nature 257:686–688, 1975.
Schwartzman RJ: Reflex sympathetic dystrophy. Curr Opin Neurol Neurosurg 6:531–536, 1993.
Schweitzer MF, Mandel S, Schwartzman RJ, et al: Reflex sympathetic dystrophy revisited: MR imaging findings before and after infusion of contrast material. Radiology 195:211–214, 1995.
Taniuchi M, Clark HB, Johnson EM Jr: Induction of nerve growth

factor receptor in Schwann cells after axotomy. Proc Natl Acad Sci U S A 83:4094–4098, 1986.

Verdugo R, Ochoa JL: Reflex sympathetic dystrophy. Neurology 45:1236–1237, 1995.

Walz MA, Price RW, Notkins AL: Latent ganglionic infection with herpes simplex virus types 1 and 2: Viral reactivation in vivo after neurectomy. Science 184:1185–1187, 1974.

Webster GF, Schwartzman RJ, Jacoby RA, et al: Reflex sympathetic dystrophy. Occurrence of inflammatory skin lesions in patients with stages II and III disease. Arch Dermatol 127:1541–1544, 1991.

Webster GF, Iozzo RV, Schwartzman RJ, et al: Reflex sympathetic dystrophy: Occurrence of chronic edema and non-immune bullous skin lesions. J Am Acad Dermatol 28:29–32, 1993.

Wybran J, Appelboom T, Famaey JP, Govaerts A: Suggestive evidence for receptors for morphine and methionine-enkephalin on normal human T lymphocytes. J Immunol 123:1068–1070, 1979.

# Infections of the Lower Extremity

# 20

*Russell J. Stumacher*

## GENERAL PRINCIPLES AND PATHOPHYSIOLOGY

Infections involving the lower extremities manifest themselves as local inflammatory changes associated, to varying degrees, with systemic responses, including fevers, tachycardia, and changes in blood pressure. Potential sites of involvement include the skin, subcutaneous tissue, fascia, muscle, synovium and joints, bones, and regional lymph nodes.

Specific clinical presentations depend on the site of involvement, species of infecting pathogens, inoculum size, and specific toxins as well as other virulence factors of responsible microorganisms.

β-Hemolytic streptococci, including group A *Streptococcus pyogenes* as well as Lancefield group B, C, and G serotypes, produce exotoxins, such as hyaluronidase, fibrinolysins, NADases, and deoxyribonucleases A and B. These exotoxins are antiphagocytic and enhance the spread of infection, resulting in rapid proximal extension of soft tissue erythema at a rate of approximately 1 cm/h, a notable clinical characteristic of streptococcal soft tissue infections.

Erythrogenic toxins of group A streptococci are responsible for scarlet fever, whereas other streptococcal toxins produce toxic shock–like syndromes produced by staphylococcal enterotoxin F or exotoxin C (toxic shock syndrome toxin 1). Different exotoxins found in specific serotypes of group A streptococci appear to contribute to the development of necrotizing fasciitis and myositis.

β-Hemolytic streptococci also have a propensity to invade regional lymphatics, producing lymphangitis, which is recognized clinically by erythematous, linear streaking extending proximally from primary site of infection, a pathognomonic sign of infection with these organisms.

Lastly, certain M types (e.g., 2, 4, 12, 36, 49, 50, 51) and "Red Lake," all major producers of deoxyribonuclease B, are so-called nephritogenic strains of *S. pyogenes* that may engender postinfectious acute poststreptococcal glomerulonephritis by deposition of streptococcal antigen-antibody complexes in renal glomeruli.

*Staphylococcus aureus*, by contrast, produces coagulase, catalase, and clumping factor, as well as dermonecrotic and other toxins that promote abscess formation and localize infectious foci. Other staphylococcal toxins inhibit qualitative neutrophilic function. Leukocidins, in particular, are lethal to polymorphonuclear leukocytes. Catalase also qualitatively impairs killing of certain phagocytosed bacterial species (e.g., *S. aureus* and aerobic gram-negative bacilli) by degrading bactericidal hydrogen peroxide produced by these organisms.

Staphylococcal enterotoxin F or exotoxin C (toxic shock syndrome toxin 1) acts as a superantigen that activates monocytes, macrophages, neutrophils, and endothelial cells to produce cytokines and other endogenous mediators (e.g., tumor necrosis factors, interleukins, β-endorphins, endothelial relaxation and platelet-activating factors, kinins, and the complement and cyclooygenase systems). These by-products, in turn, produce fever, myocardial depression, shock, diarrhea, diffuse organ system failure, and the diffuse erythema with desquamation characteristic of toxic shock syndrome.

Lastly, exfoliating toxins (e.g., exfoliatin) lead to blister formation and the so-called staphylococcal scalded skin syndrome of infancy and childhood.

Other toxin-producing bacteria include *Clostridium perfringens* and other clostridial species whose phospholipases, lecithinases, and other toxins, in the setting of severe circulatory impairment, contribute to tissue necrosis, toxemia, and the delirium typical of clostridial myonecrosis (i.e., gas gangrene). The toxins of *Vibrio vulnificus* contribute to necrotizing myositis secondary to seawater exposure. Exotoxin A of *Pseudomonas aeruginosa* contributes to the development of ecthyma gangrenosum, the septic venulitis responsible for this pathognomonic peripheral manifestation of *P. aeruginosa* sepsis.

Host factors are also important determinants of lower extremity infection, including underlying disease, circulatory status, previous surgery, the presence of foreign bodies, vascular grafts, artificial prostheses, and prior chemotherapy, including corticosteroids, immunosuppressive therapy, cancer chemotherapy, and antibiotics.

The incidence, clinical presentation, and outcome of leg infections, like those of infections elsewhere in the body, also depend on the effectiveness of the patient's immunologic resistance and responses to infection. Certain underlying diseases have intrinsic propensities to impair specific host defenses.

Diabetes mellitus, cirrhosis, chronic renal insufficiency, corticosteroid therapy, and acute lymphatic and myelocytic leukemias, for example, qualitatively impair polymorphonuclear leukocyte and monocyte chemotaxis, phagocytosis, and killing of ingested microorganisms. These defects heighten both the frequency and severity of resulting infections.

Patients with human immunodeficiency virus (HIV) infection, Hodgkin's disease or other forms of lymphoma, organ transplantation, or corticosteroid treatment have impaired cellular immunity, predisposing to infections with intracellular pathogens such as *Listeria*, salmonella, mycobacteria (tuberculous and atypical species), herpesviruses such as simplex and zoster, and fungi such as *Cryptococcus neoformans* and *Histoplasma capsulatum*. With the exception of *Listeria monocytogenes*, all of these microorganisms may produce focal infections involving the lower extremity.

In like manner, insulin-dependent diabetics, intravenous drug abusers, and patients receiving chronic hemodialysis are frequent skin and nasal carriers of *S. aureus* and exhibit increased frequencies of localized and systemic infections related to apparent inoculation of these bacteria during procedures or the administration of medications, insulin, or narcotics.

Other patient-related factors contributing to lower extremity infections include foreign bodies, artificial grafts, and artificial joints, which promote morbidity by reducing the inocula of microorganisms necessary to induce infection, providing sanctuaries for pathogens against host defenses and antimicrobial agents, and precluding cure by antibiotics alone without removing these devices. Venous and lymphatic edema, pressure sores resulting from immobility related to hemiplegia or paraplegia, sensory impairment caused by peripheral neuropathy, diffuse skin disease such as eczema or psoriasis, and the adequacy of the patient's arterial circulation each may predispose to and facilitate infection.

Arterial insufficiency, either of large vessels in atherosclerosis obliterans or microangiopathy in diabetes mellitus, is of particular importance. Resulting ischemia, tissue necrosis, and gangrene augment sensory neuropathies that reduce pain and other sensations, thus facilitating bacterial invasion. Leg ulceration as well as gas-forming, notably anaerobic and coliform infections of soft tissue, fascia, or muscle are additional important clinical by-products of these events.

Exogenous factors also contribute to leg infec-

tion. Blunt and penetrating trauma, insect and animal bites, burns and other forms of tissue necrosis, incisions and other surgically induced breaks in the cutaneous barrier to infecting agents, and coinfection with other pathogens, notably superficial dermatophytic fungi and herpesviruses, all permit the entry of potential pathogens into soft tissue.

## Pathophysiology

The initial step in the development of leg infections is the entry of pathogens into soft tissues. Direct inoculation appears to be the most important mechanism in this regard. This may occur as a result of scratches; penetrating trauma by thorns, nails, or splinters; mosquito, tick, or animal bites; inoculation intra- or postoperatively; and contamination during dressing changes or by soil, if in the setting of trauma.

Other mechanisms of bacterial invasion include hematogenous seeding by microorganisms from remote infections elsewhere in the body. Examples include septic emboli emanating from endovascular infections such as infective endocarditis, in turn producing metastatic abscesses; gangrene of digits if the emboli are bland; macular lesions involving the palms and soles (e.g., Janeway's lesions in the setting of acute bacterial endocarditis with *S. aureus*), and the lower extremity and trunk with disseminated candidiasis; and seeding of joints, especially the hip, knee, or ankle, leading to septic arthritis, or the metaphyses of the femur and tibia, producing hematogenous osteomyelitis.

Systemic diseases characterized by sepsis and disseminated intravascular coagulation, such as meningococcemia or pneumococcal sepsis in splenectomized patients, may produce widespread purpuric lesions in addition to septic shock and almost prohibitive mortality.

Immunologic responses (e.g, exuberant delayed hypersensitivity) in primary infections with *Mycobacterium tuberculosis* or fungi such as *H. capsulatum* or *Coccidioides immitis*, as well as noninfectious diseases (e.g., sarcoidosis and inflammatory bowel disease) may lead to the formation of tender, reddish purple nodules over the upper anterior tibial regions characteristic of erythema nodosum.

Finally, infections may spread locally from the inside out and vice versa. Examples include cellulitis, abscesses, and fistulas emanating from osteomyelitis and, contrariwise, the development of small-bone osteomyelitis by the extension to bone of overlying soft tissue foot infections in patients with arterial insufficiency, diabetic microangiopathy, sensory neuropathy, or pressure sores.

## CLINICAL PRESENTATIONS

The general manifestations of lower extremity infections are those of inflammation, stemming from inflammatory cytokines and/or toxin release, that is, erythema (rubor), swelling (tumor), pain and tenderness (dolor), and increased warmth (calor) of the involved areas. In addition, abscess formation, purulent wound drainage, fistulous tracts, subcutaneous nodules, crepitus or radiographic demonstration of gas in soft tissues or both, regional adenopathy, a variety of rashes, localized bone tenderness, or painful, swollen, virtually immobilized joints with effusion may occur, depending on the inciting pathogen and the site of involvement. If blood stream invasion by pathogens and/or sufficient inflammation or cytokine release is present, fevers, tachycardia, rigors, sweats, hemodynamic instability, altered central nervous system function, and other manifestations of sepsis occur.

In a few specific instances, the clinical presentation of infections, particularly the appearance of the extremity, may suggest specific pathogens. Erysipelas and/or lymphangitis is virtually pathognomonic of infection with group A or other Lancefield groups of β-hemolytic streptococci (i.e, B, C, or G). Ecthyma gangrenosum indicates *P. aeruginosa* or *Aeromonas hydrophila* septicemia. Erythema chronicum migrans is pathognomonic of the first stage of Lyme disease.

For the most part, however, clinical manifestations of leg infections are too nonspecific and/or overlapping to permit definitive diagnosis in and of themselves. Furthermore, noninfectious conditions may mimic infections. For example, deep vein thrombosis of the lower extremity may mimic cellulitis. Charcot neurogenic arthropathy may mimic osteomyelitis. Large necrotic skin ulcers related to ulcerative colitis–associated pyoderma gangrenosum, factitious self-administered trauma, or arterial insufficiency may mimic syphilitic gummas or mycobacterial or fungal infection. Bullae and blebs in toxic epidermal necrolysis, an extreme form of drug hypersensitivity, may mimic findings in staphylococcal scalded skin syndrome.

These overlapping presentations necessitate additional diagnostic maneuvers. These include Gram stains and cultures of wound drainage; needle aspirates of the advancing edge of cellulitis for Gram stain and culture; radiographs and radionuclide scans to rule out gas-forming infection or osteomyelitis; computed tomographic (CT) or magnetic resonance imaging (MRI) scans to detect suppurative myositis or osteomyelitis; arthrocenteses for suspected joint infections, with cell counts and white blood cell (WBC) differential, Gram stains and cultures, and joint fluid examination using polarizing microscopy to detect urate or calcium pyrophosphate crystals; blood cultures; various serologic tests; and lastly biopsies of skin lesions, bones, or abnormally enlarged lymph nodes for routine as well as special cultures and for special microbial tissue stains and histopathologic analysis.

## CLINICAL SYNDROMES

### The Discolored, Swollen, Painful Leg

It is important to recognize and then eliminate the possibility of infectious disease mimics. The most important of these is deep vein thrombosis, especially involving the saphenous vein in the calf. Manifestations of this condition include circumferential, usually nonerythematous, often pitting edema, associated with pain on manual compression, and often a positive Homans sign (i.e., calf pain on dorsiflexion of the great toe). Temperatures as high as 102.4°F may occur. Diagnostic confirmation depends on noninvasive tests (Doppler ultrasonography or contrast venography).

The onset of pain, localized muscle swelling within specific fascial compartments of the anterior or lateral lower leg, diminished arterial pulses, and paresthesias after trauma, burns, or use of tight surgical dressings may suggest an acute compartment syndrome. If it is not diagnosed quickly, that is, within 4 hours of onset, irreversible motor neuropathy and ischemic changes may evolve. The diagnosis is confirmed by measurement of interstitial compartment pressure. Readings of 30 torr or greater are strongly suggestive of the diagnosis. This condition is considered a surgical emergency and requires immediate surgical decompression and fasciotomy.

Erythema chronicum migrans, a cutaneous manifestation of primary Lyme disease, may mimic cellulitis and sometimes involve the lower extremity. The disease tends to occur between May and September, the period of maximal disease vector prevalence. Circumferential involvement of the leg does not occur. The lesion's characteristic early morphology is that of a small, indurated, reddened papule at the site of an *Ixodes dammini* (deer tick) bite. This species of tick is the primary vector for *Borrelia burgdorferi*, the etiologic agent of Lyme disease.

The initial lesion eventually progresses to a large annular plaque with a reddish blue border and a clear center. Multiple lesions are frequent. Concomitant fever, fatigue, malaise, headache, stiff neck, arthralgias, and myalgias may sometimes occur. *Borrelia* may be detected in biopsies of lesions with special stains or via specific DNA probes. Specific antibody tests with enzyme-linked immunosorbent assay (ELISA) and confirmatory Western blot methodology are frequently negative, although they eventually become positive. Early antibiotic treatment, however, may abort the development of antibodies.

Therapy of erythema chronicum migrans entails 21-day courses of doxycycline, 100 mg orally every 12 hours; amoxicillin, 500 mg orally three times daily, plus probenecid, 500 mg by mouth twice daily; or clarithromycin, 500 mg orally twice daily.

The most common cause of swelling, erythema, pain, and tenderness of the leg, however, is cellulitis. As mentioned earlier, the most common etiologic agents are β-hemolytic streptococci and S. aureus. Usual sites of bacterial entry are those of prior trauma or skin breaks, although the actual site of inoculation may often be inapparent. Recurrent bouts of cellulitis may complicate chronic lymphedema caused by prior cellulitis, malignant lymphatic obstruction, or filiariasis or may occur in legs from which saphenous vein segments have been harvested for coronary artery bypass grafting.

Erythema, warmth, tenderness, and swelling associated with cellulitis tend to occur over specific areas without circumferential involvement of the leg. As noted, streptococcal infections tend to remain localized to the initial infectious site.

Erysipelas, a painful, bright red, sharply demarcated lesion with raised, rapidly advancing edges and frequent associated high fevers and rigors, strongly suggests group A S. pyogenes infection, although, as noted earlier, cases have also been associated with group B, C, or G streptococci. Erysipelas has been a rare manifestation of P. aeruginosa infection in immunocompromised hosts and has been seen in 10% to 45% of cases of familial Mediterranean fever. In the latter, failure to respond favorably to systemic antibiotics, the periodicity of recurrences, and the Mediterranean ethnicity of patients have pointed to the diagnosis.

Soft tissue infections with S. aureus classically take the form of folliculitis, superficial abscesses or pyoderma, furunculosis (multiple boils), or deeper seated abscesses known as carbuncles or ecthyma. Diagnosis may be established by Gram stains and cultures of pus, wound drainage, or aspirates of lesions or abscesses.

Diffuse, poorly localized staphylococcal cellulitis may also occur and significantly overlap on clinical presentation with β-hemolytic streptococcal infections. Staphylococcal cellulitis tends not to progress rapidly (i.e., 1 cm/h) in contrast to streptococcal cellulitis. Given the degree of clinical overlap between these two conditions, antibiotic therapy should be directed against β-hemolytic streptococci and S. aureus.

Staphylococcal penicillinase production should be presumed. For the non–penicillin-allergic patient, intravenous (IV) semisynthetic, penicillinase-resistant penicillins should be selected, for example, nafcillin or oxacillin, 1.5 g IV every 6 hours. Oral outpatient therapy should include dicloxacillin, 500 mg to 1.0 g orally every 6 hours, either 0.5 hour before or 2 hours after eating to ensure maximum gastrointestinal antibiotic absorption as well as therapeutic serum antibiotic concentrations.

For the penicillin-allergic patient whose allergy is not immunoglobulin E (IgE) mediated (i.e., who has an immediate hypersensitivity reaction such as giant urticaria, anaphylaxis, or angioneurotic edema), parenteral cefazolin, 1.0 g IV every 8 hours, may be used, with cephalexin or cephradine at 500 mg by mouth every 6 hours (again on an empty stomach) when oral therapy is warranted.

In the event of immediate hypersensitivity to penicillins or if methicillin-resistant S. aureus is a consideration, vancomycin at 19 mg/kg IV every 12 hours is the agent of choice when creatinine clearance (Clcr) equals or exceeds 60 mL/min, every 24 to 36 hours for Clcr 41 to 59 mL/min, every 36 to 48 hours for Clcr 31 to 40 mL/min, and every 48 to 72 hours for Clcr 20 to 20 mL/min.

Potentially useful oral alternatives include clindamycin, 300 mg by mouth four times a day for penicillin-resistant, methicillin-sensitive strains (methicillin-sensitive S. aureus, [MSSA]) but not methicillin-resistant S. aureus (MRSA). Trimethoprim-sulfamethoxasole, 300 or 1600 mg (two double-strength tablets) twice daily, is useful for susceptible MRSA. Another potential oral alternative antibiotic for MRSA may be minocycline, 200 mg as a loading dose followed by 100 mg by mouth twice daily, for strains with demonstrable susceptibility to this antibiotic.

The usual duration of antimicrobial therapy for cellulitis, assuming a satisfactory clinical response to treatment, is approximately 7 to 10 days. Additional measures that abet treatment include rest and elevation of the involved leg, frequent applications of moist heat, débridement of necrotic tissues, and drainage of abscesses.

An enlarged, swollen, tender leg after immersion in seawater, frequently with superficial hemorrhage, bullae, and toxemia, suggests cellulitis and/or myositis caused by V. vulnificus, a halophilic, saltwater, gram-negative vibrio that gains access to soft tissues through breaks in the skin. This infection tends to be rapidly progressive, leading to extensive skin, soft tissue, and muscle necrosis. In patients with Laennec's cirrhosis or diseases associated with iron overload (e.g., chronic hemolytic anemias) or recipients of multiple blood transfusions, bacterial invasion of the blood stream with sepsis and/or shock may occur. Intravenous tetracyclines (e.g., doxycycline, 100 mg every 12 hours) are antibiotics of first choice. Early and extensive soft tissue and muscle débridement may be necessary as well.

Cellulitis after prolonged immersion in fresh water may be due to *A. hydrophila*, an aerobic gram-negative bacillus. In this case, quinolones (i.e., ofloxacin or ciprofloxacin) or aminoglycosides are required.

Cellulitis occurring in splenectomized patients with recent dog bites may be due to DF-2 bacillus, now *Capnocytophaga canimorsus*. Sepsis frequently complicates this infection. Antibiotics likely to be effective against this organism include clindamycin, ampicillin-sulbactam IV or ampicillin-clavulanate by mouth, and quinolones (e.g., ciprofloxacin).

Suppurative myositis, or pyomyositis, is another consideration, especially when muscle pain and tenderness are detected, evolving to woody induration of involved muscles and eventual fluctuation in some cases. The pathophysiology of this entity is thought to involve hematogenous seeding of preexisting focal areas of damaged muscle (hematomata). Cases were originally restricted to tropical, underdeveloped regions, especially in undernourished individuals. Ninety-five percent are due to *S. aureus*. Cases have begun to appear in the United States with increased frequency, especially in patients with advanced human immunodeficiency virus infection or intravenous drug abusers.

Elevated serum creatine phosphokinase levels are rarely noteworthy in pyomyositis. Magnetic resonance scans of involved areas, with guided aspiration of demonstrable collections for Gram stains and cultures, are necessary to establish the diagnosis. Bacteremia occurs in 5% to 15% of cases and mandates blood cultures as well. Therapy involves parenteral antistaphylococcal antibiotics as noted earlier, as well as incision, drainage, and débridement, if necessary, of involved areas.

## Cutaneous Abscesses

Cutaneous abscesses are among the most common infections encountered in clinical medicine. *S. aureus* is by far the most frequently encountered pathogen. Infections with mixed bacterial flora may also occur (i.e., anaerobic gram-positive and gram-negative bacteria, aerobic gram-negative bacilli, aerobic streptococci, and staphylococci in varying combinations), especially when abscesses are located in the perineum or over bony promontories, such as the sacrum, greater trochanters, knees, heels, and ankles. The latter abscesses are frequently associated with and may be due to underlying osteomyelitis.

The most common abscesses, however, are furuncles or "boils," which originate from *S. aureus* infections of sebaceous glands or of obstructed hair follicles (e.g., folliculitis) that coalesce to form the furuncles. Localized findings include inflammatory changes with ultimate fluctuation. Fever and constitutional findings are rare.

Antibiotics are unnecessary for furunculosis in the normal host, and therapy entails topical moist heat applications to facilitate localization of the abscess, followed by incision and drainage with immediate Gram staining and culture.

Empirical antibiotic therapy with antistaphylococcal antibiotics should be administered, however, for folliculitis or furunculosis in high-risk patients: patients with diabetes mellitus, malignancy, or other immunocompromising underlying diseases; those receiving hemodialysis; patients with preexisting valvular heart disease or valvular or other prosthetic devices; or those in whom concomitant cellulitis, osteomyelitis, fever, or signs of sepsis are present.

IV vancomycin should be used whenever MRSA is a possibility or has been isolated in cultures. For non–penicillin-allergic patients with MSSA, IV nafcillin or oxacillin or oral dicloxacillin is preferred, with IV cefazolin for non-IgE penicillin allergy or clindamycin IV or by mouth when IgE penicillin allergy is present.

The differential diagnosis of folliculitis includes drug hypersensitivity eruptions; viral exanthems such as varicella or various enteroviral infections; infestations such as scabies (although this condition usually develops on the trunk, hands, upper extremities, and pubic areas); and *P. aeruginosa* folliculitis secondary to immersion in poorly chlorinated hot tubs or spas, although lesions in this disorder are typically confined to areas covered by bathing suits (i.e., the hips, buttocks, lateral torso, and axillae). Furunculosis may itself raise the possibility of septic emboli from infective endocarditis or IV catheter–associated septic thrombophlebitis.

Carbuncles and ecthyma reflect coalescence of multiple adjacent furuncles; are more deep-seated; are erythematous, warm, and tender; and are often accompanied by fever and other systemic signs. Bacteremia may be induced by self-manipulation of the lesions. The infecting pathogen is invariably *S. aureus*. Systemic antistaphylococcal antibiotics are often necessary, in addition to incision and drainage with Gram staining and culture.

Abscesses located over "pressure points" (the sacrum, hips, knees, ankles, or heels) require incision and drainage with Gram stains and culture, both aerobic and anerobic. Antibiotics may be selected on the basis of Gram staining and culture results, unless substantial surrounding cellulitis or signs of sepsis are present. Gram stains are especially important, as anaerobic or microaerophilic bacteria may be visualized microscopically but fail to grow. Positive aerobic cultures may incompletely or inaccurately depict true infecting flora.

A variety of single or multiple drug regimens are available for potential mixed-flora abscesses, with selection based on how acutely "sick" the patients appear, as well as other factors such as drug hypersensitivity and antibiotic susceptibility patterns of nosocomial aerobic bacteria. In general, antibiotic coverage should encompass staphylococci, streptococci, gram-positive and gram-negative anaerobic bacteria, and/or aerobic gram-negative bacilli.

For nontoxic patients, potentially useful drug regimens include IV ampicillin-sulbactam, ticarcillin-clavulanate, piperacillin-tazobactam, and imipenem.

For penicillin-allergic patients, clindamycin is useful for coverage of staphylococci and nonenterococcal and anaerobic gram-positive and gram-negative bacteria, as is cefoxitin when non–IgE-mediated penicillin allergy is present.

Aminoglycosides (e.g., gentamicin, tobramycin, and amikacin) provide aerobic gram-negative bacillary coverage when patients are septic or when antibiotic resistance of aerobic gram-negative bacilli to nonaminoglycoside agents is prevalent.

Neither quinolones (e.g., ofloxacin or ciprofloxacin) nor trimethoprim-sulfamethoxasole is reliably active against aerobic streptococci or *S. aureus*, and these agents are inactive against anaerobic flora. These antibiotics, however, may be useful agents for treatment of aerobic gram-negative bacilli, when speciated and tested for susceptibilities.

## Cellulitis with Bullae

The occurrence of bullae or blisters overlying areas of cellulitis is highly suggestive of underlying necrosis of fascia, soft tissue, or muscle. Soft tissue accumulations of gas, a more common accompaniment of such processes, may not be detected by palpation and are more commonly detected radiographically, especially employing cross-table lateral plain radiographs of suspicious areas, or MRI scanning.

Preexisting arterial insufficiency may be suggested by the absence of arterial pulses, history of insulin-dependent diabetes mellitus, intermittent claudication and/or rest pain, loss of hair over the lower leg, or gangrenous changes.

A history of recent immersion of the leg in seawater, especially with concomitant penetrating trauma or bites by marine life such as jellyfish or Portuguese men-of-war, points to possible *V. vulnificus* infection, as noted previously. Patients with intact circulation and a prodrome of nonspecific

cellulitis, skin scratches, or penetrating skin trauma may have necrotizing group A *S. pyogenes* infection.

A history and evidence of human or animal bites, especially venomous reptile or brown recluse spider bites, should be sought.

The use of "super" vaginal tampons or a history of posterior nasal packing or surgery may point to toxic shock syndrome.

Specific anatomic sites of involvement are determined most often at surgical exploration with incision, drainage, and excision of necrotic tissues, which should be performed immediately. Toxemia and impairment of mentation most often accompany primary involvement of fascia (e.g., necrotizing fasciitis) or skeletal muscle, for example, in clostridial myonecrosis (gas gangrene), anerobic myositis, group A *Streptococcus* myonecrosis (gas gangrene), anerobic myositis, group A *S. pyogenes* myositis, or *V. vulnificus* myositis.

Other infectious causes of bullae include staphylococcal or streptococcal toxic shock syndrome, staphylococcal impetigo, infected second-degree burns, and complications of bite wounds especially from bites by humans, venomous reptiles, or arachnids (brown recluse Spiders).

Parenteral antibiotic therapy is best determined by results of intraoperative Gram staining and subsequent aerobic cultures and susceptibility tests. Antibiotics may prevent spread of infection, as well as prevent or treat potential blood stream invasion by bacteria, but have no effects against toxins such as those elaborated by *C. perfringens*.

Parenteral therapy should be started empirically to treat septic patients preoperatively. Potentially useful agents are those mentioned in the previous discussion of mixed-flora cutaneous abscesses, that is, β-lactamase inhibitor penicillins or clindamycin, in combinations with aminoglycosides. Tetracyclines are agents of choice for *V. vulnificus* infections.

Antitoxins, on the other hand, may be ineffective, in particular polyvalent clostridial antitoxins in the treatment of clostridial myonecrosis. Specific antivenins, however, may have some use early in the course of infections associated with brown recluse spider or snake bites. Success with hyperbaric oxygen chambers has been claimed anecdotally but never proved in randomized prospective clinical trials. To date, surgical débridement constitutes the primary line of defense. If the amount of devitalized tissue to be removed would leave a functionless extremity, amputation is in order and should not be delayed, especially in gas gangrene.

Other syndromes in the differential diagnosis include staphylococcal scalded skin syndrome and toxic epidermal necrolysis (TEN). The former is seen almost exclusively in infants and young children and develops as a result of a toxin, exfoliatin, elaborated by specific phage groups of *S. aureus*, especially phage group II types 70 and 71, which disrupts desmosomal bridges between cutaneous epithelial cells as well as between the epidermis and subcutaneous tissues. Clinical manifestations are pemphigus-like blebs and bullae usually surmounting areas of apparent cellulitis. The latter stems from drug hypersensitivity (e.g., to thiazide or loop diuretics, antibiotics, allopurinol) with resulting separation of the epidermis from the dermis. Cases of TEN tend to occur primarily in adults.

Otherwise, both entities resemble each other exactly at the bedside, including the presence of positive Nikolsky's signs, that is, the ability to remove sheets of normal epithelium adjacent to bullae merely by rubbing the skin. The age of patients and medication history are helpful distinguishing points clinically. A definitive distinction between scalded skin syndrome and TEN can be made by microscopy of skin biopsy frozen sections. In the former, cleavage planes are noted intraepithelially as well as between the epidermis and dermis. Cleavage planes in TEN are located solely between the dermis and epidermis. Scalded skin syndrome is treated with antistaphylococcal antibiotics. Both syndromes may respond to large doses of corticosteroids.

## Vesicles

Vesicular lesions on the lower extremity generally reflect contact reactions to vesicants of plants (e.g., poison ivy, oak, or sumac) or viral eruptions (primarily herpes simplex, herpes zoster, or varicella). Coxsackie A viruses may produce papulovesicular lesions on the feet, buttocks, and trunk of children, in addition to pharyngitis, fever, and occasionally aseptic meningitis (e.g., hand-foot-and-mouth disease).

Zoster lesions tend to distribute dermatomally and are frequently accompanied by neuritic pain. Varicella lesions are part of a generalized eruption involving the face, trunk, and upper extremities and are usually accompanied by fever and other constitutional symptoms. Herpes simplex lesions tend to favor the upper femurs and buttocks.

Tzanck's smears, Giemsa-stained scraping of the base of lesions, demonstrate characteristic Cowdry's type A inclusions of herpesvirus infections. A definitive viral diagnosis may be established by rapid fluorescent antibody stains or viral cultures of vesicle fluid.

Treatment of herpes simplex lesions is with acyclovir, 200 mg orally five times daily for 10 days. Treatment for herpes zoster may be with acyclovir, 800 mg orally five times a day; famciclovir, 500 mg orally thrice daily; or valacyclovir, 1000 mg by mouth thrice daily, each for 7 to 10 days. Treatment of varicella is with acyclovir, 500 mg orally five times daily for 10 days. Immunocompromised patients should require 10-day courses of IV acyclovir, 5 mg/kg at 8-hour intervals for disseminated herpes simplex infections or 12.2 mg/kg every 8 hours for varicella-zoster virus infection.

Corticosteroids, 60 mg/day by mouth with progressively decreased dosages, may help shorten the duration of acute pain in herpes zoster infection when combined with antiviral agents but are of no benefit in preventing postherpetic neuralgia and may promote viral dissemination.

Papulovesicular lesions or reddish papules surmounted by central pustules or vesicles, generally few in number and associated with wrist pain caused by tenosynovitis, polyarthralgias, and fever, are manifestations of systemic infection with *Neisseria gonorrhoeae* (the gonococcal arthritis-dermatitis syndrome). This diagnosis is aided by positive blood cultures or calcium alginate swabs of urethral discharge, cervical drainage, rectal mucosa, or oropharynx on Thayer-Martin medium. When multiple joints are involved with sterile joint aspirates, characteristic skin lesions, and tenosynovitis of the wrist, blood and other cultures are frequently negative. In culture-negative cases, a favorable clinical response to 3 days of antigonococcal IV therapy, e.g., ceftriaxone, 1.0 g/day, is highly suggestive of the diagnosis of *N. gonorrhoeae* infection and is, in fact, a diagnostic test. IV ceftriaxone should be given for a 7-day course. Patients with β-lactam antibiotic allergy may be treated with ofloxacin, 400 mg IV or orally every 12 hours for 7 days.

Bullous impetigo is an unusual form of *S. aureus* infection characterized by bullae 0.5 to 3.0 cm in diameter and generally flaccid that arise from normal-appearing skin. Bullae contain fluid that varies in appearance from translucent to cloudy or purulent and are surrounded by thin rims of erythema. Lesions often rupture spontaneously, leaving a flat, thin, varnish-like coating over denuded skin. Blister fluid cultures are invariably pure cultures of *S. aureus*, often phage type 71. Lesions tend to favor the lower extremities in patients beyond the neonatal period. Therapy involves systemic antistaphylococcal agents either orally in mild cases or parenterally in more extensive variants.

## Crusted Lesions

Superficial impetigo is the most common skin infection seen in children, often as an epidemic in warm, humid weather. Classical superficial impetigo is a well-tolerated, indolent infection, often present up to 3 weeks before medical assistance is sought. Lesions occur on exposed areas of the skin, especially the upper and lower extremities as well as the face. After local trauma, such as abrasions or insect bites, erythematous papules appear that evolve into thickly crusted, amber- or honey-colored lesions that exude amber-colored serous fluid after crusts are removed.

Cultures reveal group A *S. pyogenes* with or without *S. aureus*. Streptococci have traditionally been considered the agents of primary etiologic significance. Nonetheless, therapy should be directed against both streptococci and staphylococci, utilizing either oral antistaphylococcal antibiotics (e.g., dicloxacillin, cephalexin-cephradine, or clindamycin) or thrice-daily applications of topical mupirocin ointment to lesions after mechanical crust removal with chlorhexidine scrubs.

Impetigo due to *S. pyogenes*, M types 2, 4, 31, 36, 49, 55, 56, and Red Lake, may be associated with acute poststreptococcal glomerulonephritis, as previously mentioned. Antibiotic therapy of impetigo, although curative of acute infection, does not prevent the latter complication.

## Puncture Wounds of the Foot

Three percent to 15% of puncture wounds of the foot may become infected, and 0.6% to 1.8% lead to osteochondritis, pyoarthrosis, or osteomyelitis. The most common clinical scenario is that of a patient who recently stepped on a nail while wearing sneakers or athletic shoes with penetration of the shoe and puncturing of the skin of the sole. Bacteria, especially *P. aeruginosa*, may be found in cultures of the interior of rubber footwear soles. Not surprisingly, *P. aeruginosa* is the etiologic agent of complicating infections in up to 95% of cases.

Erythema, warmth, and tenderness of the soles of the feet suggest cellulitis. Point tenderness suggests osteochondritis, osteomyelitis, or pyoarthrosis, which may be confirmed with plain films or scans of hexamethyl-propyleneamineoxime (HM-PAO)–tagged WBCs, which disclose uptake of labeled WBCs in bone. The bacterial etiology of osteomyelitis may be confirmed by needle biopsy of involved bone, with culture and antibiotic sensitivity determinations.

Such wounds should be considered tetanus prone. A history of tetanus toxoid immunization as well as the date of the patient's last booster dose should be ascertained. Individuals with booster vaccination within 5 years do not require repeated booster injections with tetanus toxoid–diphtheria toxoid. If the patient has not been previously immunized against tetanus, 250 units of human tetanus immune globulin should be given intramuscularly, and a full three-dose course of tetanus toxoid should be started immediately. Individuals with the last tetanus toxoid dose within 10 years but more than 5 years, should receive a single booster tetanus toxoid dose.

Initial antibiotic therapy should consist of a parenteral aminoglycoside, such as gentamicin or tobramycin, with a concomitant second agent such as oral ciprofloxacin or IV ceftazidime, ciprofloxacin, or imipenem. If osteomyelitis of the foot is diagnosed, this regimen should be continued for 2 weeks. In the event of a favorable response to treatment and antibiotic sensitivity of the patient's isolate to this agent, monotherapy with ciprofloxacin, 750 mg by mouth twice daily, can be used to complete a 6-week therapeutic course.

## Leg Ulcers

Commonly encountered cutaneous ulcerative lesions of the lower extremity include diabetic foot ulcers and ulcers related to arterial or venous insufficiency.

Diabetic foot ulcers tend to occur in far-advanced diabetes mellitus, generally in association with local circulatory failure and sensory neuropathy resulting in diminished or absent pain sensation. Antecedent events usually involve trauma, often penetrating, which eventually leads to superficial necrosis of skin at the site of wounding and/or cellulitis. Cellulitis may vary in degree from minimal (extending less than 2 cm from the edge of the ulcer) to extensive (extending more than 2 cm beyond the ulcer margin), with the potential for gas formation, sepsis, and death.

Extension of soft tissue infection to bone may occur, leading to the development of small-bone osteomyelitis of the foot.

Cutaneous ulcers and bone involvement, on the other hand, may be merely neuropathic as opposed to infectious. Charcot's neuropathic arthropathy of the foot may mimic osteomyelitis radiographically. Cellulitis is usually absent, however, when neuropathic ulcers are present.

Foot radiographs may be negative early in the course of small-bone osteomyelitis. When bone is involved, triple-phase technetium pyrophosphate bone scans show focally increased areas of isotope uptake in the third or delayed phase of the scan. Scans of HM-PAO–tagged WBCs are positive in osteomyelitis, exhibiting focal WBC accumulation in bone, but fail to show such uptake in Charcot's arthropathy.

Infections of bone underlying chronic diabetic foot ulcers are often polymicrobial and may include varying permutations and combinations of β-hemolytic and other streptococci, *S. aureus*, Enterobacteriaceae, anaerobic gram-positive cocci, clostridia, and bacteroides species, especially *Bacteroides fragilis*. Bacteriologic diagnosis depends on Gram stains and cultures of pus, blood, bone obtained by needle biopsy through uninvolved skin, or material obtained by bone curettage at the time of surgery.

A variety of antibiotic regimens may be used for initial treatment. If available, initial microbiologic culture and antibiotic sensitivity data, together with data from accompanying Gram stains, help narrow and sharply focus antibiotic selection. If infections are mild, in patients with recent antibiotic therapy, or neither life nor limb threatening, outpatient therapy with clindamycin, 300 mg, or either cephradine or cephalexin, 500 mg, orally four times daily is a reasonable choice in the absence of Gram stain or culture results.

When adjacent cellulitis is present, parenteral agents—cefazolin, 1.0 g IV every 8 hours, plus metronidazole, 500 mg by mouth thrice daily; or ampicillin-sulbactam, 3.0 IV every 6 hours; or clindamycin, 900 mg IV every 8 hours—as monotherapy are reasonable first choices.

If concomitant sepsis is present or the infection is thought to be life or limb threatening, an aminoglycoside (e.g., gentamicin, 6 mg/kg/day every 24 hours for Clcr equal to or greater than 60 mL/min, every 36 hours for Clcr between 35 and 59 mL/min, or every 48 hours for Clcr between 20 and 34 mL/min) should be added, pending blood cultures and any wound Gram stain and culture-sensitivity results. If MRSA is a concern, add IV vancomycin in dosages mentioned earlier.

Other regimens that may be effective include cefoxitin, 2.0 g IV every 6 hours; ticarcillin-clavulanate, 3.1 g IV every 4 hours; clindamycin, 900 mg IV every 8 hours, plus ofloxacin, 400 mg IV every 12 hours; and imipenem, 500 mg IV every 6 hours.

Initial surgical management includes unroofing encrusted areas, débriding necrotic tissue or purulent exudates, and probing wounds to determine their extent. Wounds that extend directly to bone are highly predictive of underlying osteomyelitis.

Edema is treated with bed rest and elevation of the involved extremity, with diuretic agents if necessary.

The exact nature of concomitant vascular insufficiency, that is, large versus small-vessel disease, may be determined by Doppler ultrasonography and/or contract arteriography. Large-vessel arterial obstruction may be amenable to angioplasty and/or vascular bypass surgery. If arterial circulation and sufficiency can be reestablished, infection treated, and diabetes adequately controlled, lower extremity cutaneous ulcer healing can occur. Ancillary topical application to ulcers of platelet-derived growth factors, which stimulate fibroblast proliferation and tissue repair, may help to accelerate ulcer healing.

Contaminated wounds caused by occupational injuries, that is, factory or farm related, reflect different bacteriology. Both types of injuries are tetanus prone. Anaerobic gram-positive cocci or bacilli are much less likely, and gram-negative bacilli such as *P. aeruginosa* and *Xanthomonas maltophilia* (especially in farm settings) are seen more commonly, in addition to the usual staphylococci, streptococci, and/or clostridia.

Ulcers are also common manifestations of advanced arterial and venous insufficiency. Ulcers associated with arterial insufficiency have a proclivity for the lateral aspect of the lower extremities because of relatively sparse blood supply to that area. Surrounding cellulitis is uncommon, although the ulcers themselves are usually painful. Osteomyelitis of underlying bone may be ruled out by radiographs and radionuclide scans. Secondary infection is rare, although superficial wound cultures are frequently positive for various bacterial species, including pathogenic variants. These positive cultures generally represent superficial wound colonization. Systemic antibiotics are not warranted. Successful ulcer therapy depends on restoration of the lower extremity arterial blood supply. If this is accomplished, topical application of platelet-derived growth factor may augment wound healing.

Ulcers associated with venous insufficiency, by contrast, are located over the medial aspect of the lower extremity, in particular, the medial malleolus or lower tibia, and occur in the setting of long-standing venous insufficiency and/or prior episodes of lower extremity deep vein thrombosis. Residual edema and stasis pigmentation commonly occur adjacent to venous stasis ulcers.

Antibiotic therapy of complicating cellulitis should be directed against *S. aureus* and β-hemolytic streptococci, with IV nafcillin, oral clindamycin, or IV vancomycin (for β-lactam allergy or suspected MRSA).

Primary therapeutic modalities, however, involve elevation of the leg, treatment of edema, and topical therapy such as Unna's boot applications or topical platelet-derived growth factor.

Cutaneous ulcers of the lower extremity may also be seen in patients with factitious self-administered trauma, pyoderma gangrenosum associated with inflammatory bowel disease, and squamous cell carcinoma. Infectious cutaneous ulcers include syphilitic gummas and those associated with inoculation with unusual pathogens (e.g., atypical mycobacteria such as *Mycobacterium haemophilum* or *M. marinum* in Australian locales, *Nocardia* species, and fungi such as *C. neoformans* in compromised hosts or *Blastomyces dermatiditis* in the American southeast and upper midwest), recent brown recluse spider bites, and cutaneous leishmaniasis when patients give histories of *Phlebotomus* (sandfly) bites occurring in tropical South America or the Middle East. Diagnoses are suggested by history, geography, insect bites, serum antibody testing (e.g., rapid plasma reagin [RPR] test), and biopsies of ulcer edges with special stains and cultures for acid-fast bacilli and fungi.

## Fistulas

Fistulous tracts overlying bone generally denote chronic osteomyelitis, which can be detected with plain films or magnetic resonance imaging scans. Microbiologic etiologies are best determined by cultures and sensitivity testing of bone biopsy specimens. Cultures of material from nondraining fistulas are unreliable, and positive growth of bacteria probably reflects colonization from the outside in.

In tropical areas or the American south, fistulous tracts draining sulfur granules, associated with swelling and induration of the foot, suggest cutaneous nocardiosis, as in Madura foot secondary to infection with *Nocardia brasiliensis*. *Nocardia* species are weakly acid fast on smears and require weak decolorization with 0.1% $H_2SO_4$ in order to be detected. Successful growth may also be seen with special stains of histopathologic sections of soft tissue or bone.

Treatment of Madura foot is with trimethoprim-sulfamethoxazole, two double-strength tablets orally twice daily; or combination of parenteral Amikacin 15 mg/kg once daily IV (for Clcr equal to or greater than 60 mL/min.), every 36 hours (for Clcr of 35 to 49 mL/min.), or every 48 hours (for Clcr of 20 to 24 mL/min.) with ceftriaxone, 1 g IV every 24 hours. Prolonged treatment (i.e., for 6 months) with either regimen is necessary for cure.

Draining fistulas, hemorrhage from surgical incisions, and cellulitis and/or dehiscence of surgical wounds may point to infection of underlying vascular prostheses. This diagnosis may be confirmed by WBC scans with HM-PAO or indium 111, ultrasonography, or MRI scans of the suspicious graft, with Gram stains and cultures of draining wounds as well as blood cultures. Infecting microflora are usually *S. aureus, S. epidermidis*, or aerobic gram-negative bacilli including *P. aeruginosa*.

Antimicrobial treatment of vascular graft infections can be chosen on the basis of microbiologic data. Presumptive antimicrobial therapy should be initiated on the basis of Gram stains of wound drainage if the patient is hemorrhaging, has extensive cellulitis, or is septic. Therapy should be directed against presumed MRSA and methicillin-resistant *S. epidermidis* (vancomycin IV) and resistant gram-negative aerobic bacilli, including *P. aeruginosa* (IV aminoglycosides—gentamicin, tobramycin, or amikacin), in combination with ceftazidime, imipenem, aztreonam, or ciprofloxacin. Excision of all prosthetic graft material is necessary for cure.

## The Swollen, Painful, Warm, Immovable Joint

The differential diagnosis here essentially includes septic arthritis or crystalline arthropathy (e.g., gout or pseudogout). Arthrocentesis, with cell count and differential, Gram stain, polarizing microscopy for detection of crystals, and culture and sensitivity results, is diagnostic.

Normal synovial fluid is viscous with good mucin clot formation, as exhibited by formation of a tenacious "string" when the fluid is allowed to drip from the bottom of a pipette (a positive string test). Cell counts are less than 60 cells/mm$^3$ with mononuclear cell predominance and no more than 2% neutrophils.

Infected synovial fluid, by contrast, is notable for WBC counts ranging from 6000 to 250,000 cells/mm$^3$ but most often greater than 50,000 cells/mm$^3$ with WBC differentials of at least 90% neutrophils. Similar synovial WBC glucose concentrations are often depressed in arthritis because of infection with pyogenic organisms, rheumatoid arthritis, gout, and pseudogout. Synovial fluid glucose concentrations in bacterial arthritis are more likely to be 40 mg/dL or more below concomitant blood glucose levels.

When synovial fluid is examined by polarizing microscopy, negatively birefringent crystals are composed of urate and are diagnostic of gout, whereas positively birefringent crystals indicate calcium pyrophosphate crystals pathognomonic of pseudogout. If crystals are not detected, infection should be expected, especially with pyogenic bacteria. Synovial fluid Gram stains are positive in 35% to 65% of cases. Synovial fluid cultures yield bacteria in 25% to 80% of cases and blood cultures are positive in up to one third of cases, depending on the species of infecting pathogens. In 10% of cases, positive blood cultures may be the only means of establishing microbial etiologies.

*N. gonorrhoeae* should be a primary etiologic consideration in sexually active patients and is the cause of septic arthritis in up to 94% of patients 15 to 45 years old. Two syndromes occur, with biologic and metabolic differences and different degrees of invasiveness of infecting strains. The first is an isolated, culture-positive, classical septic monoarthritis, usually involving the knee, ankle, or shoulder. The second is the gonococcal arthritis-dermatitis syndrome (i.e., polyarthritis), which is characterized by negative cultures, tenosynovitis of the wrist, and sparse, acrally distributed maculopapular skin lesions surmounted by vesicles or pustules.

The most common causes of septic arthritis in patients younger than 14 and older than 45 years of age are *S. aureus* (90% of cases) and β-hemolytic streptococci of various Lancefield groups. Septic arthritis may arise through hematogenous seeding of joints from remote infections, direct extension from nearby infections, or direct or inadvertent manipulation of joints (e.g., contaminated intra-articular injections).

*P. aeruginosa* and *Serratia* species tend to occur in IV drug abusers, hemodialysis patients, or individuals with long-standing vascular access catheters as a result of vascular catheter infection.

Sickle cell anemia predisposes to salmonella as well as pneumococcal infections, including septic arthritis and osteomyelitis. Autosplenectomy, caused by multiple sickle cell–induced splenic infarcts, destroys the spleen's ability to produce critical components of the alternative complement pathway system necessary for nonspecific opsonization of newly encountered bacterial strains to which the patient is immunologically naive. Iron overload of hepatic Kuppfer cells and other components of the reticuloendothelial system resulting from chronic hemolysis of any etiology likewise reduces the ability of the reticuloendothelial system to phagocytose and kill salmonellae and other intracellular pathogens.

Pneumococcal septic arthritis may also occur in the setting of pneumococcal pneumonia as well as other predisposing conditions, such as cirrhosis, prior splenectomy, multiple myeloma, chronic lymphocytic leukemia, hypogammaglobulinemia, or IgG subclass deficiency, wherein the ability to make specific immune opsonizing antibodies to pneumococci is impaired.

*Haemophilus influenzae* type B is usually hematogenous in origin and occurs in early infancy, before receipt of *H. influenzae* B vaccine.

*Escherichia coli* and other coliforms may produce septic arthritis in the setting of prior urinary tract, biliary, or other gastrointestinal infections.

IV antibiotics in large doses and daily arthrocenteses are the foundation for treating septic arthritis. Treatment should be started empirically before receipt of culture and antibiotic sensitivity results. Parenteral antibiotics achieve more than adequate synovial fluid concentrations to inhibit infecting bacteria. Direct antibiotic injections into infected joints achieve no better synovial antibiotic levels or clinical results. Indeed, intra-articular antibiotic administration is hazardous to the patient by producing chemical synovitis, which may be clinically as severe as or worse than the joint infection.

In sexually active patients, ceftriaxone, 2.0 g IV every 24 hours, should be started presumptively for gonococcal infection, with ofloxacin, 400 mg IV every 12 hours, reserved for β-lactam antibiotic–allergic patients. IV vancomycin is the drug of choice for *S. aureus*, including MRSA, and methicillin-resistant *S. epidermidis*. Aminoglycosides (e.g., gentamicin, tobramycin, or amikacin) are indicated for coverage of gram-negative bacilli. Vancomycin covers *Streptococcus pneumoniae*, including highly resistant strains, and ceftriaxone or ofloxacin covers ampicillin-resistant *H. influenzae.*

Initial open joint drainage is mandatory for septic arthritis of the hip because of the relative inaccessibility of this joint to repeated closed arthrocenteses. For other joints, open drainage is indicated for inadequate response to antibiotics and closed daily arthrocenteses. Infected prosthetic joints require removal for cure.

Tuberculous, fungal, and other granulomatous infections tend to be more indolent than bacterial arthritis and have predilections for large, weight-bearing joints (i.e., the hips or knees). Tuberculous synovial effusions may exhibit a neutrophilic predominance, in contrast to tuberculous infections of the pleura, meninges, and peritoneum, wherein lymphocytic predominance is the rule. Acid-fast and fungal smears of synovial fluid are usually negative. In tuberculosis, 85% of intermediate-strength (5 tuberculin units) purified protein derivative skin tests are positive, although chest radiographs fail to disclose suggestive findings in approximately 50% of cases. Synovial fluid cultures for acid-fast bacilli may be negative in up to 20% of cases of tuberculous arthritis, and the diagnosis may depend on stains and cultures of synovial biopsy specimens. Tuberculosis requires multidrug antituberculous chemotherapy: isoniazid in combination with ethambutol, rifampin, and pyrizinamide for the first 2 months, followed by isoniazid plus rifampin for the remaining 6 to 9 months. Individuals with tuberculous arthritis should be screened for concomitant human immunodeficiency virus infection.

In otherwise normal patients with granulomatous synovitis and histories of travel to or residence in endemic areas, infections with geographic fungi, especially with *C. immitis*, or *B. dermatiditis* should be suspected and are best diagnosed by special fungal staining of synovial biopsy and fluid samples, demonstrating the classical morphology of these agents, or by positive fungal cultures. Fungal cultures may be delayed, and fungal serology is useful for coccioidomycosis but of no value for blastomycosis. Therapy, when the diagnosis is established, may be with prolonged IV amphotericin B or oral itraconazole.

Candidal septic arthritis tends to be a hematogenous complication of systemic *Candida* infections in immunocompromised patients, intravenous drug abusers, or patients with prolonged hospitalization, multiple prior infections and courses of antibiotic therapy, and/or prior total parenteral nutrition. Diagnosis is established with Gram stains and/or cultures. Therapy is with prolonged courses of either intravenous amphotericin B or IV or oral fluconazole for *Candida* species other than *glabrata* or *krusei*, which are intrinsically fluconazole resistant.

Viral arthritides may accompany the prodrome of hepatitis B, influenza, measles, varicella, HIV or Epstein-Barr virus (EBV) infection, arboviruses, rubella; may be a complication of rubella vaccination in women; or may be an isolated manifestation of parvovirus B19 infection (fifth disease). Arthritis is often polyarticular, associated with rashes, and with mononuclear predominance in joint effusions. Specific diagnoses are suggested by concomitant clinical syndromes, vaccination histories, or epidemic exposures.

Infectious prepatellar bursitis may mimic acute septic arthritis of the knee. The usual clinical presentation is that of pain and swelling of the bursa, usually after recent minor trauma, sustained or intermittent pressure to the patella related to occupations (e.g., housekeepers, carpet installers, carpenters, gardeners, or plumbers), antecedent gout or rheumatoid arthritis, or recent intrabursal corticosteroid infections. Fever occurs in 50% of cases. In contrast to that in septic arthritis of the knee, the knee joint is freely movable. The prepatellar bursa is frequently red, warm, tender, and swollen. Overlying cellulitis and tender inguinal adenopathy are often present.

Diagnosis depends on aspiration of bursal fluid with Gram stains (positive in 65% of cases) and cultures. Polarizing microscopy reveals no urate or calcium pyrophosphate crystals, which excludes gout or pseudogout. Blood cultures may occasionally be positive as well.

*S. aureus* is the responsible pathogen in more than 90% of cases. Therapy includes needle drainage of the bursa, as well as oral antistaphylococcal antibiotic for MSSA (i.e., dicloxacillin, cephalexin-cephradine, or clindamycin). Parenteral agents (nafcillin, cefazolin, or clindamycin) should be used in the presence of severe disease and/or underlying immunocompromising illnesses. IV vancomycin should be used for suspected or confirmed MRSA infection.

### Focal Bone Pain, Tenderness, and Drainage

Of the many causes of focal lower extremity bone pain and tenderness, osteomyelitis is the primary infectious entity to be considered. Types of lower extremity osteomyelitis include childhood osteomyelitis (i.e., prepubertal hematogenous osteomyelitis of the metaphyses of long bones—the femur, tibia, and fibula); posttraumatic osteomyelitis complicating compound or compound-comminuted fractures with or without open reduction and internal fixation, infected internal fixation devices, or prosthetic joints; small-bone osteomyelitis of the foot related to arterial insufficiency; osteomyelitis related to overlying infected cutaneous decubitus or vascular ulcers; and osteomyelitis complicating prior bone infarcts in sickle cell disease.

Diagnosis of osteomyelitis, once considered, may be established by plain films, magnetic resonance imaging scans, and triple-phase technetium pyrophosphate and/or HM-PAO–labeled WBC scans. Microbial etiology may be determined with blood cultures and aerobic and anerobic cultures as well as gram staining of purulent wound drainage or of bone curettage or biopsy samples. Cultures representing dry sinus tracts overlying sites of chronic osteomyelitis are notoriously unreliable and tend to reflect colonization of these fistulas rather than infection per se.

*S. aureus* is the usual pathogen responsible for hematogenous long-bone osteomyelitis, although group B *Streptococcus agalactiae* and *E. coli* may occur in the neonatal period. *H. influenzae* type B in childhood, and *Salmonella* species in sickle cell disease. Blood cultures are frequently although not invariably positive in this form of bone infection.

Posttraumatic osteomyelitis, particularly after open fractures, is generally due to *S. aureus*. Diagnosis depends on bone biopsy cultures; blood cultures are invariably negative.

Osteomyelitis associated with orthopedic hardware is most often due to *S. aureus* or *S. epidermidis*, although gram-negative bacilli including *P. aeruginosa* and fungi such as *Candida* species may be seen, especially in recurrent disease associated with infected orthopedic hardware and/or infected fracture nonunions.

Small-bone osteomyelitis of the foot or leg in association with circulatory impairment and osteomyelitis concurrent with decubitus ulcers are generally polymicrobial, including anaerobic bacteria, aerobic gram-negative bacilli, staphylococci, and streptococci in varying permutations and combinations. Blood cultures are again usually negative, and etiologic diagnosis depends on bone biopsy cultures.

Antimicrobial therapy of osteomyelitis can often be deferred until Gram stain and culture and sensitivity data are available. Empirical antibiotic therapy, however, is indicated for hematogenous osteomyelitis or osteomyelitis associated with cellulitis, sepsis, or other potential life- or limb-threatening complications. In the latter settings, the choice of therapeutic agents depends on the spectrum of likely pathogens as well as their antibiotic susceptibilities and resistances. Specific drugs of choice for these agents have been delineated in earlier sections of this chapter.

Infected hardware requires removal for cure, with the significant exception of devices for open reduction and internal fixation, which should be retained until fracture healing has occurred, at which time removal is indicated. Removal of these devices before complete fracture healing leads to infected fracture nonunions.

## BIBLIOGRAPHY

Bisno AL, Stevens DL: Streptococcal infections of the skin and soft tissues. N Engl J Med 334:240, 1996.

Chartier C, Grosshans E: Erysipelas. Int J Dermatol 29:459, 1990.

Finch R: Skin and soft tissue infections. Lancet 1:164, 1988.

Fine JD: Management of acquired bullous skin diseases. N Engl J Med 333:1475, 1995.

Fitzgerald RH Jr, Cowan JD: Puncture sounds of the foot. Orthop Clin North Am 6:956, 1975.

Gemmell G: Staphylococcal scalded skin syndrome. J Clin Microbiol 43:318, 1995.

Gentry LO: Diagnosis and management of the diabetic foot ulcer. J Antimcrob Chemother 32(Suppl A):72, 1993.

Goldenberg DL: Septic arthritis and other infections of rheumatologic significance. Rheum Dis Clin North Am 17:149, 1991.

Goldstein EJC: Bite wounds and infection. Clin Infect Dis 14:363, 1992.

Gulli B, Templeman D: Compartment syndrome of the lower extremity. Orthopedics 8:1106, 1984.

Hafner J, Bounameaux H, Burg G, Brunner U: Management of venous ulcers. Vasa 25:161, 1996.

Ho G Jr, Mikolich DJ: Bacterial infection of the superficial subcutaneous bursae. Clin Rheum Dis 12:437, 1986.

Holloway GA Jr: Arterial ulcers: Assessment and diagnosis. Ostomy Wound Manage 42:46, 1996.

Klontz KC, Lieb S, Schreiber M, et al: Syndrome of *Vibrio vulnificus* infections: Clinical and epidemiologic features in Florida cases, 1981–1987. Ann Intern Med 109:318, 1988.

Laughlin RT, Wright DG, Mader JT, Calhoun JH: Osteomyelitis. Curr Opin Rheumatol 7:315, 1995.

Lewis TT: Necrotizing soft tissue infections: Infect Dis Clin North Am 1:635, 1987.

Musher DM, McKenzie SO: Infections due to *Staph. aureus.* Medicine (Baltimore) 56:383, 1977.

Nadelman RB, Wormser GP: Erythema migrans and early Lyme disease. Am J Med 98(Suppl 4A):15S, 1995.

Naides SJ: Viral arthritis, including HIV. Curr Opin Rheumatol 7:337, 1995.

O'Brien JP, Goldenberg DL, Rice PA: Disseminated gonococcal infection: A prospective analysis of 49 patients and a review of pathophysiology and immune mechanisms. Medicine (Baltimore) 62:395, 1983.

Piano G: Infections in lower extremity grafts. Surg Clin North Am 75:789, 1995.

Rolston KU: Infections involving the skin and soft tissues of the lower extremities. J Foot Surg 26(Suppl 1):S25, 1987.

Semel JD, Trenholme G: *Aeromonas hydrophila* water-associated traumatic infections: A review. J Trauma 30:324, 1990.

Walling DM, Kaelin WG Jr: Pyomyositis in patients with diabetes mellitus. Rev Infect Dis 13:797, 1991.

# The Lower Extremity in Vascular Disease

# 21

*Mark B. Kahn and Rodney Bell*

When interviewing a patient who complains of leg pain, it must be kept in mind that an accurate history and physical examination allow an accurate diagnosis 90% of the time. It is important to determine the exact location of the pain, whether it is in the lower back, buttock, thigh, calf, foot, or toes. Does the discomfort occur spontaneously, with a certain position, or with exercise? Is the patient complaining of pain, numbness, or both? Is the pain bilateral or unilateral? Is one side worse than the other?

The issue that must be addressed quickly is the acuteness of the complaint. The patient with a severely ischemic limb of acute onset may have a surgical emergency that needs to be addressed within a few hours to prevent permanent injury or perhaps limb loss. Symptoms with a duration of a few days or weeks may be managed relatively easily via a percutaneous route by intra-arterial lytic therapy and/or balloon angioplasty but only if the diagnosis and referral to a vascular surgeon are made quickly enough. If evaluation of these acute or subacute nonemergency problems is delayed too long, what may have been treated percutaneously may require surgical intervention. If in doubt about the possibility of an acute change in a patient's vascular system, do not hesitate to refer immediately to a vascular specialist. Fortunately, the evaluation of most patients with leg pain is not urgent and is easily accomplished in the office situation.

## SYMPTOMS

### Acute Ischemia

Classically, a patient with an acutely ischemic limb presents with the five Ps: pain, pallor, pulselessness, paresthesias, and paralysis. The patient complains of sudden onset of severe pain and/or weakness. In the nontraumatic situation this usually results from an embolus originating in the patient's heart, frequently because of atrial fibrillation, or a mural thrombus that forms after a myocardial infarction. The embolus usually lodges at the femoral bifurcation, suddenly occluding blood flow to the limb. In most patients the primary complaint is pain, but in approximately 10% to 20% of patients the numbness and paresthesia may overshadow the pain. The symptoms may subside somewhat over the next few minutes or hours, depending on the patient's ability to recruit collateral channels of blood flow and whether any vasospasm resolves.

On physical examination the patient has a cool leg and foot. There may or may not be a palpable femoral pulse, and popliteal and pedal pulses are usually not present. The characteristic signs of severe chronic arterial occlusive disease are usually not present. Frequently, the opposite leg has a normal pulse examination. The degree of motor and sensory loss present is thought to correlate with the ultimate prognosis, even after adequate surgical revascularization.

Occasionally, a large saddle embolus to the aortic bifurcation causes sudden onset of paraplegia as the blood supply to the spinal cord is compromised. This diagnosis is not difficult to make if the examiner thinks of it. The legs are usually cool and pale, frequently described as cadaveric. Femoral pulses are absent. One must think of associated problems such as renal or visceral ischemia as well.

Paralysis indicates advanced ischemia that may be irreversible and demands prompt surgical attention. Even with advanced ischemia the limb may be salvaged, but the neurologic deficits may prove to be permanent and debilitating. Reperfusion of a profoundly ischemic limb may have serious metabolic effects, as acid and potassium are released into the systemic circulation.

### Chronic Ischemia

Chronic leg and foot pain caused by arterial occlusive disease does not often present as a surgical emergency unless complicated by infection. The diagnosis can almost always be made by history and physical examination. There are two common presentations of chronic leg and foot pain caused by arterial occlusive disease: intermittent claudication and rest pain.

*Intermittent claudication* related to ischemia (vasculogenic claudication) occurs when a muscle group that is pain free at rest develops pain as its metabolic demands increase with exercise. Arterial occlusive disease prevents the muscle group from receiving the blood flow it needs to supply oxygen and remove metabolic by-products such as lactic acid during exercise. Because of this, the muscle starts to cramp or ache. The location of the discomfort may vary depending on the location of the arterial disease.

Buttock claudication and thigh claudication usually result from iliac artery disease. Frequently, these patients complain of aching and weakness and report that their hip or thigh may "give out" while walking. Cramping or aching of one or both calves with exercise is associated with disease of the superficial femoral artery supplying the calf and foot.

The hallmark of both of these vasculogenic claudication syndromes is the reproducible nature of the symptoms. The symptoms do not usually vary, and they occur every time the patient walks or exercises a certain, constant distance. They typically do not occur while the patient is standing, sitting, or lying down. They are relieved when the patient stops walking and rests, even if the patient remains standing.

*Rest pain* is associated with advanced arterial occlusive disease and occurs because the metabolic needs of the foot are not met even at rest. The patient complains of pain in the toes or over the metatarsal heads. This pain usually occurs at night, awakening patients from sleep. Frequently, it is relieved by hanging the foot over the side of the bed in a dependent position or by rubbing the foot and walking around. Some patients can sleep only with the foot in a dependent position, resulting in a swollen foot at the time of presentation.

## Venous Disease

Pain associated with venous disease is usually described in a more vague and inconsistent fashion than that associated with arterial disease. Patients with venous insufficiency frequently complain of leg "heaviness" and fatigue that is worse as the day goes on and the longer they stand on their feet. This discomfort is usually relieved by elevating their legs.

## PHYSICAL EXAMINATION

The pulse examination is the mainstay of the physical examination in patients with vascular disease. Although various grading systems have been proposed to characterize the strength of pulses, by definition these are subjective and have poor interobserver reproducibility. Generally, it is important to note whether a pulse is present or absent and whether there is a significant difference between the right and the left.

Approximately 10% of the normal population lack one or the other of the pedal pulses. It must be emphasized that it is not unusual for elderly patients, especially with risk factors for cardiovascular disease such as smoking, hypertension, or diabetes, to have an abnormal pulse examination while they are completely asymptomatic. This is because the arterial occlusive disease progressed slowly enough to allow the development of collateral circulation sufficient to prevent symptoms. In addition, many elderly patients live comparatively sedentary lives and do not stress their leg muscles enough to cause symptoms. If there is no pulse, simply record that finding. It is not helpful for later examiners if you assume that there is a pulse and record that it is a "weak" one. The presence or absence of a pulse is important only in the overall context of a patient's complaints and physical examination.

The abdomen should be carefully palpated for the presence of an abdominal aortic aneurysm, and the presence of an abdominal bruit may signify aortic or iliac vascular disease. The femoral pulses are usually located halfway between the middle of the pubic ramus and the anterior superior iliac spine. In obese patients they may be difficult to locate. The presence or absence of a bruit should be noted in this location as well. Popliteal pulses are best felt by grasping the supine patient behind the knee and supporting the relaxed leg, palpating the middle of the popliteal space. Popliteal pulses are sometimes difficult to appreciate, and if they are easily felt the presence of a popliteal aneurysm should be suspected. The posterior tibial pulse is usually felt in the hollow behind the medial malleolus, and the dorsalis pedis pulse is felt along the dorsum of the foot over the first and second metatarsals or just lateral to the tendon of the extensor hallucis longus.

Loss of hair on the toes and thickened toenails are common signs of advanced chronic arterial occlusive disease. As the disease progress, the skin may become scaly, shiny, and atrophic. Delayed capillary refill may be present, but this is an unreliable and inconsistent finding. Buerger's sign, cadaveric pallor when the leg is elevated and rubor when it is dependent, is common in patients with rest pain. Ischemic ulcers are usually found distally on the foot, either between the toes or on the tips of the toes. They are usually clean, with poor granulation, and frequently painful and/or associated with rest pain.

Patients with pain secondary to venous insufficiency may have swollen legs as well as brawny edema, stasis dermatitis, and perhaps ankle or lower leg ulceration. The pain associated with varicose veins is usually localized to the veins themselves, and patients rarely have more generalized complaints of leg pain unless deep venous insufficiency is present.

## DIAGNOSIS

Patients with arthritis may describe discomfort similar to that with claudication, especially hip or thigh claudication. Careful questioning usually reveals that the discomfort, although it may be worsened by exercise, does not occur at constant, reproducible distances and is not consistently and rapidly relieved by rest.

Spinal stenosis (pseudoclaudication, neurogenic claudication, cauda equina syndrome) may also mimic vascular claudication. Patients usually complain of numbness and paresthesias as well as weakness. Symptoms are frequently reproduced by having the patient stand, lie down (usually when the patient straightens his or her back), or walk. Symptoms associated with walking are usually reproduced at more variable distances than those associated with true claudication. Relief is obtained only by sitting or lying down, not merely resting. Relief usually occurs after 5 to 10 minutes, rather than 2 to 3 minutes as with vascular claudication.

The pulse examination is frequently helpful in differentiating between vascular and other forms of leg and buttock pain. Although it is not unusual for elderly patients to have an abnormal pulse examination, it would be unusual to find severe buttock and thigh claudication with a normal femoral pulse examination and no iliac or femoral bruit.

Rest pain associated with arterial occlusive disease may be difficult to differentiate from pain secondary to a peripheral neuropathy. The differential diagnosis includes diabetic neuropathy, which is usually bilateral and frequently symmetric. Neuropathic pain is usually constant and not relieved by dependency. True rest pain is associated with severe arterial occlusive disease, and the patients frequently cannot walk far because of their overall health status and frequently have the stigmata of severe arterial occlusive disease such as dependent rubor and/or ischemic ulcers. Whereas diabetic patients with a neuropathy may have pedal pulses, patients with rest pain never have pedal pulses.

## ISCHEMIC NEUROPATHY

Ischemic neuropathy is an injury of a peripheral nerve that is caused by a reduction of blood supply. The metabolic needs of the large nerves of the legs are met by the intraneural blood vessels, the vasa nervorum; the small nerves are supplied by diffusion from the surrounding tissue. The vasa nervorum originate from the large arteries and supply the nerve trunks at multiple levels generally around the joints. The epineural arteries branch and penetrate the perineurium to perfuse the endoneurium. This provides a complete terminal network of capillaries through the perineurium providing blood supply to the nerve. This network is at some distance from the nutrient arteries and constitutes an extensive collateral network of blood supply to the major nerves. Because of this collateral circulation, it is difficult to damage a major nerve by occlusion of one or even several nutrient arteries.

However, the pattern of epineural vessels varies in different nerves, and in some instances a single nutrient artery provides the major blood supply to a length of nerve. For example, the sciatic nerve receives an arterial branch from the inferior gluteal artery and the distal tibial and peroneal nerves receive their blood supply from popliteal branches. Between these levels, the distal sciatic and proximal tibial and peroneal nerves receive a variable blood supply from the deep femoral artery. In the popliteal fossa the popliteal artery supplies the sciatic nerve. The tibial nerve is intimately related to the posterior tibial artery, which supplies a large number of direct nutrient arteries. The peroneal nerve, however, diverges from the main vessels and receives its blood supply from small adjacent arteries in the region of the fibular head. At this point, the major intraneural arteries occupy a superficial and exposed position and are vulnerable. In the calf, the posterior tibial and peroneal nerves receive branches from the anterior and posterior tibial arteries. The intraneural arterial pattern in the buttock and thigh contains several arterial channels of large caliber, but below the knee one major vessel is usually dominant. The peroneal nerve at the knee and the more distal parts of the peroneal and posterior tibial nerves are more liable to ischemic damage.

The sympathetic nerve fibers innervate the blood vessels in the epineurium and perineurium. High sympathetic tone can decrease the blood flow by 90%. Sympathetically mediated vasoconstriction may be important in the chronic pain of reflex sympathetic dystrophy.

Experimental studies have shown that severe ischemia for 10 to 15 minutes produces a rapid decrease in the action potential and conduction is blocked. With restoration of blood flow, recovery begins in 1 to 2 minutes and is complete in 10 minutes. The mechanism of the ischemic effect involves loss of ionic gradients and fast axoplasmic transport. The block of fast axoplasmic transport becomes irreversible after 6 to 8 hours of total ischemia. Thus, short periods of ischemia are reversible, the nerve's metabolic needs being met by diffusion from surrounding tissue. Ischemia lasting longer than 6 hours produces irreversible damage.

The incidence of neurologic deficits in chronic peripheral vascular disease is unknown but is probably underestimated because the symptoms of pain, sensory changes, and weakness may easily be confused with those of claudication or ischemic rest pain. Neuralgic changes that have been described include painful burning and reflex loss, muscle wasting, and weakness. In patients with severe atherosclerotic disease with claudication at 100 yards, impaired sensation can occur in as many as 88%, weakness in 50%, and decreased reflexes in about 50%. Slowed conduction may be found in an even higher percentage of patients, but many of the studies are confounded by the presence of diabetes.

Symptoms of burning pain in the foot aggravated by rest, with paresthesia and distal muscle weakness, should suggest the diagnosis. The Achilles reflex is depressed or absent, and there may be wasting of the small muscles of the foot. There may be a stocking-glove sensory loss extending a variable distance into the calf involving all primary sensory modalities, including touch, pain, temperature, vibration, and position sense.

The problem with considering this a distinct clinical entity is that many of these features are not specific for ischemia but are also seen in diseases that affect blood vessels, such as diabetes. Asymmetry in the clinical and electrodiagnostic examination should alert the clinician to the possibility of a chronic ischemic neuropathy. The prognosis is guarded in that even with revascularization procedures the changes are generally not reversible, at least at 12 months. Acute arterial occlusion caused by embolism, thrombosis, or arterial injury is frequently associated with acute neural dysfunction. Motor signs occur in about 20% and sensory symptoms in one half of the patients. The chief complaint is one of a burning pain that is frequently worse with rest and at night. The foot is frequently perceived to be cold when in fact it is warm. Weakness in the small muscles of the foot and a depressed Achilles reflex are often observed. A unilateral stocking-glove sensory deficit to vibration is common. Electrical studies show unilateral loss of motor potential amplitude from the small muscles of the foot, reduced distal sensory potential amplitudes, and evidence of denervation of the small muscles of the foot.

Treatment of the burning pain associated with ischemic neuropathy is largely ineffectual, although some relief has been reported with carbamazapine and gabapentin.

Acute ischemic mononeuropathy often occurs in association with vasculitis and diabetes. Femoral and peroneal neuropathies are common. The lumbosacral plexus may also be involved. Diseases such as periarteritis nodosa, rheumatoid vasculitis, Churg-Strauss syndrome, and Wegener's granulomatosis can affect the endoneural arteries and produce a mononeuritis with nerve infarction.

## HEMORRHAGIC COMPRESSIVE NEUROPATHIES

Hemorrhagic compressive neuropathies are focal nerve injuries that result from the pressure of an expanding hematoma. Disruption and stretching of nerve fascicles by blood dissecting between the fascicles may also play a role. Iliopsoas hemorrhage or hemorrhage into the retroperitoneal space can occur as a complication of hemophilia, trauma, rupture of aortic or iliac aneurysms, fibrinolytic therapy, and anticoagulation. The femoral nerve originates from the second through fourth lumbar nerves and emerges along the lateral margin of the psoas muscle. It courses inferiorly in a groove between the psoas and iliacus muscles, crossing into the thigh under the inguinal ligament. The iliacus fascia is firmly adherent to the iliac crest, the brim of the true pelvis, and the posterior margin of the inguinal ligament ventral to the nerve and forms a compartment in which the femoral nerve can be compressed. At the inguinal ligament this fascial compartment is particularly indistensible. Dissection of blood into this compartment or hemorrhage within the psoas or iliacus muscle can result in nerve compression. Bleeding distal to the ilioinguinal ligament generally does not cause a compressive neuropathy.

The patient frequently experiences pain in the groin and hip that spreads to the inner thigh. Hypoesthesia develops along the medial aspect of the thigh in the distribution of the medial femoral cutaneous nerve. Hip extension exacerbates the pain, and a position of flexion and external rotation of the hip is usually assumed for comfort. Progression produces quadriceps paralysis, and patellar reflexes are diminished or lost. The diagnosis is confirmed by computed tomography, which shows an enlarged psoas or iliacus muscle of variable density consistent with a hematoma.

Treatment of the retroperitoneal hemorrhage is generally nonoperative. Correction of any coagulopathy, restoration of blood volume, hip flexion, analgesics, bed rest, and later physical therapy are the mainstays of therapy. Surgical decompression can be used for a rapidly progressive paralysis.

## COMPARTMENT SYNDROME

Chronic compartment syndrome can cause leg pain, usually in younger individuals. A mild case of this problem is commonly known as "shin splints." Symptoms occur when the blood flow to a muscle compartment increases with exercise, causing the muscle group to enlarge. If the fascial envelope surrounding the muscle is too tight, pressure builds up within the compartment, causing pain. The elevated intracompartmental pressure may become high enough to cause not only pain but also, in severe, acute cases, muscle, artery, and nerve compression and necrosis. This may result in permanent damage within a few hours if not diagnosed and treated promptly.

The typical chronic case occurs in an otherwise healthy person who complains of anterior or lateral lower leg pain about 10 to 20 minutes after beginning exercise. The pain may be in one or both legs and is usually a dull aching discomfort in the anterior and/or lateral compartments of the affected leg. The intensity of the pain varies from a dull ache to severe pain. The superficial peroneal nerve coursing through the lateral compartment may become compressed as well, causing paresthesias over the dorsum of the foot and the medial four toes. The patient may complain of a mild footdrop and inability to dorsiflex the foot. In chronic cases the pain usually resolves after a few minutes of rest. Physical examination while the patient is asymptomatic is generally unremarkable, with a normal pedal pulse and sensory examination.

The diagnosis is usually made from the typical history and physical examination. In a difficult case, compartment pressures may be measured before and after exercise. If rest and alteration of training habits do not resolve the problem, treatment usually consists of anterior compartment fasciotomy.

Acute compartment syndrome frequently occurs after an episode of trauma, fracture, crushing, or revascularization. The trauma or reperfusion injury causes intracompartmental muscle swelling, as compared with a normal increase in perfusion with exercise in the chronic syndrome. The pathology is the same—compression of the muscle, nerve, and arteries within the fascial compartment—but is usually not as severe in the chronic syndrome.

Although any muscle compartment may develop an acute compartment syndrome with sufficient trauma, the most commonly affected area is the anterior and lateral compartment of the lower leg, as in the chronic compartment syndrome. The acute syndrome is characterized by pain out of proportion to the physical findings, particularly with passive plantar flexion of the foot and toes. This action stretches the muscles of the anterior compartment, causing pain. Hypoesthesia in the web space of the first and second toes, representing the sensory distribution of the deep peroneal nerve, is a classical finding. Loss of the dorsalis pedis pulse is a late finding, usually associated with irretrievable loss of nerve and muscle function despite decompression. The patient may complain immediately after the injury or after swelling has continued for several days. Placement of a cast that becomes too tight as the limb swells may contribute to the problem. A high index of suspicion must be maintained for this injury, especially in patients suffering from multiple trauma, who may have an altered mental status. The diagnosis may be aided by measuring intracompartmental pressures. Frequently, the anterior compartment is tender, although this may be difficult to evaluate in patients with a fracture; a late finding is shiny or red skin over the compartment, suggesting cellulitis.

Treatment is urgent surgical fasciotomy. If it is performed in a timely fashion, the patient may suffer no permanent harm. If it is performed too late, permanent footdrop and even extensive myonecrosis of the affected compartment may result.

## NONINVASIVE ARTERIAL EVALUATION

Although the diagnosis of leg pain secondary to vascular disease can usually be made on the basis of the history and physical examination, noninvasive vascular laboratory techniques can be helpful. The ankle pressure can be determined by placing a blood pressure cuff proximal to the medial malleolus and using a Doppler probe to listen for flow while the cuff is inflated. To correct for blood pressure variations between examinations and between individuals, the result is usually reported in terms of the ankle-brachial index (ABI). This value is derived by measuring the ankle pressure and dividing by the brachial blood pressure. Typical normal values are 1.0 to 1.2. Patients with claudication commonly have ABI values between 0.5 and 0.9. Patients with rest pain frequently have ABI values less than 0.5.

Unfortunately, there is considerable variability between patients and the ABI can be used only as a rough guide. Patients with diabetes mellitus frequently have calcified, poorly compressible blood vessels, which tend to elevate the ABI artificially even in patients with significant arterial occlusive disease.

In order to increase the accuracy of the ABI, the ankle and brachial pressure measurements are frequently accompanied by pulse volume recordings. These tracings are derived from transducers attached to air-inflated cuffs placed around the patient's thigh, calf, ankles, and feet. As the arteries become more and more diseased, the tracings become flatter and blunter.

Noninvasive laboratory techniques are most useful for patients with an atypical history or examination. Patients with stenosis of the common iliac arteries may have normal pulses and ABIs at rest, but the values may drop with exercise as the peripheral resistance in the distal vasculature drops. Patients whose symptoms sound much like those of claudication but who have normal pulses may benefit from having the ABI determined after exercise.

## INITIAL MANAGEMENT, OUTCOME, AND DISABILITY

After the diagnosis of claudication is made, patients should be counseled regarding lifestyle changes such as cessation of smoking, introduction of a fat-free diet, and increase in exercise. Multiple authors have demonstrated that cessation of smoking improves the prognosis of patients with arterial occlusive disease. A regular walking program can increase walking distance greatly, although the increase in distance has varied from 36% to 234%. The only drug approved by the Food and Drug Administration to treat claudication is pentoxifylline (Trental). When pentoxifylline was combined with a regular exercise program in a multicenter, prospective, randomized trial in the United States, a statistically significant increase in walking distance after 24 weeks was noted in those who received pentoxifylline compared with those who received a placebo. Most consider the benefit of pentoxifylline compared with exercise alone to be of unclear clinical significance and reserve use of pentoxifylline for those in whom a trial of exercise and smoking cessation is unsuccessful.

It is unlikely for claudication to progress to the point at which revascularization is required in most patients. The usual indications for intervention are the following:

1. Tissue loss such as with gangrene or nonhealing ulcers.

2. Rest pain, which is usually regarded as a pregangrenous condition.

3. Disabling claudication. This is a subjective indication: claudication at 50 feet may be disabling to a 45-year-old who delivers mail but not to

an 85-year-old who has just suffered a third myocardial infarction.

In the absence of rest pain or tissue loss, most patients are reassured to know that claudication is usually a benign disease. Of patients with documented claudication secondary to arterial occlusive disease who have sought medical advice, only about 25% to 30% ever need revascularization and only about 5% come to amputation. In epidemiologic studies the risk of amputation is even lower, 1.6% after 8 years.

## SUMMARY

The signs and symptoms of acute and chronic lower extremity ischemia as well as the natural history and differential diagnosis have been reviewed. Other causes of lower extremity pain such as venous disease, compartment syndrome, and neurogenic claudication have also been discussed.

## BIBLIOGRAPHY

Clifford PC, Davies PW, Hayne JA: Intermittent claudication: Is a supervised exercise class worthwhile? Br Med J 280:1503, 1980.

Daube JR Jr, Dyck PJ: Neuropathy due to peripheral vascular diseases. In Dyck PJ, Thomas PK, Lambert EH, et al (eds): Diseases of the Peripheral Nervous System. Philadelphia, WB Saunders, 1984, pp 1458–1478.

Durham JD, Rutherford RB: Hemorrhagic compressive neuropathies: Nerve injury without direct trauma or regional ischemia. Semin Vasc Surg 4:26–30, 1991.

Ekroth R, Dahllof AG, Gundevall B, et al: Physical training of patients with intermittent claudication: Indications, methods and results. Surgery 84:640, 1978.

Ferguson FR, Liversedge LA: Ischemic lateral popliteal nerve palsy. Br Med J 2:333–335, 1954.

Jurgens IL, Barker NW, Hines EA: Arteriosclerosis obliterans: A review of 520 cases with special reference to pathogenic and prognostic factors. Circulation 21:188, 1960.

Lundborg G: The intrinsic vascularization of human peripheral nerves—Structural and functional aspects. J Hand Surg 4:34–41, 1979.

Lundborg G: Ischemic nerve injury. Experimental studies on intraneural microvascular pathophysiology and nerve function in a limb subjected to temporary circulatory arrest Scand J Plastic Reconstr Surg 6(Suppl):3–113, 1970.

McDaniel MD, Cronenwett JL: Natural history of claudication. In Porter JM, Taylor LM (eds): Basic Data Underlying Clinical Decision Making in Vascular Surgery, 1st ed. St. Louis, Quality Medical Publishing, 1994, p 129.

Passini L, Pastorelli F, Beerman M, et al: Peripheral neuropathy associated with ischemic vascular disease of the lower extremity. Angiology 47:569–577, 1996.

Sundrland S: Nerve and Nerve Injuries. Edinburgh, Churchill-Livingstone, 1978.

Turley JJ, Johnston KW: Ischemic neuropathy. Semin Vasc Surg 4:12–19, 1991.

Watson JT: Compartment syndrome. In Young JR, Graor RA, Olin JW, Bartholomew JR (eds): Peripheral Vascular Diseases, 1st ed. St. Louis, Mosby Year Book, 1991, p 553.

# Chronic Pain in the Lower Extremity

# 22

*Mitchell J. M. Cohen*

## FROM NOCICEPTION TO CHRONIC SUFFERING

Pain begins as nociception, the neural activity involved in the transmission of pain, and becomes pain only when it is perceived and given a weighting of negative emotion. With this and associated losses and changes in the patient's life, or suffering, nociception becomes pain. As pain becomes chronic, it begins to dominate mental life. All activities are seen through the lens of chronic pain, and many may be avoided because of fear of pain itself or further injury. Pain is a signal of tissue injury and danger. Patients often come to see their lives as shaped fundamentally by their chronic pain, which defines their present and future. Such a psychologic position is evidenced by statements such as, "Because of my pain, I must do this, I don't do that, I'll never change this." Whereas this pain focus is critical to survival in acute injury and focus on pain is "wired into" the central nervous system and appropriate in the short term, it becomes a component of the pathology over time, serving little constructive end.

It is critical neither to overinterpret pain on psychologic grounds nor to pursue it endlessly medically, ignoring mental life issues. Adolf Meyer's psychobiologic approach is an ideal to aspire to, although difficult to achieve fully. Meyer advocated a balanced interest in the routing of mental life events in medical pathophysiology at the same time that their individual meanings and life context are considered.[1]

## NEUROBIOLOGY OF CHRONIC PAIN AND CLINICAL IMPLICATIONS

Knowledge of the neurophysiology and neuroanatomy of pain has increased greatly since 1965, when Melzack and Wall published the gate control theory, which provided a model for major modulation of nociception centered in the dorsal horn and substantia gelatinosa of the spinal cord. This theory provided a neurobiologic mechanism whereby nociception could be modified in various ways, leading to different levels of perception, suffering, and ill-

ness behavior. The gate control theory made understandable the clinical observation that the same lower extremity disease or injury could lead to different levels of suffering. Perhaps a "golden age" of the development of knowledge was 1965 through 1980. After the gate control theory, which has been significantly refined since 1965, endogenous opiates and their receptors throughout the central nervous system were discovered, and through the late 1970s neuropathways capable of producing analgesia were better described.

Our knowledge of pain transmission has actually proceeded from the periphery of the nociceptive apparatus proximally toward the brain. It could be argued that detailed knowledge of the pain system decreases from the dorsal horn of the spinal cord upward or cephalad. We know least about central processing and integration. Our current level of understanding of the pain system predicts the complex, variable presentations of lower extremity pain that we see in patients. Major components of our current understanding are as follows:

1. There are multiple levels of modulation throughout the central nervous system and peripheral nervous system, including "gating" at the substantia gelatinosa as well as descending modulation through the midbrain, medulla, and spinal cord.
2. There is an endogenous analgesic system that involves endorphins and enkephalins as well as various neurotransmitters of major significance in mental life, such as serotonin and norepinephrine.
3. There is tremendous plasticity within the pain system. The system changes when it is provoked or activated. Nociceptors become sensitized and may change structurally if constantly activated. The spinal cord may "accelerate" pain transmission over time with chronic pain through neurophysiologic windup. Location, frequency, duration, and other parameters of noxious stimuli determine how the system changes with nociceptive input.
4. Plasticity may account for the observation that the efficacy of successful treatments often wanes over time.

5. Stimulus-independent factors such as baseline mental state at the time of nociception, environmental and life context, and individual meanings of symptoms affect pain transmission.

In evaluating chronic pain in the lower extremity, the features of pain transmission lead to important practical points in determining the lower extremity pain generator. Basic questions that must be asked in the initial formulation include the following: Is the chronic pain generator an external driver to the nerve fibers, a *nociceptive* pain (e.g., coming from an ongoing noxious stimulus through mechanical or myofascial forces on afferent fibers, ischemia to the nerve, continuing trauma, constriction of scar tissue, compression with movement)? Is the chronic pain generator reflective of intrinsic nerve damage, a spontaneous internal driver to nerve fibers, a *neurogenic* or *neuropathic* pain (e.g., sustained damage and altered function in the afferent fibers related to infection, major or minor trauma, degenerative neurologic disease)? Beyond the local pain generators, what psychologic, behavioral, social, and physiologic factors might be altering modulation of the pain experienced from the pain generator? Is the patient sleeping, exercising, engaged interpersonally with others, bored, or angry? Is there antagonism with caregivers, insurance carriers, lawyers, or employers?

## PSYCHIATRIC COMORBIDITY IN CHRONIC PAIN

### Depression

As a mental life syndrome, depression, like pain, is complicated to assess, and the prevalence in chronic pain varies from 23% to 88%.[4] The relationship between pain and depression is complicated and has involved controversy, including the question of whether a depressive syndrome can be clearly teased apart from the dysphoric phenomenology of pain itself.[2, 3] The vast majority of evidence suggests that the syndromes can be separated and that there is value in doing so.

Most evidence suggests that the majority of patients with chronic pain do not have a past history of depressive illness[4]; more often, depression develops after or simultaneously with pain. The minority of patients who do have personal or family histories of affective disorder before pain may develop particularly difficult pain and mood problems. The most critical point regarding depression is that it is treatable but often undertreated or missed entirely, especially when it presents with chronic medical illness.[5–7] The hallmarks of a significant comorbid depression fall into four major categories appreciated through examination of the patient's mental state: (1) low reported and outward mood, (2) diminished self-attitude, (3) impaired sense of physical and mental vitality, and (4) hopelessness or suicidal ideation. Patients with pain who develop significant comorbid depression report anhedonia, crying spells, apathy, and loss of initiative. Outwardly, they may appear restricted in their range of emotional show, either overtly sad in appearance or stilted and "flat," lacking emotional reactivity and spontaneity. Self-attitude becomes colored by guilty concerns over loss of productivity, burdening family members, or being "crippled" or worthless. Depressed patients feel sickly and weak and have difficulty with memory and concentration.[8] Unlike the common personal helplessness of depression in other settings, pain patients may describe "universal" helplessness, that is, ascribing blame more to failure of the medical community than to personal inadequacies. This feature can lead clinicians to miss the depression or feel personally attacked. Depressions in chronic pain may also lack the diurnal mood variation (mood worst in the morning) of classical major depression.[8]

The first line of treatment for a depressed patient with pain should be a selective serotonin reuptake inhibitor such as fluoxetine (Prozac) 20 mg/day or paroxetine (Paxil) 20 mg/day. If the pain is neuropathic in etiology, a secondary-amine tricyclic such as nortriptyline (Pamelor, Aventyl) or desipramine (Norpramin) should be considered. Secondary-amine tricyclics are better tolerated than the older tertiaryamine tricyclics, such as amitriptyline (Elavil), in terms of anticholinergic and antihistaminergic side effects, and they appear essentially as effective with neuropathic chronic pain. Tricyclics in general have specific analgesic effects for some neuropathic pains. Evidence that mood and analgesic effects can be separated has emerged. Risk of undertreatment argues for titration of these drugs toward full therapeutic dosages for full trials, the equivalent of 75 to 150 mg of nortriptyline for 6 to 12 weeks with serum level monitoring.

Newer selective serotonin reuptake inhibitors such as fluoxetine (Prozac) and sertraline (Zoloft) have superior side effect profiles in most patients, are easier to dose, safer in overdose, and are becoming first-line treatment for standard depressed patients. Although they may perform equally well in relieving mood symptoms, to date there are only limited reports of their analgesic efficacy in chronic pain and results are conflicting.[9, 10] Selective serotonin reuptake inhibitors may also not as reliably normalize the disturbed sleep common in patients with lower extremity pain problems, and serum level ranges have not yet been correlated with therapeutic response.

## Anxiety Disorders

Severe posttraumatic stress disorder (PTSD) involves vivid relivings of the leg injury or accident by the patient, intrusive fear of being hurt again, panic episodes with autonomic elevations (e.g., increased pulse, blood pressure, flushing), and nightmares with content evocative of the feelings and circumstances surrounding the original injury. Generalized anxiety disorder (GAD) would present as a tendency to "worry about everything": family, work, litigation, further injury, and so forth in a ruminative, nonproductive manner. GAD is the most vague and difficult to diagnose of these syndromes. Panic disorder can present in patients with pain as part of PTSD or as an independent syndrome. Panic episodes can involve intense anxiety, subjective dread, the autonomic changes mentioned, chest pain, and exacerbated chronic lower extremity pain. Such attacks disable patients, magnifying fear of reinjury, increasing emergeny room and office visits, and fueling progressive activity reductions, even leading to the full confinement of agoraphobia.

PTSD and panic disorder can respond to serotonin-selective reuptake inhibitors, tricyclic, or monoamine oxidase inhibitor antidepressants. Again, secondary amines are preferred among the tricyclics. Tranylcypromine (Parnate, therapeutic dose 10 to 15 mg three times a day) is among the best tolerated monoamine oxidase inhibitors. PTSD, panic episodes, and GAD can also respond quite dramatically to benzodiazepines.

## Personality Issues

It is best to think in terms of individual vulnerabilities rather than disorders in assessing personality problems in patients with chronic pain.[11] Trait vulnerabilities that most often complicate chronic pain include dependent, passive-aggressive, histrionic, paranoid, antisocial, and obsessive-compulsive dimensions.[12–14] Long and colleagues noted the difficulty in categorically assigning a personality disorder, assigning mainly "mixed" personality diagnoses to 59% of their patients with failed back syndrome and noting primarily antisocial, histrionic, and dependent traits. The "pain-prone" composite put forth by Engel[15] and modified by others[16] is one that clinicians have recognized in individual patients with pain in whom medical or surgical treatments were unsuccessful, although it is difficult to validate. Pain-prone patients in this personality characterization are described as blue-collar, unusually hard-working before to injury ("ergomanic"), perhaps frequently punished as children, and uncomfortable with expression of negative emotion. These historical and trait features are often complicated by

mood disorder.[15, 16] One aspect of this characterization, the lack of openness to emotional or psychologic issues, has been given the special designation *alexithymia,* literally meaning inability to put one's feelings into words.[17] As a result, such individuals tend to express their psychic distress behaviorally, some of them in the form of reports of magnified lower extremity pain or poor progress in treatment.

## Opioid Therapy and Substance Abuse

Opioid therapy is an evolving area of practice, with limited useful data addressing the issue. It continues to be a controversial area, but the growing number of anecdotal, open, and uncontrolled trials suggest that opioids have a treatment role,[18–21] although better data are needed. Across many pain contexts (oncology, burn units, and noncancer pain centers), clear opioid addiction appears rare.[18, 22–24] With the recognition that opioids may have legitimate analgesic utility and underdosing is common and can provoke overcompliance or "drug seeking,"[25, 26] defining substance abuse becomes complicated. Because there is accumulated clinical experience that narcotics and opiates become problematic in a subpopulation of patients with chronic pain, it is probably best to formulate some overarching principles for treatment. First, opiates should not be categorically withheld because of clinicians' fears of relatively rare substance use disorders. Second, opioid treatment must be highly individualized and should be only one component of treatment. Third, patients who receive opiates need careful monitoring by a physician and family members, assessing for continuing benefit and signs of misuse or impairment longitudinally. Finally, greater vulnerability to substance use problems can be expected in patients with significant current psychic distress, a family or personal past psychiatric history, and particularly past substance abuse.[12]

The small group of pain patients who are illicit or recreational substance abusers are a difficult subset who often have substance abuse histories, antisocial traits antedating their pain problem,[4] and often have poor treatment outcomes.[27] The most commonly abused drug is alcohol,[4] and these patients with pain are more likely to have family histories of substance abuse and mood disorder.

## Abnormal Illness Behavior

Abnormal illness behavior has received considerable focus as a form of psychopathology encountered in patients with chronic pain, despite the rarity of the most serious forms of abnormal illness behavior, such as somatization disorder (prevalence in studies varies from none[13] to as high as 8.1% definite cases). Abnormal illness behavior is physical and verbal behavior that communicates distress in excess of what would be expected on the basis of the objective findings or discoverable etiopathogenesis or beyond what is needed to obtain an appropriate helping response.[28] When formally studied, frank malingering and factitious illness diagnoses (consciously feigning illness for external or emotional gain) were found to be quite rare in patients with chronic pain,[10, 13] with a prevalence at 2% or less.[14] Symptom amplification, a much less serious form of illness exaggeration, often occurs in these patients, frequently because they fear that clinicians do not believe them or are not successfully reducing their pain or because they sense that friends and family are distancing themselves. The symptom amplification is, of course, counterproductive and raises suspicion of frank factitious illness in clinicians, payers, friends, and family. Data have not always supported the clinical concern that disability and insurance concerns drive much pain behavior,[29, 30] although this can be quite relevant in individual cases.

### Bereavement, Interpersonal Relationships, Role Changes

Patients with chronic pain are often grieving the loss of their former healthy selves, and they cannot come to terms with the losses because the diagnosis, treatment, and prognosis are often not clear.[11] These patients really cannot be fully satisfied because no intervention can return them to the days before chronic pain, which they have idealized and on which they are often still focused. Striking anger and frustration are experienced by patients with chronic pain generally.[31] Sources of anger in these patients are many: "wired-in" arousal and irritability from paleospinothalamic and spinoreticular tracts in the ascending pain system, the grief response, disappointment over an unclear diagnosis or unsuccessful treatment, and social pressure to resume function. Anger can be the most prominent component of emotional suffering in some patients with chronic pain.[32] Anger can also cause distress in their families.[33]

Patients with pain are often struggling in relationships with health care professionals at the same time they are negotiating derailments in other major interpersonal spheres. Although patients often receive initial compassion, support, and even enabling of illness behavior, the real burdens of this help eventually become clear to those providing it. Initial understanding in the patient's interpersonal circle can give way to impatience, frustration, questioning the legitimacy of symptoms, and emotional distance. Shifts in relationships and roles with spouse, children, friends, and neighbors occur as everyone tries to find some balanced way to interact in the presence of the painful illness and impairment.

## TREATMENT PRINCIPLES EMERGING FROM PAIN CENTERS

Pain treatment center approaches vary among facilities, but they do share emphasis on provision of longitudinal care as opposed to definitive cure, which is often unavailable. Pain center approaches represent a "buckshot" method, aimed at attacking the problem from various angles simultaneously: working in physical therapy to increase strength, range of motion, and confidence; working in occupational therapy to develop novel approaches to the accomplishment of tasks, given physical limitations, and learning to pace activities appropriately; identifying connections between stress and pain and learning stress management and relaxation techniques; identifying major associated anxiety and depression and treating it with indicated medications and psychotherapy; evaluating the responses of the family and employer to the patient's pain and intervening in positive ways; and treating the pain with all available appropriate direct procedures.

Outcome research from pain centers is fraught with methodologic problems because of the multifaceted nature of the treatment.[34] It has been difficult to determine which components of the approach are critical when positive effects have been demonstrated. Recognizing limitations of study design, a large number of outcome studies have been conducted and reviewed in large meta-analytic studies. The body of data suggests that reductions in emotional distress, functional impairment, and medical utilization occur as a result of the pain center's care versus cure, rehabilitative approach. Trials of transcutaneous electrical nerve stimulation, biofeedback, hypnosis, relaxation training, stress management, and complementary medicine (e.g., acupuncture, nutrition teaching) have been undertaken in various pain centers, but the individual value of these approaches has not been determined clearly. Narcotic detoxification has been a component in most pain centers, but its value remains an open question, as alluded to earlier. The clinical belief that opioid drugs have little utility in treating chronic pain was one of the orthodoxies that rose out of the pain center experience of the first two decades of the past quarter-century.[22] This has begun to change dramatically. It is clear that the risks of addiction, although real, have been greatly overestimated. Certainly, the state of current knowledge does not justify categorical exclusion of opioid use in treating chronic lower extremity pain.

Comprehensive formulations of patients' suffering appear more effective than narrowly focused symptomatic treatment. Rigorous treatment of comorbid depression, anxiety, and substance abuse has also contributed to some of the positive outcome data. Involvement of the family has been reported to promote progress and the promise of longitudinal attention and practical treatments has reassured patients, whereas promises of dramatic interventions and improvements and simplistic psychologizing (e.g., "It's all in your head" or "Just live with it") have been unsuccessful. Ultimately, the clinician's task is to develop a practical pathway for improvement.

## REFERENCES

1. Rutter M: Meyerian psychobiology, personality development, and the role of life experiences. Am J Psychiatry 143:1077–1087, 1986.
2. Pelz M, Merskey H: A description of the psychological effects of chronic painful lesions. Pain 14:293–301, 1982.
3. Pilowsky I, Chapman CR, Bonica JJ: Pain, depression, and illness behavior in a pain clinic population. Pain 4:183–192, 1977.
4. Atkinson JH, Slater MA, Patterson TL, et al: Prevalence, onset and risk of psychiatric disorders in men with chronic low back pain: A controlled study. Pain 45:111–121, 1991.
5. Katon W: Depression: Somatic symptoms and medical disorders in primary care. Compr Psychiatry 23:274–287, 1982.
6. Katon W: The epidemiology of depression in medical care. Int J Psychiatry Med 17:93–112, 1987.
7. McCombs JS, Nichol MB, Stimmel GL, et al: The cost of antidepressant drug therapy failure: A study of use patterns in a Medicaid population. J Clin Psychiatry 51(6 Suppl):60–69, 1990.
8. Davidson J, Krishnan R, France R, Pelton S: Neurovegetative symptoms in chronic pain and depression. J Affect Disord 9:213–218, 1985.
9. Conroy JM, Kee WG, Harden N, Williams A: Fluoxetine in the treatment of chronic low back pain. American Pain Society 11th Annual Scientific Meeting, San Diego, 1992, p 78.
10. Eisendrath SJ, Kodama KT: Fluoxetine management of chronic abdominal pain. Psychosomatics 33:227–229, 1992.
11. Cohen MJ: Psychosocial aspects of evaluation and management of chronic low back pain. *In*: Physical Medicine and Rehabilitation: State of the Art Reviews. Philadelphia, Hanley & Belfus, 1995, pp 726–746.
12. Fishbain DA, Goldberg M, Meagher BR, et al: Male and female chronic pain patients categorized by DSM-III psychiatric diagnostic criteria. Pain 26:181–197, 1986.
13. Gatchel RJ, Polatin PB, Mayer TG, Garcy PD: Psychopathology and the rehabilitation of patients with chronic low back pain disability. Arch Phys Med Rehabil 75:666–670, 1994.
14. Reich J, Tupin JP, Abramowitz SI: Psychiatric diagnosis of chronic pain patients. Am J Psychiatry 140:1495–1498, 1983.
15. Engel GL: "Psychogenic" pain and the pain-prone patient. Am J Med 26:899–918, 1959.
16. Blumer D, Heilbronn M: The pain-prone disorder: A clinical and psychological profile. Psychosomatics 22:395–402, 1981.
17. Catchlove RFH, Cohen KR, Braha RED, Demers-Desrosiers LA: Incidence and implications of alexithymia in chronic pain patients. J Nerv Ment Dis 172:246–248, 1985.
18. France RD, Urban BJ, Keefe FJ: Long-term use of narcotic analgesics in chronic pain. Soc Sci Med 19:1379–1382, 1984.
19. Portenoy RK: Chronic opioid therapy in nonmalignant pain. J Pain Symptom Manage 5(1 Suppl):S46–S62, 1990.
20. Taub A: Opioid analgesic in the treatment of chronic intractable pain of non-neoplastic origin. *In* Kitahata LM, Collins D (eds): Narcotic Analgesics in Anesthesiology. Baltimore, Williams & Wilkins, 1982, pp 199–208.
21. Zenz M, Strumpf M, Tryba M: Long-term oral opioid therapy in patients with chronic nonmalignant pain. J Pain Symptom Manage 7:69–77, 1992.
22. Bouckoms AJ, Masand P, Murray GB, et al: Chronic nonmalignant pain treated with long-term oral analgesics. Ann Clin Psychiatry 4:185–192, 1992.
23. Perry S, Heidrich G: Management of pain during debridement. A survey of U.S. burn units. Pain 13:267–280, 1982.
24. Porter J, Jick H: Addiction rare in patients treated with narcotics. N Engl J Med 302:123, 1980.
25. Ferrell BR, Eberts MT, McCaffery M, Grant M: Clinical decision making and pain. Cancer Nursing 14(6):289–297, 1991.
26. Marks RM, Sachar EJ: Undertreatment of medical inpatients with narcotic analgesics. Ann Intern Med 78:173–181, 1973.
27. Finlayson RE, Maruta T, Morse RM, Martin MA: Substance dependence and chronic pain: Experience with treatment and follow-up results. Pain 26:175–180, 1986.
28. Mechanic D: Social psychologic factors affecting the presentation of bodily complaints. N Engl J Med 286:1132–1139, 1972.
29. Dworkin RH, Handlin DS, Richlin DM, et al: Unraveling the effects of compensation, litigation, and employment on treatment response in chronic pain. Pain 23:49–59, 1985.
30. Mendelson G: Chronic pain and compensation: A review. J Pain Symptom Manage 1:135–144, 1986.
31. Fernandez E, Turk DC: Anger in chronic pain patients: A neglected target of attention. Am Pain Soc Bull 3(4):5–7, 1993.
32. Fernandez E, Milburn TW: Sensory and affective predictors of overall pain and emotions associated with affective pain. Clin J Pain 10:3–9, 1994.
33. Schwartz L, Slater MA, Birchler GR, Atkinson JH: Depression in spouses of chronic pain patients: The role of patient pain and anger, and marital satisfaction. Pain 44:61–67, 1991.
34. Aronoff GM, Evans WO, Enders PL: A review of follow-up studies of multidisciplinary pain units. Pain 16:1–11, 1983.

# Rehabilitation: The Lower Extremity and Neurologic Impairment

# 23

*Ernest M. Baran*

Neurologic impairment of the lower extremity may present with neuromuscular deficits, and the manifestations of these deficits present with functional and mobility problems for the patient. The primary neurologic injury may present with mobility deficits, pain, weakness, and impaired sensation; however, the patient may also develop secondary musculoskeletal problems. Not only must one have an understanding of the neurologic impairment, but also a comprehensive functional-musculoskeletal evaluation is needed so that all soft tissue and joint problems are accurately identified.

## APPROACH TO THE PATIENT

The rehabilitation examination consists of a thorough functional evaluation of the patient, including the history and physical examination and the disability that has resulted from the neurologic impairment. Assessment of the patient's remaining functional capabilities is essential in formulating a strategy for optimizing the patient's functional outcome. An analysis of the activities of daily living should be performed, including a functional history, ambulation status, ability to drive or use public conveyance, personal hygiene, dressing, feeding, environmental control (e.g., patient's ability to control household appliances), communication, recreation, homemaking, and workplace functions.

In addition to the conventional history (chief complaint, history of present illness), a functional history (activities of daily living) should be obtained. The analysis of symptoms should include the following: date of onset, character and severity, location and extension, time relationships, associated complaints, aggravating and alleviating factors, previous treatment, and effects and progress, noting remissions and exacerbations.

In evaluating patients with neurologic impairment of the lower extremities, special attention to analysis of posture, balance, and gait is mandatory. It is important to observe sitting balance, ability to transfer from a sitting to a standing position, stand-ing balance, and ambulation. Observations for fixed or abnormal postures and inadequate, excessive, or asymmetric movements of body parts should be noted. Observation for head and trunk listing or tilting, shoulder dipping, elevation, protraction, and retraction is important. Protective positioning or posturing and observation of the pelvis and hip should be made to identify hip hiking, drooping (Trendelenburg symptom), or lateral thrust. Inspection for knee genu valgum (outward angulation), varum (inward angulation), or recurvatum (excessive extension) and excessive foot-ankle inversion or eversion should be made. It is important to observe ambulation factors such as cadence (rate, symmetry, fluidity, and consistency), stride width (narrow or broad based, knee-ankle clearance), stride length (short, long, or asymmetric), stance phase (normal heel strike, foot flat, push-off; knee stability during all components of stance phase and coordination of knee-ankle movements), and swing phase (adequate and synchronized knee and ankle dorsiflexion during swing abduction or circumduction) so that gait training can be directed to specific deficits.

## REHABILITATION ASPECTS OF TREATMENT

### Identification of Goals

When the neurologic impairment and functional deficits have been identified, a systematic analysis of the rehabilitation tools for achieving the objectives should be made.

### Therapeutic Exercise

#### Range of Motion

Before prescribing therapeutic exercise, knowledge of range of motion of the hip, knee, ankle, and lumbosacral spine must first be ascertained. If limited range of motion of any joint is present, active, active- assisted, or passive range-of-motion exercises may be needed to restore full movement, pending analysis of the reason for limitation of joint movement. Range of motion may be lost for many reasons, including deficits in the articulating surface (intra-articular loose bodies—bone or cartilage, excessive fluid or contracture). A contracture may be produced by soft tissue (skin, joint capsule) or the muscle-tendon system. Common physical causes of contracture include inflammation, resulting from disease or trauma; spasticity; and decrease in motion resulting from pain, paralysis, or externally applied appliances (casts, splints). Contractures become functionally significant when they restrict ambulation, self care, or attendant care or cause skin ulcers. For example, a hip flexion contracture can cause excessive lumbar lordosis by realigning the center of gravity when the patient is standing upright.

### Exercise

Exercise has immediate effects and late (adaptive, training) effects on the localized area undergoing exercise as well as systemic effects.

#### Systemic and Acute Effects

Systemic effects of exercise are dependent on the type of activity (e.g., walking, cycling), specific muscle groups involved in the exercise, and percentage of maximum force used to exercise. Initially, there are increases in heart rate, cardiac output, blood pressure, and vasodilatation. Muscle contraction increases venous return. Hormonal changes occur and include decreased insulin production; increased glucagon production; an increase in circulating catecholamines; increases in growth, adrenocorticotropic, thyroid-stimulating, and posterior pituitary hormones; and an increase in androgens, usually with periods of exercise greater than 20 minutes. Endurance exercise decreases triglyceride, increases high-density lipoprotein, and decreases low-density lipoprotein concentrations for 1 to 2 days depending on the intensity of exercise. The cardiovascular responses to exercises consist of increases in oxygen uptake, minimum heart rate, maximum stroke volume, and peripheral vascular resistance. Syncope can occur after vigorous exercise and is secondary to hypotension resulting from blood pooling in the extremities. This stimulates catecholamines, increasing the risk of cardiac ischemia and dysrhythmia in susceptible patients. Therefore, a cooldown period is important after vigorous exercise.

Upper extremity exercise increases systolic and diastolic blood pressures and heart rate more than lower extremity exercise. Upper extremity exercise requires higher oxygen uptake than lower extremity exercise. A combination of arm and leg endurance exercises has been shown to be most effective for cardiovascular fitness because of the greater number of muscle groups involved.

In the muscle being exercised, there is a linear increase in oxygen consumption with the intensity of exercise. An increase in carbon dioxide production is also seen, and vasodilatation occurs in the exercising muscles. During isometric contraction, there is complete occlusion of blood flow at 70% of maximum voluntary contraction. Strengthening programs benefit the muscles being exercised and have little systemic effect other than increasing absolute left ventricular wall thickness and left ventricular hypotrophy. Endurance training increases aerobic capacity of the muscles being exercised, and there is also an improvement in cardiovascular adaptation. Therefore, there is a reduced resting heart rate at a given level of exercise, increase in stroke volume, increase in left ventricular end-diastolic volume, increase in maximum ventilatory ability, and increase in blood volume and hemoglobin with endurance training.

### Exercise Prescription

Before a prescription for exercise can be written, several factors have to be taken into consideration: goals to be achieved, type of exercise, and medical status of the patient.

#### Goals

Patients have different goals and objectives depending on the neurologic deficit of the lower extremity, medical status, and the type of lifestyle the patient would like to achieve with the therapeutic exercise program. Common objectives include an increase in strength or endurance, improvement in range of motion, increase in motor control and coordination of the lower extremities, and increase in the ability to relax muscles. The patient's general fitness and conditioning must also be considered in the prescription goals. Communication between the physician and therapist is critical in achieveing the best outcome with any therapeutic exercise program within the framework of the patient's medical status.

#### Specific Considerations

**Clinical Status.** After the neurologic deficit is identified, type of exercise (passive range of motion, active assisted range of motion, active, isotonic, isometric); coordination; angina; congestive heart failure; arrhythmia; joint contracture; previous spine, limb, or joint surgery; febrile illnesses; pulmonary disorders (e.g., asthma, chronic obstructive pulmonary disease); age; and body habitus should be taken into consideration before the prescription is formulated. Age-predicted maximum heart rates are an important guide before prescribing the intensity of exercise. If there may be questions concerning the status of the cardiovascular condition, monitoring or prior stress testing is useful. Effective cardiac drugs must also be considered in the contort of exercise. Exercise increases glucose utilization; therefore, a balance should be achieved between the amount of insulin being taken by a patient and the exercise prescription to avoid hypoglycemia. Injection of insulin into a muscle that is to be exercised increases the insulin absorption rate and may produce earlier or faster hypoglycemia. Heavy exercise in diabetes may cause dehydration and ketosis. Intraocular hemorrhage is a concern during isometric exercise, and peripheral neuropathy may facilitate injury in areas of impaired sensation when involved limbs are undergoing exercise.

There may be a risk of precipitating attacks in asthmatics with exercise; therefore, pre-exercise medication may have to be used. Patients with chronic obstructive pulmonary disease have to be evaluated for problems of hypoxia, pulmonary hypertension with resistance to right ventricular output, and air trapping. Supplemental oxygen may be necessary for these patients.

In patients with neuromuscular disease, strengthening attempts may result in increased muscle weakness. Excessive exercise involving partially denervated or reinnervated muscles may interfere with reinnervation. For patients with lower motor neuron lesions, including primary muscle disease, the amount of exercise and change in the muscle strength may have to be monitored with the use of muscle enzymes to ensure no adverse effects of exercise.

**Timing of Exercise Program.** How soon a specific exercise program should be started must be considered to avoid injury of the muscle groups or aggravation of a medical condition. Therefore, the number of exercise sessions per week, length of the exercise period, number of repetitions, and rest periods are important considerations in an exercise prescription. It is important to achieve a balance between the stress of the exercise to stimulate muscle strength and endurance, and adequate rest for adaptation to the exercise.

**Environment.** Factors such as temperature, altitude, and humidity are important in the exercise prescription. In general, temperatures between 60 and 70°F with low humidity are ideal for exercise, but this is dependent on multiple considerations including the medical status, age, and neurologic status of the patient. Adequate hydration before exercise ensures a safe exercise program.

**Warm-Up and Cooldown.** A warm-up period with stretching is recommended even for patients with neurologic injuries to produce a gradual increase in body temperature, circulation, and flexibility and minimize cardiovascular stress. A cooldown period is important to prevent postexercise syncope.

**Specificity of Instructions.** The physician should make the diagnosis specific enough that the therapist knows which part of the body is to be exercised. Substitution of muscle groups should be avoided so that the involved muscles can be properly strengthened. An appropriate follow-up by the physician is necessary to determine whether the exercise goals and objectives are being achieved, and modification of the exercise program may be necessary to optimize the exercise prescription.

## Type of Exercise (Passive, Active Assisted, Active, Aerobic or Subaerobic, Coordination, Motor Control)

### Passive Range of Motion

Passive range of motion of the individual limb or joint may be needed if the patient has no motor control of the limb or joint. Care must be taken in performing passive range-of-motion exercises to avoid joint, capsule, or muscle injury.

### Active Assisted Exercise

If a patient has partial motor control of a joint or limb, the involved extremity can be assisted through the range of motion with the patient partially contracting the muscle to assist in movement. This activity not only improves range of motion but also aids in strengthening the involved muscle groups. The exercise can be performed by a therapist or physical therapy assistant. A water program would also be beneficial in achieving assisted movement because the buoyancy of water assists movement.

### Active Exercise

Active exercise can be achieved with isotonic exercise (volitional movement through a range of motion) or isometric exercise (contraction of a muscle in a static position without movement).

Active exercise programs using progressive resistance with 10 repetitions at 25%, 50%, 75%, and 100% of maximum capability for successive efforts

(DeLorme's strengthening program) are effective. Two minutes of rest are allowed between repetitions, and the weight is increased weekly after redetermining the maximum weight that a patient can lift 10 times.

Isometric exercise consists of a least five maximum contractions per session held for several seconds with 2 to 3 minutes between maximum contractions to allow recovery. Strength gains of 5% per week are reported with this method of contraction.

Eccentric exercise consists of lengthening a muscle while it is contracting; however, this type of exercise involves a higher risk of muscle damage, particularly to type II muscle fibers.

### Endurance Exercise

Strengthening exercises of the lower extremities for neurologic injuries do not usually involve an aerobic protocol, but they may be used in selected situations. Aerobic exercise involves at least 50% of the body muscle mass and should last for 15 to 20 minutes. The patient's heart rate should be 60% to 70% of the age-predicted maximum, and the exercise should be performed at 60% to 70% of maximum oxygen uptake. Any patient older than 30 years should have a cardiac stress test so that a maximum heart rate can be determined to avoid cardiac injury when exercising.

### Coordination and Motor Control Exercises

These exercise programs are designed for patients with ataxia, incoordination, or impaired control of movement. The patients usually have upper motor neuron lesions (e.g., cerebral palsy, incomplete spinal cord injury, CVA), but some patients with lower motor neuron lesions (e.g., polio, peripheral neuropathy, radiculopathy) may require such a program. The goal of control and coordination exercises is to develop sensory engrams and motor programs that can be stored in the central nervous system for future activities. These exercises attempt to reactivate neuronal pathways that may have been inhibited because of central nervous system lesions. In patients with upper motor neuron lesions, there may also be disuse weakness that can benefit from strengthening programs so that coordination and motor control are optimized. Gait and upright-sitting balance training are important in achieving coordination and motor control objectives. Gait and balance training should be directed to correction of specific gait or balance deficits; however, if these corrections are not amenable to training, compensa-

tory strategies can be used to achieve optimal ambulation.

## PHYSICAL MODALITIES USED TO ACHIEVE REHABILITATION GOALS

Physical agents are an important part of the armamentarium in treatment of neurologic deficits and enhancement of exercise programs for the lower extremities.

### Contractures

If a contracture is associated with a neurologic injury (joint contracture resulting from weakness), heat and stretching may be beneficial in augmenting movement. A prolonged stretch on a contracture that has been preheated with ultrasound or moist heat can prove effective in achieving more movement. Ultrasound can produce a joint temperature elevation of as much as 8 to 10°C; therefore, soft tissue extensibility is enhanced with this modality.

### Transcutaneous Electrical Nerve Stimulation

Analgesia can be introduced with a transcutaneous electrical nerve stimulation (TENs) unit. A painful muscle or joint can be treated during or before therapeutic exercise to improve the patients participation in the exercise program. The stimulating electrodes must be placed in different locations to optimize the analgesic effect of the TENs unit. The frequency, intensity, and waveform of the stimulating current have to be adjusted for optimal induction of analgesia.

### Electrical Stimulation of Muscle

Surface stimulation of muscle has been shown to be effective in strengthening muscle. Atrophic muscle increases in strength with electrical stimulation, and stimulation of denervated muscle can prevent atrophy and loss of oxidative enzymes. Terminal sprouting in lower motor neuron lesions has occurred with electrical stimulation of muscle. The method and characteristics of stimulation have not been optimized; therefore, this modality should be used by someone who has had experience in optimizing the adjustment of the electrical stimulation. This modality can be helpful when conventional exercise programs have had limited usefulness or when pain or other causes of reduced muscle activity prevent the voluntary contraction of muscle.

## LOWER EXTREMITY ORTHOTICS, GAIT AIDS, AND WHEELCHAIRS

Orthotics are devices (braces, splints) that immobilize a joint or body segment, restrict movement, control mobility, assist with movement, or reduce weight-bearing forces. An orthotic device provides support to a weak or paralyzed extremity. Before a physician prescribes an orthosis, the anatomy, neuromuscular status, and functional-biomechanical deficits should first be clearly understood.

### Materials

Advances in synthetic materials (thermoplastics) have provided lightweight, durable, and flexible orthotic devices with cosmetic features. Ankle-foot orthoses (AFOs) and knee-ankle-foot orthoses (KAFOs) are available for impairment or weakness of ankle and knee musculature. These devices provide support for weight bearing, and the AFOs can be constructed to assist in ankle dorsiflexion. The traditional AFOs (brace consisting of metal uprights attached to a shoe with T straps) are also commercially available for patients who need more mechanical ankle support.

### Ankle-Foot Orthoses

These devices are prescribed for muscle weakness involving the ankle and subtalar joints. AFOs can also affect the stability of the knee by varying the degree of plantar flexion or dorsiflexion at the ankle. An AFO fixed in dorsiflexion induces flexion at the knee, thereby preventing excessive knee extension (genu recurvatum). An AFO fixed in plantar flexion induces extension at the knee, thereby providing more stability in the knee during the stance phase of gait. Plastic AFOs are worn inside the shoe and consist of a foot plate, an upright component, and a Velcro calf strap. The plastic leaf-spring orthosis is the most commonly prescribed AFO (Fig. 23–1). Metal AFOs have medial and lateral uprights with an ankle joint mechanism. The uprights are attached to a shoe by a stirrup and secured to the calf by a padded calf band or leather strap and buckle. Orthopedic shoes are required for metal orthoses. Different joint mechanisms allow fixed, limited, or full dorsiflexion or plantar flexion. The Klenzak ankle joint orthosis assists ankle dorsiflexion by a spring in the ankle mechanism. A plantar flexion

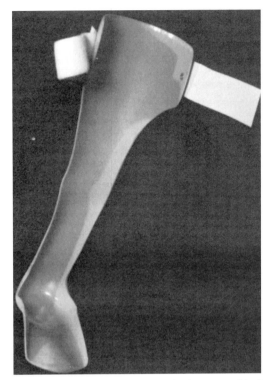

**Figure 23–1.** Custom-made posterior leaf-spring ankle-foot orthosis. (From Dyck PJ, et al: Peripheral Neuropathy, 3rd ed. Philadelphia, WB Saunders, 1993, p 1704.)

stop can be applied to induce knee flexion, and a dorsiflexion stop can be added to induce knee extension (during the stance phase of gait) to prevent excessive knee extension.

### Knee-Ankle-Foot Orthoses

These devices produce knee stability for weight bearing in addition to ankle stability. A free knee joint hinge may be used when there is adequate knee extension or flexion strength while maintaining control of medial and lateral instability. If the knee extensors are weak, a knee lock is needed (drop-ring lock). A spring-loaded lock may be added to assist in locking and unlocking the knee. Thigh uprights are connected to a soft thigh band with a closure and should clear the ischium by 1.5 inches to avoid irritation of the region. Plastic laminated KAFOs provide a lightweight brace and incorporate the standard knee mechanism and solid ankle mold. A suprapatellar support is needed for knee extension force and provides medial and lateral stability.

KAFOs are prescribed for patients with weak knee and/or ankle muscles, but these patients must have normal hip extensors, full knee extension, and no spasticity. The Swedish knee orthosis fits only around the knee and provides control of lateral, medial, and posterior knee stability and is indicated for genu valgum, varus, and recurvatum.

## Hip-Knee-Ankle-Foot Orthoses

These orthoses have the same components as described for the AFOs and KAFOs with the addition of a lockable hip joint and pelvic band to control movements at the hip. Paraplegics may benefit from these orthoses, but the devices may also increase the lumbar excursion and displacement of gravity during ambulation, thus increasing the energy needed for ambulation. A reciprocating gait orthosis provides bilateral hip-knee-ankle-foot orthoses with posterior offset knee joints, knee locks, posterior plastic ankle-foot and thigh pieces, a custom-molded pelvic girdle, and a special thrust-bearing hip joint couple together with a cable and conduit and a thoracic extension with Velcro straps. This cable coupling mechanism provides hip stability by preventing simultaneous bilateral hip flexion yet allowing free unilateral hip flexion-extension in a reciprocal fashion when a step is attempted. Two crutches or a walker is required when using this type of orthosis. This orthosis has also been tested and used in conjunction with a functional electrical stimulation system to facilitate paraplegic ambulation.

## Gait Aids (Cane, Crutches, Walkers, Wheelchairs)

Gait aids are prescribed to improve balance, decrease pain, decrease weight-bearing forces on injured or inflamed joints or muscles, and compensate for weak muscles in the lower extremities. Canes are made of wood or metal and come with a variety of hand molds to accommodate the patient's hands. All canes should have rubber tips on the weight-bearing end. Three- and four-prong canes are available to provide a wider base of support.

Crutches are indicated for patients with more severe weakness or balance deficits, but good upper extremity strength and good range of motion are required for weight bearing and propulsion on the upper extremities. Axillary, Lofstrand, and forearm crutches are available for the appropriate clinical conditions. The Lofstrand crutch consists of a single aluminum tubular shaft adjustable in length, a molded handpiece, and a forearm piece that adjusts posteriorly above the handpiece. This crutch is lightweight, easily adjustable, and allows freedom for hand activities because the handpiece can be released without losing the crutch. This crutch requires greater skills than the axillary crutch, good strength of the upper extremities, and adequate balance for safe ambulation. Forearm crutches may be prescribed when clinical conditions of the forearm, wrist, or hands prevent safe or comfortable weight bearing (e.g., in the presence of arthritis of the hand, wrist, or elbow) or in the presence of weakness of triceps or grasp.

Walkers provide the widest base of support and are prescribed for patients who require maximum assistance with balance, especially if the patients are fearful and uncoordinated. Good grasp and arm strength are needed for walkers. Walkers are available in various sizes; are adjustable in height; and come in different designs such as folding and rolling. Reciprocal and stair walkers are also available.

Wheelchairs are available for patients who are unable to ambulate. Wheelchairs come in different sizes and types and are prescribed according to the patient's needs. Electrically controlled wheelchairs or scooters are available for patients who desire a higher level of independence and are capable of controlling the device.

## BIBLIOGRAPHY

Braun SR, Fregosi R, Reddan WG: Exercise training in patients with COPD. Postgrad Med 71:163–173, 1982.

Calliet R: Knee Pain and Disability, 3rd ed. Philadelphia, FA Davis, 1992, pp 45, 47, 164, 264.

Delisa J, Gans B: Rehabilitation Medicine: Principles and Practice. Philadelphia, JB Lippincott, 1993, pp 504–506, 526–554, 671, 751, 773.

Fiatarone MA, Marks EL, Ryan ND, et al: High intensity strength training in nonagenarians. Effects on skeletal muscle. JAMA 263:3029–3034, 1990.

Jensen MD, Miles JM: The roles of diet and exercise in the management of patients with insulin-dependent diabetes mellitus. Mayo Clin Proc 61:813–819, 1986.

Lehneis HR: New developments in lower limb orthotics through bioengineering. Arch Phys Med Rehabil 53:303–310, 1972.

Milner-Brown HS, Miller RG: Muscle strengthening through electric stimulation combined with low-resistance weights in patients with neuromuscular disorders. Arch Phys Med Rehabil 69:20–24, 1988.

Saltin B, (ed): Biochemistry of Exercise VI. International Series on Sport Sciences, Vol 16. Champaign, IL, Human Kinetics Publishers, 1986.

Tyler E, Caldwell C, Ghia JN: Transcutaneous electrical nerve stimulation; an alternative approach to the management of post-operative pain. Anesth Analg 61:449–456, 1982.

Weinstein SL, Buckwalter JA: Turek's Orthopaedics: Principles and Their Application. Philadelphia, JB Lippincott, 1994, p 586.

Woodburne RT: Essentials of Human Anatomy. New York, Oxford University Press, 1961, p 530.

# AMA Guide to Functional

# Capacity Evaluation

# 24

*Richard W. Bunch*

## IMPORTANCE OF FUNCTIONAL CAPACITY EVALUATIONS

The use of a functional capacity evaluation (FCE) to assist physicians in determining disability is gaining importance. Neurologic impairment of the lower extremity can obviously cause disabilities that significantly affect a person's ability to engage effectively in activities of daily living and/or work. The clinician who must determine how such an impairment affects the client's activities must first clearly understand the difference between impairment and disability and how to measure both. Impairment, as defined in the *AMA Guidelines to the Evaluation of Permanent Impairment,*[1] is an alteration of an individual's health status. Impairment is related to the loss, loss of use, or derangement of any body part, system, or function. Disability is defined as an alteration of an individual's capacity to meet personal, social, or occupation demands or statutory or regulatory requirements because of impairment. Therefore, the inability to accomplish an activity or task, especially as it relates to employment, is referred to as a disability.[2]

Because assessment of impairment does not equate directly to disability, the clinician must be able to determine accurately to what degree, if any, an impairment translates into a disability. This is particularly true when return to work or employability is being considered. With more attention focused on ability to return to work or perform specific job tasks, case managers, insurance companies, and other health-related entities have become concerned about accurately determining the functional capacities of individuals.

With the advent of the Americans with Disabilities Act (ADA), the clinician can no longer afford to guess about a person's ability to return to work. An inaccurate assessment of abilities or false assumptions based on measured impairments alone may lead to a variety of problems. These problems, in relation to the client, can involve loss of employment or reinjury because of premature return to work or insufficient accommodations. In relation to

the employer, problems can include reduced productivity, unnecessary expenses, further injury, and litigation. Employers, in increasing numbers, are turning to physicians and other clinicians for help in accommodating tasks to the unique abilities of disabled employees. The FCE has gained increased importance in response to this growing need for objective and accurate estimation of the residual functional capacities of individuals. An FCE is probably the most useful clinical tool for providing the objective information necessary for rational design decisions for modifying workstations and assigning specific work restrictions.

## FUNCTIONAL CAPACITY EVALUATION—DEFINITION, PURPOSE, AND GENERAL GUIDELINES

An FCE is a systematic process using standardized examination procedures to analyze an individual's abilities and willingness to perform functional tasks associated with activities of daily living and/or work.[3] The examination addresses the client's current medical, physical, psychologic, and motivational status. The primary purpose of the FCE is to assess return to work capacities (Table 24–1). It is also an important evaluation in determining physical reasons for functional deficiencies and whether rehabilitation procedures such as work-hardening conditioning are appropriate. Clients are often administered an FCE to determine levels of physical functioning at the conclusion of a rehabilitation program. The results of an FCE can also provide the basis for providing accommodations for return to work. When there is litigation regarding occupational injury, the physician should always use results from an FCE, if available, in his or her estimate of disability. To summarize, the FCE has become instrumental as an evaluation tool to assist in determining:

1. An individual's capacity to return to work
2. Whether impairment translates into occupational disability

**Table 24-1    Flow Diagram of Return to Work Process Based on the Functional Capacity Evaluation**

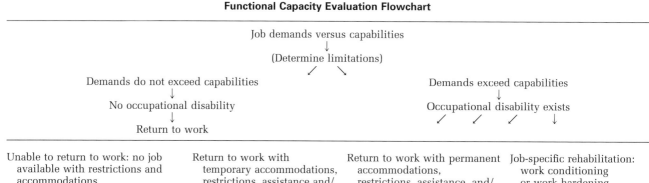

3.  The validity of disability

4.  The need for training, job modifications, or accommodations to return to work

5.  The need for further rehabilitation

Like impairment ratings, the FCE cannot be totally objective. However, the FCE provides a format for increasing objectivity and enables the clinician to evaluate and report functional capacities in a standardized manner. An FCE ranges from simple to complex and can be performed in various time formats (usually 2 to 8 hours) to test an individual's functional abilities (Table 24-2). These abilities are assessed as they relate to residual impairments, symptoms, body mechanics, safety, strength, flexibility, joint range of motion, endurance, pulmonary and cardiovascular fitness, and motivation.[4]

## THE FUNCTIONAL CAPACITY EVALUATION—REQUIREMENTS

An FCE is usually ordered by a physician. Other sources of referral include vocational counselors, insurance claim representatives, attorneys, and administrative judges. The FCE is usually best performed by a physical or occupational therapist, although other health professionals may be trained to provide this service. However, referral sources are becoming more aware of differences in the quality of FCE reports related to the qualifications of the evaluator.

Because an FCE is designed to measure maximal capacities, it is by definition a stress test. Therefore, it is imperative that the functional capacity evaluator is a skilled health professional trained in performing FCEs and that all tests are performed safely at all times. A functional capacity evaluator who

does not have medical or allied health training in the assessment of the neuromusculoskeletal system and body mechanics (kinesiology) is at a disadvantage for performing a safe and valid FCE. For example, the evaluation of an injured worker's ability to lift, carry, push, and pull weight safely is important in guiding the determination of whether the worker is capable of handling the physical demands of a job. A kinesiophysical approach to analyzing body mechanics is essential for determining reliably when a client approaches or reaches a safe biomechanical end point. Good interrater and intrarater reliability has been demonstrated among physical therapists in determining safe maximal floor-to-waist lifts during FCE testing. This supports the recommendation that physicians and other referral sources should require that an evaluator have the credentials and specialized training required for carrying out a safe FCE.

Many FCEs are based on standard protocols. However, the experienced functional capacity evaluator is able to deviate from a standard protocol to address specific questions needed to accurately determine functional capacities. Therefore, an FCE should be a dynamic evaluation process that can test job-specific criteria or abilities related to general employability.

Basic requirements for an FCE are as follows:

1.  The evaluation should be performed by a health professional who has the ability to perform a pre-FCE baseline neuromusculoskeletal evaluation and analyze and monitor body mechanics, consistency of effort, and cardiovascular responses to exertion.

2.  The purpose, procedures, and possible side effects of the evaluation should be clearly explained to the client and verification of under-

standing secured by signature of a pretest consent form.

3. The evaluation should allow accurate cross-referencing of measured impairments to measured disability.

4. All functional tests should be reproducible and have high inter- and intrarater reliability.

5. All functional tests should be valid for application to real-world situations.

**Table 24–2 Typical Functional Tests Used in a Functional Capacity Evaluation**

A. STRENGTH TESTS

1. Static lift testing
   Leg lift
   Arm lift
   Floor level
   High far
   High near
2. Dynamic lift testing
   Knuckles to waist level (level at which elbows are flexed 90 degrees)
   Knuckles to shoulder level (acromion level)
   Knuckles to overhead level (crown level)
   Floor to knuckles level
   Floor to waist level
   Floor to shoulders level
   Floor to overhead level
3. Grip strength (Jamar dynamometer): recordings of all five positions with coefficient of variations.
4. Carrying, for example, 50 feet (or job-specific distance)
5. Pushing, for example, 25 feet (or job-specific distance)
6. Pulling, for example, 7 feet (or job-specific distance)
(Note: Pushing and pulling can be done statically with a dynamometer as well.)

B. ENDURANCE TESTS

Endurance tests can involve single activities (e.g., walking on treadmill, stair climbing) performed repetitively over time or a combination of various activities (e.g., lifting and carrying repetitively in a circuit) that should be characteristic of job-specific demands. Heart rate monitors should be used throughout all functional testing. Can use psychometric tools such as the Borg rating of perceived exertion.[7]

C. PHYSICAL AGILITY AND POSTURAL TESTS

Walking, by distance or on treadmill
Bending, 25 repetitions
Squatting, 2 minutes
Sitting, may be actual test or may use client's estimate (must indicate type of data used)

D. OTHER CRITICAL FUNCTIONAL DEMANDS DERIVED FROM THE JOB ANALYSIS

Specific work simulations derived from a functional job description should always be utilized when possible, especially when results from the testing are used to determine capacities to return to work. All tests of physical performance should be analyzed for maximum voluntary effort whenever possible. Variance in effort can be quantitatively determined by calculating the coefficient of variance (CV). This is best determined utilizing isometric and/or isokinetic strength testing and range-of-motion testing.

6. All functional tests should require safe, full effort and be designed within safe medical parameters.

## COMPONENTS OF THE FUNCTIONAL CAPACITY EVALUATION FOR CLIENTS WITH LOWER EXTREMITY NEUROLOGIC DYSFUNCTION

Impairments of the lower extremity are common and often result in occupational disabilities. An FCE performed to estimate disability associated with lower extremity impairment follows the general guidelines of any FCE. The primary difference is related to focusing the neuromusculoskeletal examination and functional testing on measuring disability related to the lower extremity impairment(s).

The FCE for lower extremity impairments should follow organizational guidelines involving specific components of assessment. These components are summarized as follows:

1. Preintake interview data analysis
2. Intake interview
3. Physical examination
4. Functional testing
5. Validation
6. Results and recommendations

### Preintake Interview Data Analysis

The preintake interview data analysis involves a review of medical records, job description, work history, standardized questionnaires (e.g., psychometric, pain behavior), and symptom diagrams completed by the client. This information is important because there is a relationship between self-perceived disability, depression, anxiety, self-efficacy, and the client's performance on the FCE.[5] Clients who are depressed or angry, for example, should be monitored closely, using extreme cautionary measures to ensure that they are not accidentally or purposely injured during testing. A client with a high degree of anxiety may provide submaximal efforts during testing for fear of pain or further injury. This type of evaluee may require significantly more reassurance and instruction or demonstration than other types of clients. A client with poor motivation to return to work or who is seeking secondary gain from litigation may demonstrate submaximal and inconsistent efforts that need to be carefully documented. Such clients, when questioned during the intake interview, typically have poorly defined goals, especially in relation to employment, or goals that are totally unrealistic and not well thought out. Therefore, information related to the client's state of mind is important information for the functional capacity evaluator before actual testing.[6]

## Intake Interview

The actual one-on-one evaluation begins with the intake interview of the client, which is used to assess and document initial observations and subjective data related to symptoms, dysfunction, impairment, and self-perception of disability. Both short- and long-term goals should be assessed with questions directed toward the client's willingness and ability to return to work. The importance of the intake interview in assessing the client's attitude and level of motivation is often underestimated and the interview is, unfortunately, sometimes performed hastily.

As with any type of physically demanding test, the purpose and methods of the FCE should be explained thoroughly to the client during the intake interview with adequate time afterwards for questions and answers. This is followed by the client signing a witnessed medical release form that details the procedures of the FCE, possible side effects, responsibility for self-reporting of aggravation of symptoms, and the right to terminate participation in any procedure. The final statement on this document should indicate that the client understands the procedures and methods involved in the FCE and agrees to participate of his or her own free will.

## The Physical Examination

Baseline data related to resting vital signs, posture, gait, neurologic status, gross strength, joint range of motion, peripheral vascular status, and the characteristics and behavior of symptoms should be assessed immediately before functional testing. It is also important to assess for veracity of complaints by noting objective signs that are inconsistent with subjective complaints.

During this examination, the evaluator should assess the severity, irritability and nature of the impairment of the lower extremity. From such an evaluation, the evaluator can determine whether there are any inherent risks that should be addressed during functional testing. Special precautions or deletion of certain functional tests may have to be incorporated on the basis of the physical examination findings. The bottom line, after all, is that the FCE does not cause harm to the client and safely assesses the client's functional capacities.

## Functional Testing

Functional testing is required to determine to what degree an identified impairment translates into a disability. The clinician who performs gait analysis should be familiar with functional deficits related to the most common peripheral neuropathies of the lower extremity. For instance, peripheral nerve injuries in the hip and lower extremity can be related to a variety of causes including fractures, dislocations, compartment syndromes, tumors, and penetrating wounds. A femoral nerve injury is characterized by weakness or paralysis of the quadriceps that can lead to ineffective active knee extension characterized during ambulation as a steppage gait, or lifting the knee high and using gravity and momentum to extend the knee passively as the hip is extended. Injury to the obturator nerve, which supplies the obturator externus, adductor, and gracilis muscles, can lead to impaired function of the hip adductors and gracilis. This in turn reduces the functional capacity to adduct and externally rotate the hip and makes crossing the legs difficult. Injury to the sciatic nerve in the gluteal region results in impairment of knee flexion related to paresis or paralysis of the hamstrings and dysfunction of all the muscles in the leg and foot. This impairment is also characterized by a steppage gait as well as inability to stand on the toes or balance on the heels. Trophic and vasomotor changes are also common with sciatic nerve injury at this level. Damage to the tibial nerve can lead to clawing of the toes, and damage to the common peroneal nerve can lead to footdrop with steppage gait and foot slapping. The degree to which such impairments translate into actual disability is not always apparent. Therefore, an FCE should be utilized to demonstrate how such neurologic impairments interfere with functional activities of daily living and work.

One must remember that an identified impairment of the lower extremity (e.g., muscle weakness) may or may not cause disability. For example, a client who has paresis affecting the anterior tibialis muscle should be tested to determine whether impairment translates into compensatory movements during ambulation and walking up and down stairs because of footdrop. If not, the identified impairment has not caused disability. However, if the impairment causes the client to have difficulty walking or climbing up and down stairs, disability is identified and recommendations for accommodating this disability must be considered. Cross-referencing an impairment to expected functional deficits is also an important method for validating disability. Extraordinary disability that is out of proportion to objective signs of impairment raise suspicion of symptom magnification or illness behavior.

Functional testing also determines the impact of any deconditioning effects secondary to an injury or illness. Effects on the cardiorespiratory system or endurance of the client are important in relation to repetitive or physically demanding tasks. For example, paresis of the lower extremity may not alter the ability of the client to perform a task on an infrequent basis but may be disabling in terms of performing the task on a repetitive basis. Some lower extremity impairments may cause compensatory changes in gait and other dysfunctions that place greater demands on energy expenditure, leading to fatigue, unsafe heart rates, and/or elevated blood pressure. In such a situation, a simulated task that represents a typical work cycle can provide the physician with objective information about the client's capacities to perform the job safely.

Functional testing is directed to assess functional capacities and how such capacities are adversely affected by impairments related to strength, flexibility, sensorimotor integration (neurologic control), and cardiorespiratory function. Functional testing should be standardized for reliability and include job-simulated tasks for validity. Individuals with neurologic impairment of the lower extremity may demonstrate significant functional deficits that can adversely affect their activities of daily living and work capacities.

The most common lower extremity functional deficits secondary to neurologic pathology result from abnormal changes in joint range of motion, paresis, paralysis, and pain. FCEs of these clients should focus on the influences of lower extremity impairments on activities such as standing; balancing; walking; jumping; running; climbing; squatting; kneeling; repetitive movement of the hips, knees, and ankles or feet while standing and sitting (e.g., as in operating brake and accelerator pedals in vehicles); and material handling. Each of these activities would be targeted using functional tests that yield valid information to estimate abilities in real-world situations. Job tasks simulations may include functional test activities such as prolonged standing while working with the hands overhead; walking up and down stairs; walking while carrying weight; and repetitive lifting, pushing, and pulling of boxes and weights of various sizes. The skilled evaluator monitors body mechanics; compensatory movements; ability to maintain balance and coordination; physical and subjective expressions of pain, numbness, or other symptoms; and cardiovascular and respiratory responses to exertion.

Static and isokinetic testing of the lower extremity, although not job specific, can provide reliable information regarding strength deficits and consistency of effort. Isometric tests are performed using a dynamometer to measure the force created by the

lower extremity against fixed resistance. In this case, the lower extremity is not allowed to move through a range. Static strength can be compared with that of the contralateral limb. Isokinetic testing involves the use of a dynamometer to measure force throughout a specified range at a constant speed of motion. The dynamometer used in isokinetic testing permits accommodating resistance throughout the range, and therefore the force, or torque, generated varies at different points throughout the range. Most isokinetic tests are used to measure concentric forces of contraction (i.e., force generated by contractions that occur during shortening of the muscle) as occur in the quadriceps during knee extension. However, some isokinetic dynamometers have the capacity to measure eccentric force (i.e., contraction force during lengthening of muscle) as occurs in the quadriceps during squatting. In certain cases, residual knee problems after neurologic dysfunction are manifested by a primary eccentric weakness rather than concentric weakness. Rehabilitation focused primarily on concentric strengthening would not be effective in addressing such an impairment and could result in an inappropriate determination of permanent disability during an FCE (see Case History 1).

Repetitive tasks in an FCE should be job specific whenever possible and based on an accurate job assessment or physical demand validation. Identified work cycles or components of work cycles should be used in an FCE whenever possible. For example, a work cycle may consist of unloading 150 boxes from a truck in a 3-hour period. Each box weighs 45 pounds and measures 12 by 21 by 10 inches. The job requires walking 10 feet, climbing up three steps, loading a box on a pallet successively from 4 inches off the ground to as high as 60 inches, and then returning to the truck to repeat the process. This process should be simulated in the clinic if possible. However, to simulate the complete work cycle for 3 hours may not be practical. The work sample used in the FCE may incorporate the same frequency of lifts and carries but test for a shorter duration (e.g., 30 minutes). The results of this test can be extrapolated to the real-world situation in most cases by an experienced evaluator by carefully monitoring the client's vital signs, body mechanics, and self-perception of exertion (e.g., using the Borg scale of exertion[7]).

When performing an FCE of a client with neurologic impairment of the lower extremity, special concerns need to be considered during material-handling tests. For example, clients with motor deficits, sensory deficits, and/or dysesthesia affecting the lower extremity may use compensatory mechanisms such as shifting body weight to the uninvolved side when lifting, carrying, pushing, or pulling. Such a situation creates an unequal distribution of forces to extremity and spinal joints that can be potentially harmful to the client. Therefore, it is imperative that the evaluator monitor all material-handling tests closely for any compensatory or substitution patterns. Several FCE formats include torso lifts and dynamic lifting with reversed lordosis. Although there remains some debate about proper and safe lifting technique, it has been the experience of the author that lifting tests performed with the torso or reversed lumber lordosis are potentially harmful to the spine and should be avoided.

Impaired proprioception or balance sense resulting from neurologic impairment of the lower extremities must be analyzed carefully when the job requires working at elevated heights or walking on narrow walkways. Tests involving balance beams and body reactions to sudden changes in forces applied to the body are appropriate in this situation. Reaction time to braking in a simulated driving situation and other tests in which the reaction time of the lower extremity is measured are important components of an FCE for a client with an impaired lower extremity.

Upon completion of functional testing, the evaluator should be able to determine what functions are impaired. In addition, the evaluator should be prepared to recommend assistive devices such as ankle-foot orthoses, canes, and orthopedic shoes that may improve function and safety for return to activities of daily living and work. In some cases, the evaluator may find reason to recommend additional medical tests, rehabilitation, and/or psychologic counseling. In relation to return to work, the evaluator should also be able to recommend specific job site accommodations to assist the disabled client to return to the job safely. This requires a thorough knowledge of the physical demands and environment of the job in question. A knowledge of ergonomics can be extremely helpful when specific recommendations related to job modification appear to be reasonable accommodations that do not place an undue hardship on the employer.

## Validation

As pointed out in the *AMA Guidelines to the Evaluation of Permanent Impairment*, an FCE does not necessarily reflect what the client should be able to do but rather reflects what the client can do or is willing to do at a given time.[1] An FCE is essentially useless, especially in medicolegal cases, if no guidelines are used by the evaluator to determine the degree of validity of effort. After all, maximum effort in an FCE is highly dependent on sincerity of effort,

motivation, and other psychologic factors such as self-perceived disability, anxiety, depression, and self-efficacy. Compared with clients who gave maximum efforts during the FCE, clients who did not exert maximum effort reported considerably more anxiety and self-perceived disability and reported lower expectations for both their FCE performance and return to work.[5]

Ensuring the highest level of validity is an essential element of an FCE that enables the clinician to estimate functional capacities with a high degree of confidence. The biggest threat to validity in most FCEs, especially when the evaluation is related to a workers' compensation case, is symptom or disability magnification.[8] An FCE provides information about either the true capacities of the individual or only the level of willingness to perform. Submaximal efforts during testing must be identified and noted. Therefore, an FCE may not always be valid as an indicator of the individual's true functional capacities but, as mentioned before, may represent only what the individual is willing to do at that time. A good FCE contains methodology to determine whether the client is exerting best effort. Important information related to the level of motivation and attitude about return to work can be obtained by a skillful examiner with the intake interview and questionnaires. Cross-referencing impairments and symptom presentation during a focused physical examination with functional testing is essential. Monitoring heart rate and blood pressure continuously during the FCE can provide useful information about autonomically induced cardiovascular responses to subjective reports of sudden increases in pain.

When disability and symptom magnification is determined, the evaluator is unable to report the results of the FCE as being a valid representation of the client's true maximum functional capacities. Symptom magnification is determined when objective signs fail to support subjective complaints or when there is evidence that the subjective complaints are nonorganic in nature. Disability magnification is determined when submaximal efforts are identified during functional tests. A functional capacity evaluator may not be able to determine whether symptom and/or disability magnification represents a conscious or unconscious behavior or whether such behavior is the result of psychogenic problems. The referring physician must then determine whether psychologic testing is warranted when nonorganic signs are presented. If secondary gain is suspected and disability magnification behavior appears to be conscious game playing, the report becomes important in a court of law, especially if other methods such as surveillance reveal inconsistencies between the person's reported symptoms and disabilities and the actual functional abilities demonstrated.[9]

Maximum volitional effort testing is often used to assess whether or not the client is a providing maximum effort during the FCE. Various instruments are available to the evaluator to measure isometric or isokinetic forces generated by the extremities. These forces are reproducible and, when effort is consistent, should show low coefficients of variation (CVs) with repeated tests. To analyze consistency of effort, repeated trials (at least three) are needed to calculate the CV for both isometric and isokinetic tests. The CV is expressed as a percentage and is defined using the formula $CV = (standard\ deviation/mean) \times 100$. A low CV, generally accepted as less than 15%, indicates consistency of effort. However, the evaluator should be warned that clients can provide consistent, submaximal efforts during isometric and isokinetic tests. Therefore a clinician should not accept a low CV as a sign that the results of the FCE are based on maximum efforts. FCE tests that base validity entirely on maximum volitional effort outcomes with CV cutoffs of 15% or less are potentially exposed to great errors in judgment. For example, the author has found that a significant number of symptom magnifiers can give consistent submaximal efforts well within the 15% margin. In a review of 50 FCE reports of clients identified as symptom magnifiers, 42% demonstrated consistent maximum volitional effort with CV scores less than 15%. Twenty-two percent of this group had CV scores less than 10%, and 10% of the group had CV scores less than 5%! Therefore, a CV less than 15% cannot be accepted as the qualifier of test validity without additional cross-referencing and assessment for nonorganic signs. A high CV (above 15%), on the other hand, can be accepted as indicating either a poorly administered test or inconsistant, submaximal effort. Misunderstanding related to CV-based validity is one of the most significant errors made today by functional capacity evaluators.

## Results and Recommendations

Upon completion of an FCE, the evaluator should be able to determine the level of the client's motivation to return to work or rehabilitation. Signs and symptoms should have been validated and the estimated functional capacities delineated. On the basis of these findings, recommendations should be made regarding one or more of the following:

1. The client's capacity to return to a specific job with or without accommodations

2. The client's capacity to return to the general workforce using U.S. Department of Labor guidelines[10]

3. The need for additional medical procedures or rehabilitation

4. The need for administrative intervention

5. The need for psychologic rehabilitation

The FCE is a valid and appropriate tool for the physician to use in assessing disability. Understanding how an FCE should be structured and its validity analyzed is essential for all referral sources. As managed care attempts to reduce medical treatment and rehabilitation time, employers attempt to reduce the cost associated with lost time at work, medicolegal cases increase, and ADA issues continue to demand objective assessment of accommodations for the disabled, the role of the FCE will continue to gain increasing importance.

---

### CASE 1

A 42-year-old captain of a tugboat fell at work and fractured his left femur with resultant injury to the femoral nerve and paresis of the quadriceps. After recovering adequately from successful surgery involving open reduction with internal fixation, he underwent rehabilitation for 3 months with physical therapy primarily focused on strengthening the quadriceps. Maximum medical improvement (MMI) was determined and he returned to work. Shortly after return to work, the client had difficulty descending stairs, reporting pain and sensations of instability in the left knee. He returned to his physician for evaluation. He was taken off the job and underwent 3 more weeks of physical therapy. The physical therapist noted that the vastus medialis on the left remained atrophied compared with that on the right. At the completion of 3 weeks of additional exercise therapy, the client indicated that his knee felt stronger but that he continued to experience instability and pain in the knee, especially when descending stairs.

An FCE was ordered to determine his functional capacity to return to work as a boat captain. The FCE found that the client had the functional capacities to perform all the essential functions of the job except for activities requiring eccentric loading of the left lower extremity. The most important functional limitation related to the discomfort and instability of the left lower extremity was in walking down stairs. This was a serious disability because climbing up and down stairs on the tugboat was an essential job demand for which there was no reasonable job site accommodation. All validity tests indicated that there was no evidence of symptom or disability magnification and that the client gave reasonably safe maximum efforts.

The functional capacity evaluator recommended that the referring physician consider isokinetic assessment of eccentric strength of the quadriceps. This recommendation was followed, and the results indicated normal concentric strength in both quadriceps and a 48% deficit in eccentric strength of the left quadriceps. The physician then ordered specific rehabilitation of the left quadriceps using isokinetic and dynamic eccentric loading exercises for 6 weeks. At the end of 6 weeks, the eccentric strengths of both lower extremities were compared and found to be comparable. The client returned to work successfully.

Comments: This case demonstrates that functional testing can provide the physician with specific recommendations for further treatment that lead to successful return to work.

---

### CASE 2

A 38-year-old waitress reported a lower back injury while lifting at work. She presented with severe lower back and right lower extremity pain. She reported inability to work because she was unable to stand or walk because of the pain in the lower extremity and back. She was covered by workers' compensation and was seen by an orthopedic specialist, who found normal deep tendon reflexes and positive straight leg raise (SLR) at 20 degrees on the right. He prescribed pain medication and a nonsteroidal anti-inflammatory drug and sent the client home with instructions to walk, stay active, and avoid lifting and sitting until her return visit in 1 week.

Because of persistent pain, a magnetic resonance imaging analysis of the lumbar spine was performed. The imaging revealed mild spondylosis of L4-5 with narrowing of the L5-S1 disk. There was no evidence of nerve root or thecal encroachment.

She was referred to physical therapy, which consisted of modalities and McKenzie-based exercises. The physical therapist found a nonmechanical pattern of pain production and four out of five positive Waddell tests for nonorganic signs. Suspecting symptom magnification, the therapist had a personal conversation with the client and attempted to explain the inconsistences noted during physical therapy. The client was non responsive and denied that

she was magnifying pain. Within the subsequent 2 weeks of therapy, she reported an improvement in lower back pain but no change in the right lower extremity symptoms. After 3 months of physical therapy, the referring physician determined that she was not improving with physical therapy and that she was not a surgical candidate. The physician ordered an FCE to determine capacities to return to work.

Oswestry Low Back and Dallas Pain Questionnaires given to the client before the intake interview found that client had a self-perception of crippling disability. She indicated poorly defined goals and was not optimistic that she could return to her job. She initially rated her pre-FCE pain level as 10/10 on a scale of 0 to 10. After the evaluator repeatedly defined the scoring system and indicated that a score of 10/10 indicated pain so unbearable that she would have to be placed in the hospital, the client finally settled for a pain rating of 6/10.

During the intake interview, the client displayed anger and frustration about having to go through the FCE and indicated that she had obtained an attorney. She indicated that she could not tolerate sitting for more than 10 minutes. However, it was noted that she was able to sit without apparent signs of distress for approximately 1 hour during the intake interview. It was also discovered that she was able to drive for approximately 45 minutes to get to the clinic to take the FCE.

In the pre-FCE physical examination, the client again scored positive on four of five Waddell tests for nonorganic signs. Her gait pattern was quite abnormal and she complained of "pins and needles" throughout the entire right lower extremity as well as frequent "giving away" or buckling of the right knee. She displayed marked reduction in spinal range of motion and increased lower extremity pain as a result of all movements of the spine. Increases in pain to as high as 9/10 were reported without any significant change in heart rate (as observed on the heart rate monitor strapped to her chest). Blood pressure recordings taken at the time of reports of markedly increased pain failed to show any significant change from the resting level.

Functional testing was punctuated with repeated reports of increased pain and need for rest. Maximum lifting capacities were based on pain-limited responses and were consistent at 10 to 15 pounds regardless of the type of lift attempted. Therefore, there was no significant improvement in the client's ability to lift regardless of the mechanical advantage provided by the least physically demanding lift tests. The functional capacity evaluator determined that the client was magnifying symptoms and disability and reflected this in the summary report.

Consultation between the physician and physical therapist followed. The physician indicated that the client had reached MMI. Workers' compensation was terminated and the client was counseled on the results of the FCE and offered the opportunity to return to work. The client refused the offer and filed suit. The medical and FCE reports were entered into the trial and the court found in favor of the defendant.

Comments: This example indicates that an FCE can be used to achieve closure in a case related to symptom magnification or malingering. Employers and workers' compensation carriers are demanding accountability for the need for continued treatment, especially when a client shows no signs of improvement. There are workers' compensation claims that have lasted years without functional assessments to determine capacity to return to work and whether the disability presented is valid. The FCE is proving to be a useful tool in helping to remedy this dilemma in medicine.

## REFERENCES

1. American Medical Association: AMA Guidelines to the Evaluation of Permanent Impairment, 4th ed. Chicago, American Medical Association, 1993.
2. Luck JV Jr, Florence DW: A brief history and comparative analysis of disability systems and impairment rating guides. Orthop Clin North Am 19:839–844, 1988.
3. Hart DL, Isernhagen SJ, Matheson LN: Guidelines for functional capacity evaluation of people with medical conditions. Orthop Sports Phys Their 18:682–686, 1993.
4. Isernhagen SJ: Functional capacity evaluation. In Work Injury—Management and Prevention. Gaithersburg, MD, Aspen Publishers, 1988, p. 137.
5. Kaplan GM, Wurtele SK, Gillis D: Maximal effort during functional capacity evaluations: an examination of psychological factors. Arch Phys Med Rehabil 77:161–164, 1996.
6. Matheson L: Work Capacity Evaluation—Systematic Approach to Industrial Rehabilitation. Anaheim, Employment and Rehabilitation Institute of California, 1988.
7. Borg G: Psychophysical bases of perceived exertion. Med Sci Sports Exerc 14:377–381, 1982.
8. Matheson L: Symptom magnification Syndrome. Anchorage, National Rehabilitation Association, 1985.
9. Bunch RW: Defensive Hiring and Identification of Symptom Magnifiers. Louisiana Workers' Compensation Law. Wisconsin, Professional Educations Systems, 1994.
10. NIOSH: Work Practices Guide for Manual Lifting. Washington, DC, Department of Health and Human Services (National Institute for Occupational Safety and Health), 1981.

# Pediatric Disorders

# 25

*Lawrence W. Brown*

There is significant overlap between adult and pediatric aspects of the diagnosis and management of disorders of the lower extremity. Basic anatomy, localization of pathology, neurodiagnostic procedures, and clinical presentation are shared in common. Many of the disorders that can affect the lower extremity—from trauma to neuropathies to genetically determined neuromuscular diseases—can occur at any age. In this chapter, only selected areas with emphasis on special pediatric considerations are highlighted. These include gait evaluation in the child, chronic weakness in the young child (the floppy infant syndrome), and acute weakness of the lower extremities. The reader is referred to the other chapters in this book for discussion of other topics of relevance to children.

## GAIT EVALUATION

Walking is a complex skill requiring integration of many pathways in the nervous system. Therefore, gait disorder in children is a common finding in a variety of conditions affecting many locations in the nervous system. Basal ganglia, sensory cortex, visual receptors, cerebellum, anterior horn cell and sensory tracts in the spinal cord, peripheral nerve, neuromuscular junction, and muscle are all potential sites of involvement.

Examination may reveal developmental abnormalities whose presence is indicated by skin manifestations such as a sacral dimple, midline hairy tuft, lipoma, asymmetric gluteal folds, scoliosis, or café au lait spots. Pain or contractures may be found at the hip, knee, and ankle. For example, congenital dislocation of the hip often presents with an asymmetric thigh crease, excessive external rotation, and limited range of motion with contracture as well as pain on motion. Functional disturbances may require more careful analysis. Walking should be evaluated both in shoes and barefoot, with and without orthopedic devices (i.e., braces or orthotics), including walking and running, heel-toe gait, and climbing stairs. Additional information can be gained by ob-

serving the child walking in a circle with sudden turning and stopping. Hip girdle strength can be assessed even in the toddler by asking the child to sit from the supine position. Gower's sign, with the child pushing his hands up his legs in an attempt to stand, is the classical indicator of proximal muscle weakness. More subtle weakness can be assessed by squatting and rapidly rising. Children older than 5 years should be tested for tandem walking.

Several classical patterns of gait abnormality can be distinguished. None of these are specific in the sense that they are seen in only one syndrome or diagnostic category. Rather, they should be considered as neurologic signs that must be considered with the history and remainder of the examination to create an appropriate differential diagnosis. Because gait abnormality is the hallmark of cerebral palsy, many of the best discussions can be found in monographs on this subject.[2-5]

## Spastic Hemiplegic Gait

Unilateral cerebral disorders affecting gait result in increased tone, reduced knee flexion, abduction, and exaggerated circumdcution. Typically, the child brushes the toe and lateral sole as he or she drags the affected foot, which may be kept in the equinovarus posture. Heel walking is dramatically impaired. The time of weight bearing on the affected side is reduced. Hemiparetic gait usually includes posturing of the upper extremity as well, with decreased reciprocal arm swing. There are many causes of hemiparetic gait in childhood, including congenital anomalies of brain migration, intrauterine stroke, porencephaly, acquired cerebrovascular disease, mass lesion such as tumor or subdural hematoma, intracerebral hemorrhage, and malignant focal epilepsy (e.g., Rasmussen's encephalitis).

## Spastic Paraplegic Gait

Bilateral corticospinal tract involvement leads to a crouching posture with spasticity including hip and knee flexion, leg weakness, and dorsiflexion and equinovarus deformities of both feet. Less often, the child shows exaggerated knee extension. Young children may show scissoring resulting from excessive thigh adduction, and older children have a narrow-based gait leading to the knees brushing against one another. Walking is typically slow and deliberate with short steps. Associated findings include pathologically brisk tendon reflexes, ankle clonus, contractures, and Babinski's sign. Spastic paraparesis occurs as a result of bilateral cerebral or spinal cord lesions. Bilateral periventricular leukomalacia or consequences of intraventricular hemorrhage are seen in former premature infants. Hydrocephalus is another frequent cause because ventricular enlargement preferentially stretches leg fibers. Meningitis, encephalitis, and demyelinating diseases are other common acquired causes.

## Cerebellar Gait

Children with cerebellar dysfunction have a wide-based, unsteady gait, often with a lurching or staggering quality. Midline cerebellar lesions lead primarily to disordered balance and gait without limb dysmetria. Involvement limited to the vermis leads to titubation. Cerebellar hemisphere disease leads to ipsilateral hypotonia, dysmetria, and a tendency to veer in the direction of the abnormality. Nystagmus is an inconstant feature in children. Clinical examination should include standing, walking in a straight line, reversing direction, and walking in circles as well as tandem (heel-toe) walking. The Romberg test brings out defects in sensory input to the cerebellum resulting from posterior column disease. Other features of cerebellar disease include hypotonia, dysmetria, tremor, and scanning speech. There are many potential etiologies of cerebellar disease in childhood. Congenital lesions including the Dandy-Walker malformation (cyst of the fourth ventricle with hypoplasia of the vermis), hydrocephalus, hereditary cerebellar atrophies, metabolic disorders, posterior fossa tumors, intoxications, demyelinating disorders, and acute cerebellar ataxia are an incomplete list of some of the causes of acute, recurrent, or chronic ataxia.

## Extrapyramidal Disorders

Gait disorders resulting from involvement of the basal ganglia or rubrothalamic tracts are relatively uncommon in children except for consequences of perinatal injury. Contemporary approaches to the prevention and treatment of prematurity and isoimmunization (e.g., Rh incompatibility) have markedly reduced the incidence of bilirubin encephalopathy (kernicterus) and choreoathetoid cerebral palsy. Rigidity, bradykinesia, and decreased automatic movements are seen in extrapyramidal disorders and are similar to the forward-tilted posture, short steps, and shuffling gait of adult parkinsonism. Retropulsion and a festinating gait can be seen in childhood, although they more often point to a postencephalitic cause, drug toxicity, or a metabolic disorder than to juvenile Parkinsonism. Other movement disorders can lead to related dyskinetic gaits. Athetosis, dystonia, or chorea may predominate with unusual or bizarre gait patterns.

## Neuromuscular Weakness

Steppage gait results from weakness of the dorsiflexors of the leg and foot. This prancing gait is an attempt to compensate for peroneal and anterior tibial weakness leading to exaggerated hip and knee flexion and lifting the foot with each step. Instead of a normal heel-toe stride, the toe strikes the ground before, the heel. Causes include such disorders as Charcot-Marie-Tooth disease, Guillain-Barré syndrome, chronic myopathies, and progressive muscular dystrophies. When proximal weakness of the pelvic girdle predominates, it is characterized by a wide-based, wobbly gait with hyperlordosis. Disturbances in posture and balance are made worse by equinovarus deformities associated with progressive weakness. Chronic causes include Duchenne's muscular dystrophy and other myopathies.

## Frontal Lobe Gait

Gait disturbances resulting from bilateral frontal lobe disease can be seen in children. Initiating the walking process and completing complex motor tasks occur with rigidity, perseveration, and fluctuating resistance. These findings are seen with mass lesions or progressive dementias involving the frontal lobes.

## Miscellaneous

Finally, there are other nonneurologic gait abnormalities. Painful (antalgic) gait produces limp; it results from decreased weight support on the affected side with compensatory overemphasis on the noninvolved extremity. Conversion reactions may present as any of the previously discussed gait disturbances. Although hysterical gait can occur at any age, it is most common in children older than 10 years. Often, these psychogenic abnormalities are unsophisticated, with glaring inconsistencies between sitting and standing, eyes open and closed, and standing versus walking. Findings may include hopping well, but inability to walk with the eyes closed, lurching without ever falling, and other bizarre, nonphysiologic presentations. Hysterical gait can be diagnosed without reversion to extensive laboratory testing. Evaluation requires a multidisciplinary approach. Determining the cause of a conversion reaction in paramount, because it may derive from serious underlying psychopathology or child abuse.

## THE FLOPPY INFANT

Maintenance of normal tone requires integrity of the central and peripheral nervous systems. Therefore, hypotonia is a common sign of a disturbance anywhere in the nervous system in early childhood. Conditions as disparate as brain, spinal cord, neuromuscular junction, and muscle disorders must be considered.[6] Whereas cerebral injury in older individuals produces spasticity within days or weeks, even chronic brain lesions in infants can lead to axial hypotonia.

All floppy infants share the same appearance regardless of the location of the defect. They have reduced spontaneous activity and in the supine position assume a semiflexed posture with the hips fully abducted. Long-standing, severe hypotonia is often further accompanied by a pectus excavatum, flattening of the occiput, and hair loss over the region of contact with the crib mattress. On examination, the infant typically slides through the examiner's hands when held under the axillae, is unable to support his or her standing weight and hangs limply like an inverted "U" when held in horizontal suspension. Traction response in the supine position leads to inadequate resistance of the arms and head lag.

Congenital hypotonia may be associated with fixed contractures at birth (arthrogryposis), dislocated hips, or both. Joint contractures are probably a nonspecific reaction to reduced intrauterine movement. It is a general finding that severely affected neonates with arthrogryposis who require ventilatory assistance do not survive extubation unless the underlying diagnosis is myasthenia gravis.

Localization to a single involved area may not be possible. It is not uncommon to find more than one area of pathology. For example, severe hypoxic-ischemic encephalopathy may include both brain and spinal cord and myotonic dystrophy may combine abnormalities of muscle and brain. Furthermore, newborn infants with severe muscle disorders or spinal cord injury at birth may not make a rapid transition to extra uterine life and suffer additional consequences of perinatal asphyxia.

Central hypotonia is another term for decreased tone with a cerebral basis; it is usually an easy diagnosis to make from the history and examination. Unusual facial characteristics, encephalopathy, seizures, and other malformations all point to a central cause. Dysmorphic features, tight fisting ("cortical thumbs"), thigh adduction leading to crossed legs in vertical suspension ("scissoring"), and normal or increased deep tendon reflexes are the hallmarks of the examination. Abnormal developmental reflexes such as an exaggerated Moro response or obligatory asymmetric tonic neck reflex are also suggestive of a central basis.

There are few clues from history or inspection to point to disorders of the motor unit. Mothers may report decreased fetal movement or polyhydramnios. Occasionally, the jaw is underdeveloped or the mouth has a fishlike appearance. Decreased deep tendon reflexes proportional to the extent of weakness suggest a myopathic process, and areflexia points to neuropathy or anterior horn cell disease. Muscle atrophy is more common in motor unit disorders but can be seen with central nervous system abnormalities. Atrophy and fasciculations are the hallmarks of denervation, but it can be difficult to distinguish normal darting movements of the tongue from true fasciculations.

### Cerebral Causes

There are many cerebral causes of the floppy infant syndrome. The constellation of dysmorphic features with profound hypotonia should lead to a search for a genetic basis. One of the most common such presentations is that of Prader-Willi syndrome.[7, 8] Central hypotonia may be dramatic long before the classic childhood triad of obesity, hypogonadism, and mental retardation. Relatively minor facial features include narrow bifrontal diameter, almond-shaped eyes, cryptorchidism, and small hands and feet. Hypotonia from birth is often profound with marked hyporeflexia and feeding problems. This condition is associated with an interstitial deletion of the proximal long arm of chromosome 15 (q11-13). A specific test employing a fluorescence in situ hybridization (FISH) assay is now available.

Cerebral dysgenesis may be difficult to suspect in the absence of specific clinical signs. Abnormal head size (too large or too small), unusual head shape, dysmorphic facial features, or other sytemic malformations should raise the distinct possibility of a migrational disorder, which can be confirmed with magnetic resonance imaging (MRI).[9] Acquired brain injuries associated with hypoxia, infection, hemorrhage, or trauma are also important causes of the floppy infant syndrome. Meningitis is a possibility when a young child presents with sudden new hypotonia because the signs of illness may be masked by the infant's limited behavioral repertoire and failure to mount an adequate febrile response. Sudden hypotonia in the premature infant should also raise the possibility of intraventricular hemorrhage.

Despite the rarity of individual etiologies, it is worthwhile to consider metabolic diseases in young children with hypotonia. In particular, one must consider the peroxisomal disorders including Zellweger syndrome and neonatal adrenoleukodystrophy. Zellweger syndrome can be suspected with specific facial features, polycystic kidneys, and biliary cirrhosis.[10] Adrenoleukodystrophy is a possibility with hepatomegaly, retinitis pigmentosa, and seizures.[11] In both disorders there are abnormalities in very long chain fatty acids.

## Spinal Cord Causes

Spinal cord injury in the newborn can present as hypotonia. Usually, the history includes a complicated breech extraction during vaginal delivery.[12, 13] The prolonged and difficult delivery process may lead to the diagnosis of hypoxic-ischemic encephalopathy, and hypotonia is often attributed to asphyxia. Decreased sensation and impaired sphincter function should strongly suggest myelopathy. This is most often seen with neck hyperextension or brow presentation, but overly vigorous forceps rotation in cephalic presentations also leads to injury.

## Motor Unit Disorders

A battery of diagnostic tests and procedures can allow differentiation of pathologic disorders affecting the motor unit.[14] Creatine kinase should be determined with the knowledge that it may be markedly elevated in severely asphyxiated neonates and normal in infants with congenital myopathies such as fiber type disporportion. Electromyography (EMG) is highly predictive of a definitive diagnosis even in the smallest infants. With normal EMG studies, abnormalities are almost never found on biopsy. Primary muscle disorders and neuropathic processes are usually easily separated. Myopathies are characterized by brief small-amplitude action potentials, whereas neuropathies are characterized by denervation potentials with fibrillations, fasciculations, sharp waves, and large, prolonged polyphasic motor unit potentials. Nerve conduction studies can distinguish between axonal and demyelinating con-

ditions. Repetitive nerve stimulation can demonstrate transmission disturbances consistent with myasthenia gravis or infant botulism. Muscle biopsy is becoming a less important technique for older children with typical features of Duchenne's muscular dystrophy, but it remains an important tool in the differential diagnosis of other neuromuscular disorders. The selected muscle should be weak but still capable of contraction. Histochemical analysis is an absolute requirement. Special techniques for analyzing mitochondrial function and electron transport may be necessary. Nerve biopsy is rarely performed in infancy and early childhood unless electrodiagnostic studies point to a sural abnormality associated with hypomyelinating neuropathy.

Spinal muscular atrophy comprises a group of genetic disorders in which there is progressive loss of function of spinal cord anterior horn cells and brain stem motor nuclei. Infantile onset of spinal muscular atrophy is a relatively common etiology of severe, generalized weakness and marked hypotonia.[15, 16] Spinal muscular atrophy type I (Werdnig-Hoffmann disease) is an acute, fulminant disease with onset in the first 6 months of life. Most infants appear normal at birth unless there is supervening perinatal asphyxia. Weakness may be insidious and progressive or may appear suddenly in association with intercurrent illness with decompensating borderline respiratory function. Death occurs by 6 months of life when spinal muscular atrophy presents at birth. The course is often slower in those first showing symptoms after 3 months, although independent walking is never achieved in Werdnig-Hoffmann disease. An intermediate form of spinal muscular atrophy (type II) presents with weakness between 6 months and 2 years. Despite symmetric proximal weakness with absent or diminished tendon reflexes, most affected children appear cognitively intact. Virtually all achieve sitting, most stand, and some actually walk independently. The course is variable with slow deterioration in early childhood followed by progress and stability. The clinical diagnosis has been classically established on the basis of normal creatine kinase and consistent electrodiagnostic studies. Fibrillations and fasciculations are seen on the resting EMG with giant compound muscle action potentials, normal nerve conduction velocities, and neurogenic atrophy on muscle biopsy. There is now a commercially available direct DNA analysis capable of detecting the homozygous deletion on chromosome 5q that is present in virtually all cases of spinal muscular atrophy.[17]

## Neuropathies

Polyneuropathies are uncommon in childhood and rare in infancy. Most present with rapidly progressive motor dysfunction and gait disorder. Only congenital hypomyelinating neuropathy typically presents as the floppy infant syndrome with signs indistinguishable from those of spiral muscular atrophy type I.[18] Laboratory investigation identifies markedly delayed motor nerve conduction velocities with increased cerebrospinal fluid protein. This is one of the few indications for sural nerve biopsy, which shows bare axons without surrounding myelin. Although most infants do not respond, a course of oral steroids is indicated.

## Disorders of the Neuromuscular Junction

Infant botulism is an infection limited to children younger than 1 year of age in which spores ingested from the environment germinate and grow in the susceptible infant gastrointestinal tract.[19] After prodromal constipation and sluggish feeding, there is a progressive skeletal and bulbar weakness with areflexia and autonomic dysfunction. Relative alertness leads away from the clinical diagnosis of sepsis. Hypotonia, ptosis, dysphagia, weak cry, and sluggishly reactive pupils are among the typical early findings. Electrodiagnostic studies can be helpful, with brief, small-amplitude action potentials on EMG and a striking incremental response of the motor unit potential on rapid repetitive nerve stimulation indicating presynaptic blockade of acetylcholine release. Diagnosis is confirmed by the finding of botulinum toxin or growth of the organism from a stool sample, but toxin is rarely found in the blood. The course may be prolonged, but nearly all infants recover completely with aggressive supportive care.

Myasthenia gravis rarely presents at birth in infants of myasthenic mothers because of passive transfer of antibodies against the acetylcholine receptor.[20] Even more unusual are familial myasthenic syndromes presenting in the first year of life. Feeding difficulty and generalized hypotonia are the presenting findings. Diagnosis is established by the temporary response to neostigmine or edrophonium. Infants of mothers with the disease also demonstrate circulating antibodies.

## Primary Muscle Disease

Congenital myopathies are a group of developmental disorders that have been characterized by histochemical changes on muscle biopsy.[21] Presentations vary but usually include hypotonia, weakness, and depressed tendon reflexes. Some, such as fiber type disproportion, have characteristic dysmorphic features. Congenital muscular dystrophy is a general term used for any muscle disorder presenting in the first months of life.[22] All are probably genetically determined. Defects in muscle structure and function are still being defined, and at present the classification of this group of disorders still rests on clinical description. These muscle disorders may be associated with cerebral dysgenesis, as seen in the Fukuyama type of congenital muscular dystrophy, which is characterized by the neonatal appearance of proximal weakness, elevated creatine kinase, myopathic EMG features, and brain migrational disturbance leading to lissencephaly, polymicrogyria, or heterotopia.

Myopathies are the most common cause of chronic and progressive flaccid limb weakness in older children. The juvenile (type III) variant of spinal muscular atrophy, known as Kugelberg-Welander disease, is the only denervating condition that leads to primarily proximal weakness. Muscular dystrophies are a group of genetic myopathies that are now known or suspected to be caused by defects in structural proteins. There has been great progress in our understanding of Duchenne's and Becker's muscular dystrophies.[23, 24] We now know that they involve reduced or nearly absent production of dystrophin, a structural protein necessary for maintenance of muscle integrity by stabilization of the sarcolemmal membrane. Although the primary problem in Duchenne's and Becker's dystrophies is the deficiency of dystrophin, there is subsequent marked reduction of all dystrophin-associated proteins in muscle. The gene is located on the short arm of the X chromosome (Xp21) and is the largest gene identified to date. The size of the dystrophin gene probably accounts for the high incidence of mutation and makes gene replacement therapy more difficult. Direct DNA testing of affected boys and accurate analysis of carriers are now possible with samples of peripheral blood. Prenatal testing can be performed using chorionic villa or amniotic fluid cells.

Gait abnormality is the earliest feature in most boys with Duchenne's dystrophy. It is sometimes not noted until school age, but careful examination usually shows a problem before 3 years of age. With clumsiness, frequent falling, and toe walking. As the disease progresses, proximal weakness leads to hyperlordosis, a waddling gait, tight hip flexors and heel cords, hypertrophy of the calf muscles (actually replacement of muscle by fat and fibrous tissue), and a positive Gower sign. Motor strength declines throughout childhood with progressive difficulties in stair climbing, running, and walking leading to loss of independent ambulation by age 12 years. The progression of disease is much slower in those with partial expression of the dystrophin gene associated with the Becker variant. Other late features with both phenotypes include scoliosis, cardiomyopathy and respiratory insufficiency. Laboratory features include extremely elevated levels of creatine kinase and other muscle enzymes, which gradually decline as the disease progresses; EMG findings of myopathy (including low-amplitude polyphasic motor unit potentials, early recruitment, fibrillation potentials, positive sharp waves, and complex repetitive discharges); and characteristic muscle biopsy findings (fiber size variability, necrosis, and regenerating fibers and fibrosis). Electrodiagnostic and even biopsy features are nonspecific, and there is little role for them in the diagnosis of Duchenne's dystrophy when definitive dystrophin testing is available.

## PARAPLEGIA IN CHILDHOOD

Although the differential diagnosis of leg weakness in children and adults includes the same causes, the patterns are quite different. Spinal injuries in children are related more to congenital anomalies such as atlantoaxial dysplasia of Down syndrome and sports injuries than to gunshot wounds.[25] Cauda equina and conus medullaris syndromes are more often caused by congenital lesions or benign tumors than in adults. Children are much more prone to spinal damage without radiological abnormality.[26]

Bilateral leg weakness sparing the upper extremities points to involvement of the spinal cord or peripheral nerves. Spinal etiologies leading to paraplegia produce symptoms below the level of involvement including spasticity, hyperreflexia, and a sensory level; flaccid weakness is seen at the level of injury. Localization of conus medullaris and cauda equina syndromes in children is difficult because they often produce complex signs. EMG and nerve conduction velocities can be helpful in these circumstances. Peripheral neuropathy is usually easily recognized by distal weakness, sensory loss, atrophy, and areflexia. With cerebral causes of paraplegia, upper extremity involvement is usually present to a lesser degree. There are circumstances in which both brain and spinal cord can be affected, such as myelodysplasia with a Chiari II malformation or extensive syringobulbia and syringomyelia.

Acute or rapidly progressive paraplegia is usually caused by spinal cord compression or myelitis. Compression of the cord of any cause is a neurologic emergency requiring immediate diagnostic testing and immediate treatment.[27] Acute processes are heralded by refusal to stand or walk because of pain, weakness, or both. Slowly progressive disorders usually present with a clumsy gait. Less commonly, scoliosis is the initial finding, particularly in prepubertal girls or boys of any age.

## Diskitis

Diskitis is a unique disorder of childhood in which there is inflammation of one disk space, which sometimes spreads to adjacent vertebral bodies.[28] An initial feature is refusal to walk, usually in children younger than 3 years of age. Often, a low-grade fever and a limp that evolves over 1 to 2 days are prominent features. Older children more often complain of back pain, but rarely appendicitis is suggested by increasingly severe abdominal pain that radiates from the epigastrium to the umbilicus or pelvis. Loss of the normal lumbar lordosis and hip and back tenderness are seen at all ages. Spinal radiographs show narrowing of the intervertebral space, more often in the lumbar than in the cervical region. MRI is optimal for demonstrating disk inflammation with osteomyelitis of surrounding vertebrae. Treatment includes antistaphylococcal antibiotics and immobilization to encourage healing.

## Infection

Epidural abscesses are more often seen in children older than 10 years of age.[29] They are usually caused by hematogenous spread of bacteria, most often *Staphylococcus aureus*. Midthoracic or lower lumbar involvement is most common. First features include localized back pain, which worsens with cough and flexion of the back. Fever can help to raise the clinician's level of concern, but elevated temperature may be delayed. Meningitis can be suspected if headache, fever, and vomiting are prominent. Within days of onset, root irritation is common, usually presenting as radiating chest pain if thoracic, or groin pain if lower lumbar in origin. Signs of spinal cord compression include paraplegia and bladder disturbance. Thoracic epidural abscess leads to flaccid or spastic paraparesis with hyperreflexia; lumbar abscess produces flaccid paraparesis and reduced reflexes. Definitive diagnosis requires MRI confirmation. Antistaphylococcal antibodies should be initiated immediately when an epidural abscess is suspected. Early surgical decompression is essential if function is to be preserved.

## Transverse Myelitis

Transverse myelitis is an acute demyelinating process often associated with focal or disseminated encephalomyelitis. Devic's syndrome is applied when transverse myelitis occurs with evidence of optic neuritis.[30] Unlike the situation in adults, isolated transverse myelitis or Devic's syndrome is usually not caused by multiple sclerosis. Rather, it is thought to be an immunologic response to preceding viral infection or immunization. Clinical features in childhood typically include rapid (but not apoplectic) progression of paraparesis with thoracic sensory level over several days. Other signs include leg weakness, which can be asymmetric; neurogenic bladder; and altered reflexes, which can be increased or more often decreased. Diagnosis of transverse myelitis requires MRI of the spine to exclude acute cord compression; cord swelling and an altered signal are compatible findings seen occasionally. MRI of the brain is also important for identifying other areas of potential involvement. Treatment is an incompletely resolved issue, although many clinicians rely on a course of high-dose intravenous steroids followed by a rapidly tapering schedule of oral prednisone. The same approach is used for those with Devic's syndrome or widespread acute disseminated encephalomyelitis. Improvement often starts within 1 week, but the course can be protracted. Recovery can be incomplete even with early initial improvement. The vast majority of affected children regain ambulation and bladder control, but subtle deficits can be found in up to half.

## Spinal Trauma

Spinal cord injuries are uncommon in children and are usually caused by motor vehicle accident or sports injuries. Diagnosis and management are comparable to those for adults with few exceptions. Spinal cord concussion is more common in children.[26] A direct blow to the back can lead to a transient spinal cord syndrome including flaccid weakness, sensory level, areflexia, and urine retention. The mechanism is spinal shock with edema and recovery is usually complete within 1 week. Treatment of concussion includes intravenous methylprednisolone.

## Tethered Cord

One of the most difficult yet common pediatric cord syndromes is the tethered cord.[31] Although this condition can be considered to be related to the spinal dysraphic states, there is no dramatic skin manifestation or associated brain abnormality. During fetal life, the spinal cord ascends from L3 to achieve its final location at L1; throughout development the spinal cord must grow in conjunction with the child's overall growth. Therefore, any process that prevents the cord from retracting in utero or stretching during childhood can lead to spinal cord traction and progressive symptoms. Common causes include a thickened filum terminale, sacral lipoma,

dermal sinus, and diastematomyelia, often in association with spina bifida occulta. A dermal sinus is often heralded by a midline hairy tuft in the sacral region, port-wine stain, or subcutaneous lipoma. Shallow, blind tracts are unassociated with tethered cord, but those that extend through a spina bifida to attach to the dura can lead to progressive disability as the child grows. The midline septum of diastematomyelia can anchor the base of the spinal cord with similar disastrous effects even without any skin manifestation.

Children with tethered cord may present at any time, but most are in the pre–school age range. Symptoms include a combination of clumsy gait, deformity of the lower extremities (short leg or pes cavus), and bladder dysfunction. Those with only clumsiness or bladder problems often have normal or increased reflexes, but absent tendon reflexes are often seen with foot deformities. Clumsy gait or scoliosis is more common in older children and teenagers. Examination may show previously unrecognized, usually mild bilateral foot deformities, urinary incontinence, or constipation. Hyperreflexia and extensor plantar responses are also seen. The most effective diagnostic procedure is MRI of the spine, because radiographs are non-specific and misleading. Spina bifida occulta is common in young children, and the septa in many cases of diastematomyelia are cartilaginous and do not appear on plain films. MRI easily demonstrates the low-lying conus medullaris, presence of a connecting sinus tract, lipoma, or other pathology. Surgical treatment is essential to prevent further deterioration, but only a small minority of children actually recover any previously lost function.

## REFERENCES

1. Swaiman KF: Gait impairment. *In* Swaiman KF (ed): Pediatric Neurology: Principles and Practice, 2nd ed. St. Louis, CV Mosby, 1994, pp. 235–241.
2. Kuban KCK, Leviton A: Cerebral palsy. N Engl J Med 330:188, 1994.
3. Russman BR, Gage JR. Cerebral palsy. Curr Probl Pediatr 19:71, 1989.
4. Palmer FB, Shapiro BK, Wachtel RC, et al: The effects of physical therapy on cerebral palsy. A controlled trial in spastic diplegia. N Engl Med 318–803, 1988.
5. Park TS, Owen JH: Surgical management of spastic diplegia in cerebral palsy. N Engl J Med 326–745, 1992.
6. Dubowitz V: The Floppy Infant, 2nd ed. Philadelphia, JB Lippincott, 1980.
7. Malzac P, Moncla A, Voelckel MA, et al: Prader-Willi syndrome: Diagnostic strategy with a cytogenetic and molecular approach. Neuromusc Disord 3:493, 1993.
8. Holm VA, Cassidy SB, Butler MG, et al: Prader-Willi syndrome: Consensus diagnostic criteria, Pediatrics 91:398, 1993.
9. Aicardi J: Disorders of neuronal migration: A spectrum of cortical abnormalities. Int Pediatr 8:162, 1993.
10. Wilson GN, Holmes RG, Custer J, et al: Zellweger syndrome:

Diagnostic assays, syndrome delineation, and potential therapy. Am J Med Genet 24:69, 1986.

11. Moser HW, Moser AB, Smith KD, et al: Adrenoleukodystrophy: Phenotypic variability and implications for therapy. J Inherit Metab Dis 15:645, 1992.

12. Bresnan MJ, Abroms IF: Neonatal spinal cord transection secondary to intruterine hyperextension of the neck in breech presentation. J Pediatr 84:734, 1974.

13. Minami T, Ise K, Kukita J, et al: A case of neonatal spinal cord injury: Magnetic resonance imaging and somatosensory evoked potentials. Brain Dev 16:57, 1994.

14. Russell JW, Afifi AK, Ross MA: Predictive value of electromyograph in diagnosis and prognosis of the hoypotonic infant. J Child Neurol 7:387, 1992.

15. Russman BS, Iannacone ST, Buncher CR, et al: Spinal muscular atrophy: New thoughts on the pathogenesis and classification schema. J Child Neurol 7:347, 1992.

16. Iannacone ST, Browne RH, Samaha FJ, et al: Prospective study of spinal muscular atrophy before age 6 years. Pediatr Neurol 9:187, 1993.

17. Crawford TO: From enigmatic to problematic: The new molecular genetics of childhood spinal muscular atrophy. Neurology 46:335, 1996.

18. Balestrini MR, Cavaletti G, D'Angelo A, et al: Infantile hereditary neuropathy with hypomyelination: Report of two siblings with different expressivity. Neuropediatrics 22:65, 1991.

19. Brown, L.W: Infant botulism. Pediatr Ann 13:135, 1984.

20. Engel AG: Congenital myasthenic syndromes. J Child Neurol 3:233, 1988.

21. Sarnat HB: New insights into the pathogenesis of congenital myopathies. J Child Neurol 9:193, 1994.

22. Leyton QH, Gabreels FJM, Renier WO, et al: Congenital muscular dystrophy. J Pediatr 115:214, 1989.

23. Darras BT: Molecular genetics of Duchenne and Becker muscular dystrophy. J Pediatr 117:1, 1990.

24. Hoffman EP, Wang J: Duchenne-Becker muscular dystophies and the nondystrophic myotonias: paradigms for loss of function and change of function of gene products. Arch Neurol 50:1227, 1993.

25. Davidson RG: Atlantoaxial instability in individuals with Down syndrome: A fresh look at the evidence. Pediatrics 80:555, 1988.

26. Pang D, Pollack IF: Spinal cord injury without radiographic abnormality in children—the SCIWORA syndrome. J Trauma 29:654, 1989.

27. Childes BW, Cooper PR: Acute spinal injury. N Engl J Med 334:514, 1996.

28. Fischer GW, Popich GA, Sullivan DE, et al: Diskitis: A prospective diagnostic analysis. Pediatrics 62:543, 1978.

29. Enberg RN, Kaplan RJ: Spinal epidural abscess in children: Early diagnosis and immediate surgical drainage is essential to forestall paralysis. Clin Pediatr 13:247, 1974.

30. Jeffery DR, Mandler RN, Davis LE: Transverse myelitis. Retrospective analysis of 33 cases, with differentiation of cases associated with multiple sclerosis and parainfectious events. Arch Neurol 50:532, 1993.

31. Brophy JD, Sutton LN, Zimmerman RA, et al: Magnetic resonance imaging of lipomyelomeningocele and tethered cord. Neurosurgery 25:336, 1989.

# Evaluation of Back Pain

# 26

*Scott A. Rushton and Todd J. Albert*

The health care professionals who provide care services for patients must possess the unique talents required for the evaluation and treatment of spinal dysfunction and pain. In the case of cervical and lumbar spinal disorders, most of the patients do not require surgery, and the accurate identification of nonsurgical etiologies and timely conservative treatment help ensure a more favorable result. The goals that we initially set for ourselves in the management of this population of patients must focus on prompt return to "normal" function while decreasing the cost to society. One initial approach follows a sound understanding of the pathoanatomy and natural history of cervical and lumbar spinal disorders. This enables the practitioner to use ancillary studies efficiently.

Therefore, the task of the health care professional who evaluates the patient with neck or low back pain is to return that patient as promptly as possible to a normal functional existence. The ability to achieve this goal is dependent on the precision and accuracy of the decision-making process.

## CLINICAL SYNDROMES

Degenerative disease of the spine is not a specific diagnosis. Rather, it is an all-inclusive term describing the morphologic manifestations of progressive deterioration of a spinal motion segment. Although most clinicians confine their discussions to the manifestations of changes in the intervertebral disk, numerous other structures are influenced by aging and repetitive use. Any structure, hard or soft, that defines the spinal canal or intervertebral foramen can participate in the production of axial or radicular symptoms. The diagnostician should be familiar with the spectrum of clinical syndromes produced by cervical or lumbar spine pathology, as well as those frequently included in the differential diagnosis.

The clinical evaluation involves an appreciation of patients' physical complaints as well as the emotional and social influences that contribute to their personal experience with the pain. With the numerous medicolegal and compensation issues facing the medical community today, a dedication to the art of interviewing and examining patients is vital in the determination of appropriate management and prediction of prognosis.

## History

A careful history is essential in the evaluation of a patient with spinal disorders. Most diagnoses are made, or at least a differential diagnosis should be possible, at this stage of the encounter.

The location, quality, and chronicity of pain should be ascertained. It is important to note the temporal relationship of the pain syndrome to sleep, position of the neck and back, and Valsalva's maneuvers and activities that exacerbate the symptoms. The clinician must determine the positions of greatest discomfort from the history. For example, in patients with cervical spondylosis, extension and rotation of the head toward the side of discomfort exacerbate the symptoms. Similarly, in the lumbar spine, the pain of a disk herniation tends to be worse when the patient is seated, presumably because of the increased intradiskal pressure that occurs in this position.

In addition, back pain must be separated from leg pain, and in the cervical spine one must distinguish neck pain from arm pain. This is not only important for diagnosis but also has therapeutic and prognostic implications.

The encounter with the patient should start with a description of the symptom complex as it relates to neck or back pain, radiculopathy, and myelopathic disturbances. Classically, radiating sciatic pain extends below the knee. However, S1 and occasionally L5 irritation can be localized to the buttock or posterior thigh. The patient may describe generalized radicular symptoms, but the exact location should be sought. For example, pain radiating to the great toe, particularly the first web space, suggests involvement of the L5 nerve root. Similarly, in the cervical spine, radicular pain should be distinguished from referred sclerotomal pain.

Associated neurologic signs and symptoms should be investigated. Dermatomal sensory loss, paresthesias, and subjective sense of motor weakness suggest radiculopathy. In contrast, generalized upper and lower extremity weakness, especially in conjunction with gait disturbances and bladder dysfunction, suggests myelopathy. In the setting of myelopathy, patients may describe neck pain; numb, cold, or painful hands; decreased fine motor skills; and subtle gait disturbances. It is important to note that radiculopathy and myelopathy may coexist (myeloradiculopathy).

Disturbances of bowel or bladder function in the absence of upper motor neuron signs and symptoms demand immediate evaluation to exclude the diagnosis of a cauda equina syndrome. The presentation includes bowel or bladder dysfunction, saddle anesthesia, and variable loss of motor and sensory function in the lower extremities. However, in the presence of a frank cauda equina syndrome or truly progressive motor weakness, equivocation and procrastination are not warranted as surgical intervention is mandatory.

The examining health care professional must also differentiate neurogenic from vascular claudication. The leg pain of vascular claudication is slowly relieved by standing still, whereas in neurogenic claudication postural changes are required to produce relief. Ascending hills is poorly tolerated by patients with vascular claudication, and walking downhill is painful in neurogenic claudication. Furthermore, activities requiring spinal column flexion are typically well tolerated by patients with neurogenic claudication. A patient's walking distance is fairly constant with vascular claudication and is generally quite variable in the neurogenic population.

In the evaluation of neck or back pain, the type of work performed by the patient is important, as is any potential secondary gain associated with the condition. When orchestrating treatment of work-related injuries, the caregiver must exercise caution when recommending surgical treatment, as results of surgery are uniformly worse in the presence of worker's compensation claims. The age of the patient must also be factored into the treatment algorithm when considering specific diagnoses. For example, cervical and lumbar disk herniations are more common in adults younger than 55 years, and spinal stenosis is far more common in patients older than 60 (Fig. 26–1)

Constant, unremitting pain or night pain is suggestive of tumor or infection. Concurrent systemic symptoms may include fever, malaise, and weight loss. A history of antecedent infection, immunologic compromise, and intravenous drug use must be ascertained.

Inflammatory arthritides and seronegative spondyloarthropathies commonly involve the axial skeleton. Patients' complaints may focus on pain, as well as focal or generalized stiffness. This stiffness is typically most severe in the morning, with improvement throughout the day. It is imperative that patients with long-standing polyarticular rheumatoid arthritis be followed regularly from a neurologic standpoint for the development of myelopathic signs or symptoms.

A history of litigation, compensation, or drug dependence and a family history of spinal disorders are also important in the prediction of successful outcome. An understanding of patients' psychosocial background and their expectations or desires to return to work helps distinguish individuals with treatable pathology.

## Radiculopathy

Radiculopathy refers to the symptoms and signs of nerve root compression. Impingement may have numerous causes. In relatively young patients, soft disk herniations are more common than osteophyte or hard disk encroachment. The herniation is usually posterolateral near the entrance of the foramen. Free or sequestered disk fragments may also be found within the neuroforamen.

When patients experience a true compressive neuropathy, their history moves from a predominance of neck pain to complaints of arm pain radiating from cervical origin. There may be associated symptoms of paresthesias, dysethesias, and frank numbness along a similar distribution. The temporal relationship between neck and arm pain is often a classic reminder that compression without inflammation is not sufficient to produce radicular pain.

Classically, manifestations of sensory, reflex, and motor deficits are found within the distribution of the affected nerve root. However, despite the dermatomal charts, the degree of functional overlap between spinal nerve roots provides variable findings from patient to patient. For example, a C6 radiculopathy should cause pain or sensory complaints in the neck, shoulder, lateral arm, radial forearm, and possibly the thumb and index finger. Frequently, however, the distribution of pain is less extensive and more proximal, whereas paresthesias predominate distally. Some patients have paresthesias only in the limb, although their pain is axial, particularly in the paracervical musculature or medial scapular border. Furthermore, it is not unusual to see patients whose distributions of pain or paresthesias in the arm are sufficiently vague to defy delineation. The fact that the symptoms do not follow a particular dermatomal map does not exclude the existence of a symptomatic nerve root. We find objective motor testing to be most useful in identifying a symptomatic nerve root.

**Figure 26–1.** Anteroposterior, lateral, and axial views of the fourth-decade and older spine show significant disk degeneration, a traction spur developing into a large osteophyte, and significant hypertrophic changes occurring within the facet joints compromising the neural elements both in the canal and in the neural foramina. Markedly thickened or redundant flaval ligament is also seen contributing to this neural compromise. (From Wiesel SW, Bernini P, Rothman RH: The Aging Lumbar Spine. Philadelphia, WB Saunders, 1982, p 22.)

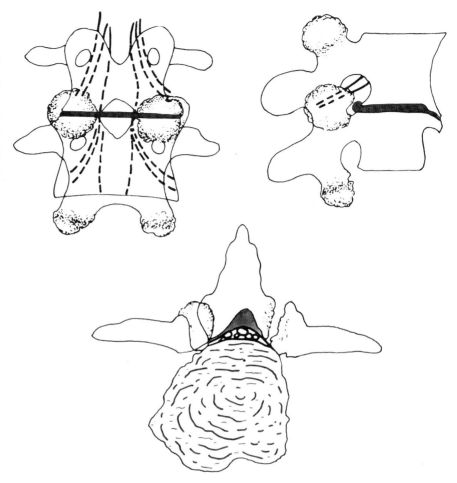

## Myelopathy

Neural compression syndromes can result from impingement on the spinal cord or can occur in combination with nerve root compression. In the absence of cervical spondylosis, a large central disk herniation may precipitate myelopathy. More commonly, myelopathy is the result of spondylotic changes superimposed on a congenitally narrow spinal canal. The net result of spinal column attrition is a multifactorial narrowing of the canal. It is a gradual process that underscores the insidious onset of myelopathic symptoms. Less commonly, symptoms are precipitated acutely by superimposition of a small disk herniation, minor trauma, or a focal inflammatory process.

A precise onset is not usually apparent to patients with myelopathic disturbances. They note a deterioration in gait or manual dexterity, generalized weakness, or urinary urgency or frequency. The legs of the patient with myelopathy may feel stiff, and patients may shuffle their feet as they walk. Patients typically lose confidence in their ability to walk and may manifest fears of falling. In contrast to that in compressive radiculopathies, pain is not a common presenting symptom. Crandall and Batz-

dorf noted radicular pain or paresthetic pain in 39% and 34% of their patients, whereas spasticity and weakness were noted in 98% and 65% of their patients. In addition, the presentation of myelopathy may be obscured by a depressed affect, which may reflect the progressive feeling of detachment from the body.

## Back Pain

Probably all adults have experienced some degree of low back pain sometime in their lives, but the lifetime prevalence ranges from 60% to 80%. Although there are wide ranges, the annual incidence is 5% but varies from 1% to more than 20% in some occupations. Many people never seek medical care, nor do they have any significant functional impairment. In addition, approximately 60% of the patients who experience back pain return to work within 1 week, and only about 10% suffer disabling back pain after 6 weeks.

It is important for health care professionals to differentiate between spine pathology, back symptoms, work-related back injury, and absenteeism. Failure to distinguish these entities may lead to inaccurate conclusions and misleading generalizations. We must recognize that in the vast majority of back problems, we are dealing with a complaint rather than a well-defined physical or pathologic entity.

There is mounting evidence that patients with compensation-related back pain respond less positively to treatment in general than those with non-compensated back disorders. Compensation is also associated with residual back pain after surgery, as well as delayed recovery with conservative treatment. Many physical and nonphysical factors influence back problems and individuals' responses to them.

## Sciatica

One important component of the low back pain syndrome is pain radiating down the legs, also referred to as sciatica. Two important factors in the development of sciatica are compression and inflammation. Compression induces impairment of the conducting properties of spinal nerve roots, and local inflammation is the nidus for referred pain. In patients, this combination is associated with sensory and motor dysfunction.

## The Lumbar Spine

The overall posture of the patient should be recorded and any deformities in the sagittal or coronal plane described. Observations of gait and generalized movements of the patient must be documented. Splinting, antalgia, circumduction, footdrop, or a Trendelenburg gait must be clinically evaluated. A sciatic list to one side may indicate a contralateral lateral disk herniation or an ipsilateral axillary disk herniation.

The overall balance of the spine should be assessed by noting the position of the head and trunk relative to the pelvis. It is important to rule out leg length inequalities before ascribing a spinal etiology. The paraspinal muscles should be palpated to detect spasm or tenderness. Pain or tenderness at the region of the sciatic notch suggests irritation of contributing nerve roots, most commonly by a disk herniation.

A complete abdominal examination is a routine part of any spinal assessment. This remains an opportunity to exclude sources of referred pain as well as to note any umbilical reflex asymmetry. The possibility of an abdominal aortic aneurysm causing the pain should always be entertained.

### Range of Motion

In the lumbar spine, the larger disk, absence of ribs, and the sagittal alignment of the facet joints allow a large flexion and extension arc, although rotation is limited. Flexion can be measured by using a goniometer or simply measuring the distance of the patient's fingertips from the floor. Extension may also be reported in a qualitative fashion.

Pain with forward flexion or hyperextension is a nonspecific finding. In the younger, active patient, pain on hyperextension may signify spondylolysis, a stress fracture in the pars interarticularis. Spondylolisthesis is rarely symptomatic as an isolated, first-time presenting entity in adults older than 40 years.

In the older patient, pain on extension may be due to spinal stenosis. A history of positional or postural relief in a flexed or seated position typifies the diagnosis of spinal stenosis. A thorough vascular examination must be performed to rule out vascular etiologies.

### Associated Tests

1. *Straight-leg raising test*: Patient is supine or sitting with the examiner lifting the symptomatic leg while maintaining knee extension and ankle dorsiflexion. A positive test reproduces radicular pain (Fig. 26–2).

2. *Lasègue's maneuver*: Straight-leg raise test with slight knee flexion and ankle dorsiflexion. A positive test reproduces radicular pain.

3. *Bowstring test*: Pressure is applied to the tibial nerve in the region of the popliteal fossa while maintaining knee flexion. A positive test produces radicular symptoms.

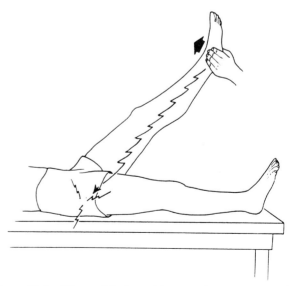

**Figure 26–2.** The straight-leg raising test. (From Frymoyer JW: Adult Spine: Principles & Practice, 2nd ed. Philadelphia, JB Lippincott, 1996, p 337.)

4. *Contralateral straight-leg raising test*: Straight-leg raising test of uninvolved lower extremity. A positive test reproduces radicular pain in the opposite (symptomatic) leg.

5. *Femoral stretch test*: With the patient prone or in lateral decubitus, extend the thigh with the knee flexed. A positive test produces radicular pain (Fig. 26–3).

6. *Cremasteric reflex*: Elevation of the scrotal sac when the skin of the ipsilateral inner thigh is scratched. Absence suggests upper motor neuron lesion.

### Neurologic Evaluation

Knowledge of the normal lumbar nerve root motor, sensory, and reflex function is essential to mastering the pathoanatomy. The nerve roots of the lumbar spine exit below the pedicle of the corresponding numbered vertebrae and above the disk that is immediately caudal. A typical posterolateral disk herniation impinges on the nerve root that traverses it, medial to the neuroforamen. For example, a disk herniation at the L4-5 level most often affects the L5 nerve root. However, a far lateral disk herniation can affect the exiting nerve root, and a central disk herniation can affect one or more caudal nerve roots. A large central herniation is a common cause of cauda equina syndrome, which mandates surgical intervention.

## ANCILLARY STUDIES

### Radiography

Radiography is an inexpensive, readily accessible starting point for the examination of patients with neck or back symptoms. In most cases, early radiographs are not indicated in the work-up of patients with neck or back pain. We obtain plain radiographs (anteroposterior lateral, flexion, extension, oblique) only with a minimum of 4 to 6 weeks of symptoms and/or worrisome signs (e.g., constitutional complaints, night pain). If indicated, the first and one of the most critical steps in evaluating the spine radiographically is to obtain high-quality screening plain radiographs.

### The Lumbar Spine

There is widespread agreement that routine radiographs of the spine are not indicated in the evaluation of patients with acute low back pain in the absence of radicular symptoms. Even for patients with sciatica, early radiographs are not needed, as many of these patients improve without treatment. The clinical examination is a better initial diagnostic tool than a lumbar radiograph.

Radiographs are recommended for patients with low back pain that continues beyond 6 weeks. This accounts for approximately 10% of the patients who present with low back pain. Radiographs are obtained to search for etiologies such as vertebral compression fractures, spondylolisthesis, spondylolysis, vertebral osteomyelitis or metastasis, degenerative changes, and spondyloarthropathies.

A number of factors would indicate earlier radiographic intervention. These include age older than 50 years or younger than 20 years, known history of a malignancy, history of serious trauma, significant weight loss, rest or night pain, fever, alcohol or drug use, corticosteroid use, and clinical suspicion of a compression fracture.

If lumbar spine radiographs are obtained, oblique views are not necessary. These views double the radiation exposure to the patient and increase the cost rather than the diagnostic yield.

Routine anteroposterior and standing lateral radiographs are sufficient to diagnose degenerative changes, sagittal instability, or fractures. In the setting of mechanical symptoms or presumed instability, lateral flexion and extension views should be obtained.

## Myelography, Computed Tomography, and Magnetic Resonance Imaging

Because of concern about the diagnostic value of plain radiographs, attention has focused on other diagnostic modalities. These include myelography, computed tomography, and magnetic resonance imaging.

### The Lumbar Spine

#### Myelography

The lumbar cistern is the site of the best visualization and greatest variation noted by myelography. Variation in the distal thecal sac is in part responsi-

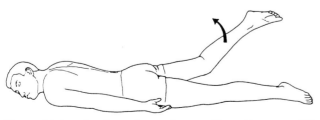

**Figure 26–3.** The femoral stretch test. (From Frymoyer JW: Adult Spine: Principles & Practice, 2nd ed. Philadelphia, JB Lippincott, 1996, p 337.)

ble for the relative insensitivity of myelography for detecting lesions in the lumbosacral space. The subarachnoid space extends laterally into dural root pouches. These pouches can extend to the medial border of the pedicles; therefore, pathology affecting the midforaminal zone is not recognizable by conventional myelography.

The variation in the level of origin and the length of the dural root pouches as well as the asymmetry of the thecal sac compromises the myelographic assessment of the involved segments. Scarring resulting from prior myelography or surgical insult can also compromise the interpretation.

Computed tomography (CT) remains comparable to myelography in the evaluation of disk prolapse. However, myelography combined with CT has provided a better understanding of spinal stenosis, disk herniation, and spondylosis. Currently, CT scanning is performed with the patients supine, which has the disadvantage of no axial load distributed to the spine. In contrast, functional myelography of the lumbar spine provides the ability to evaluate the effect of loading with erect flexion, extension, and lateral bending maneuvers, an advantage over both CT scanning and magnetic resonance imaging (MRI). For this reason, functional assessment should be routinely incorporated in the myelographic study of the lumbar spine.

However, because of the superior soft tissue resolution with modern MRI, myelography can no longer be considered a primary imaging modality for the evaluation of lumbar spine pathology. Its use should be reserved for specific cases determined on an individual basis.

### Computed Tomography

Multiplanar CT still provides the greatest amount of information in the evaluation of spinal central and intervertebral canal stenosis. It has also been accurate in the diagnosis of frank disk herniation with nerve root compression and facet joint arthrosis. In addition, with the advent of multiplanar reformation, the exact etiology of the stenotic process can be defined, thereby guiding surgical versus nonoperative treatment.

Although MRI has surpassed CT in the diagnosis of many spinal disorders, including diskitis, osteomyelitis, and disk herniation, the major role of CT in the present-day management of back pain is in evaluating spinal stenosis, primarily because of its excellent delineation of osseous abnormalities. In addition, CT with multiplanar reformation remains the preferred initial examination in the evaluation of patients who have had fusion or instrumentation and are presenting with persistent or recurrent back pain. We prefer CT examination after instillation of intrathecal contrast material.

### Magnetic Resonance Imaging

MRI has added considerably to the body of information provided by high-resolution CT and myelography. It remains an invaluable diagnostic adjunct to CT in the study of the lumbar spine. MRI has proved most useful in the differentiation of soft tissue abnormalities, such as spinal neoplasm, infection, and hematoma. MRI remains the procedure of choice in differentiating recurrent herniation from fibrosis in the study of postoperative patients.

MRI allows direct visualization of not only the pathologic processes affecting the spine but also the direct effect these lesions may have on the nerve roots and thecal sac. Together with CT, it provides clear images of the bony spinal canal and intervertebral nerve root canal as well as the soft tissues occupying these areas.

## Laboratory Evaluation

In the setting of unremitting neck or back pain, night pain, a history of malignancy, or high clinical suspicion of vertebral infection or metastasis mandates a judicious laboratory evaluation. This phase of the evaluation is commonly referred to as the metabolic work-up.

The laboratory studies routinely employed for metabolic evaluation include any combination of those shown in Table 26–1, depending on the clinical presentation.

## DIFFERENTIAL DIAGNOSIS

This section highlights the major clinical conditions that should be considered in the differential diagnosis of patients presenting with symptoms referable to the neck, arm, back, or leg. Intrinsic and extrinsic conditions of the spine include degenerative, inflammatory, neoplastic, infectious, and miscellaneous conditions of the upper and lower extremity that may have clinical presentations similar to those of degenerative conditions of the spine. One must keep in mind that many of these conditions may coexist with cervical or lumbar spondylosis.

## Rheumatoid Arthritis

Rheumatoid arthritis frequently affects the cervical spine, and the majority of patients with this disease have cervical involvement. The pathophysiology is similar to that in peripheral joints with a synovial disease process that results in destruction of bone, cartilage, and ligaments.

**Table 26–1  Metabolic Laboratory Studies to Evaluate Spinal Disorders**

| | | | | |
|---|---|---|---|---|
| Complete blood count, differential | Urinalysis | Urinary protein electrophoresis | Serum protein electrophoresis | Erythrocyte sedimentation rate |
| CRP | Electrolytes | Urine culture | Lyme titer | Antinuclear antibodies |
| Rheumatoid factor | Liver function test | Rapid plasma reagin test | Blood culture | Human immunodeficiency virus |

Clinical presentation is varied, from complaints of neck pain to frank myeloradiculopathy mandating surgical intervention. Patients may also present with few clinical complaints. Associated complaints of visual disturbances, dysphagia, tinnitus, and vertigo may be part of a cervical syndrome or a separate symptom complex.

Treatment should focus on detection and prevention of the progressive spinal instability characteristic of this disease process. Neurologic monitoring is essential, with close attention paid to the development of upper motor neuron signs.

## Neoplastic Conditions

Primary spinal tumors are rare and account for less than 1% of primary bone tumors. Spinal lesions in older patients are most frequently malignant. Benign spinal lesions include hemangioma, osteochondroma, osteoid osteoma, osteoblastoma, and giant cell tumor. Malignant spinal tumors include chordoma, myeloma, osteosarcoma, and chondrosarcoma.

Spinal metastases are by far the most common spinal malignancy. Approximately 75% of vertebral metastases originate from carcinoma of the breast, prostate, lymphoma, thyroid, and myeloma.

The clinical presentation of patients with neoplastic disease includes localized pain, unremitting night pain, and possibly rest pain. Headaches, upper and lower extremity pain, and radicular complaints are common. Extramedullary lesions may also produce radicular motor and sensory symptoms.

## Infection

Spinal sepsis accounts for a small portion of all cases of skeletal infection with a pyogenic organism. Spread to the epidural space occurs in up to one third of patients. Antecedent infection can be identified in only a minority of patients.

Clinical presentation includes tenderness, guarding, and limited motion. Pain may be increased with axial compression or percussion over the spinous processes. Radiculopathy and myelopathy might coexist because of structural instability or epidural extension.

## The Lumbar Spine

Back pain remains a significant problem in our society. The lifetime prevalence in adults for an episode of low back pain alone has been reported to be 51.4% to 80%. In idiopathic low back pain, 90% of patients return to work within 6 weeks, and the 4% to 5% who do not return to work within 3 months account for 70% to 80% of the dollars spent on back injury. Only a small percentage of cases progress to surgical intervention. As a result, conservative management of the lumbar spine is often employed in the care of these individuals.

### *Active Modalities*

#### Exercise

Physical performance or fitness is determined by capacity for energy output, neuromuscular function, joint mobility, endurance, and psychologic factors. Movement is beneficial to the nutrition of the intervertebral disk and influences the neurophysiologic perception of pain. Adequate mobility is proposed to improve function. Exercise may be either active, passive, or resistive. The exercise program must include stretching, strengthening, extension, flexion, and aerobic exercise.

There have been numerous randomized, prospective studies concerning exercise and spinal rehabilitation. Despite some evidence of no benefit, most of the research in the literature seems to support the efficacy of exercise, although there is often disagreement about the most suitable form. Two separate investigations found weakness in back extension in individuals with a history of chronic or severe low back pain.

There is continuing debate with regard to flexion versus extension exercises. One study supported the use of flexion over extension exercises in the treatment of chronic back pain, whereas another study found no significant difference in outcome between the two modalities.

It has been suggested that caution be used with both active and passive extension, which can load the disk, approximate the facet joints, and narrow the intervertebral foramen. In addition, exercise may be contraindicated for patients with acute disk prolapse, multiple back operations, and such pathologic conditions as spinal stenosis, malignancy, infection, and spondylolisthesis. We tailor our prescription to the problem: flexion programs for those with spinal stenosis and extension programs for those with herniated disks or degenerative disk disease.

In summary, exercise appears to be a beneficial form of intervention; however, use of preprinted exercise regimens that essentially assume all back disorders to be the same should be discouraged. Support has been shown for conditioning, strengthening, and flexibility exercises; however, there is no indication that one particular type is consistently better than another, as improvements have been demonstrated with a variety of exercise programs.

### Education

Back schools have become popular in the management of spinal disorders. Some of the proposed advantages include improved efficiency and economics of health care as result of group delivery compared with individual attention; camaraderie and motivational benefits derived from a group setting; and a focus on improved attitude, wellness, maintenance, and prevention.

Many attempts have been made to determine the efficacy of back schools. Unfortunately, many of the studies have basic design flaws. Also, a wide array of variables have been used to assess change, making comparison of studies difficult.

Although the concept of back school has some teleologic appeal, there are not enough prospective, controlled studies with consistent data to draw firm conclusions regarding its efficacy. At this point, incorporation of education regarding posture, body mechanics, and ergonomics as part of a progressive exercise program appears justified. More studies are needed to assess the benefit of back school and its place in rehabilitation.

### Biofeedback

Biofeedback refers to the use of equipment that reveals the state of internal physiology, both normal and abnormal, in the form of auditory or visual signals so that individuals can increase self-awareness of their physiologic state. Once recognition is mastered, the goal is to alter these neuromuscular signals for symptomatic improvement, including relief of autonomic as well as somatic symptoms.

Although there is empirical evidence for the use of biofeedback, current overall conclusions in the literature are in agreement with those of the Quebec Task Force, which found no specific studies to support the efficacy of biofeedback in the treatment of the spine.

### Passive Modalities

### Bed Rest

Bed rest is a frequently implemented form of treatment. The current trend is to favor minimizing bed rest. Two separate studies found significant losses of bone mineral content in the lumbar spine with bed rest. In examining the effect of both training and rest on muscle strength, Muller observed a significant decrease in muscle strength with inactivity, as well as improved strength with exercise.

The importance of rest in the setting of a septic condition has merit, but in the presence of a mechanical or aseptic inflammatory condition the role of early mobilization cannot be overemphasized. Appropriate movement helps decrease swelling, avoid adhesions and contractures, and promote the formation of a strong organized scar. Deyo found 2 days of rest to be at least as good as 7 days for patients suffering from acute episodes of back pain. In addition, diminished rest time may decrease potential adverse effects of deconditioning. Furthermore, increased activity has the advantage of facilitating recovery by promoting bone and soft tissue strength, improving disk and cartilage nutrition, and increasing endorphin levels.

At this time, it appears that bed rest does not alter the natural history of back pain and, in fact, can be detrimental to optimal recovery and to minimizing return-to-work time in some instances. This is particularly true for individuals who are not neurologically impaired; however, even in the presence of a herniated disk or neurologic involvement, in some instances early, controlled activity with a good understanding of the underlying biomechanical dysfunction may be beneficial. It appears that bed rest is rarely indicated for any period of time beyond a few days.

### Heat, Cold, and Ultrasound

There are several forms of heat treatment, some of which are hydrotherapy, moist heat, and ultrasound. The major effect of heat treatment is vasodilatation, which leads to an increased metabolic rate and increased clearing of local metabolites. It is intended to decrease muscle spasm, improve soft tissue extensibility, and induce a feeling of relaxation. The contraindications for heat therapy in the lumbar spine are identical to those in the management of cervical spine dysfunction.

Cold, or cryotherapy, is applied to the lumbar spine in several forms, including ethyl chloride spray, ice massage, ice packs, and ice baths and are directly applied to the injured area and can be used in conjunction with other modalities. When used alone, cryotherapy has no efficacy in the treatment of spinal dysfunction.

In general, there is a paucity of literature supporting the usefulness of ultrasound in the care of back disorders. It is of empirical value in the treatment of persistent pain after sprains and in treatment of nerve roots or sympathetic ganglion, reflex sympathetic dystrophy, and Raynaud's phenomenon. Ultrasound may be used adjunctively in combination with exercise.

### Electrical Stimulation

If transcutaneous electrical nerve stimulation (TENS) is to be used at all in the management of low back pain with or without a radicular component, it appears best utilized as an ancillary device for symptom control to facilitate exercise and return to function. However, the Quebec Task Force concluded that pain relief has been observed with the use of TENS, but this has not been shown to accelerate return to work or to a usual level of function.

### Mechanical Traction

The intended purposes of traction include mobilization of soft tissues or joints, nerve root decompression, unloading of the disk or facet joints, and reduction of herniated disks. This can be accomplished by many different methods, which should be administered on the basis of a thorough assessment of each patient.

A number of controlled, prospective studies have failed to demonstrate efficacy of traction for treatment of the vertebral column. Several authors have found autotraction to be efficacious in the management of back pain and sciatica, but these studies lack controls. The Quebec Task Force has concluded that although lumbar traction is used frequently, there is no scientific evidence for its efficacy.

### Orthoses

Orthoses are prescribed for several conditions, including trauma, scoliosis, and fractures, and for perioperative support. Proposed theories justifying their use include increased intra-abdominal pressure resulting in decreased muscular activity and compressive forces, decreased spinal motion, warming of the underlying tissues, and postural correction.

It has been shown that intradiskal pressure can be decreased and intra-abdominal pressure increased with an inflatable corset. From these observations, it was postulated that corsets helped decrease the requirement for extensor muscle action and diminished load on the vertebral column. Other studies have demonstrated increased intra-abdominal pressure with the use of corsets, but the relationship between this observation and altering the natural history of back pain is not clear.

Although braces tend to decrease movement, none can fully immobilize the lumbar spine. In addition, with the use of long back supports, there is a tendency to increase lumbar spine movement in flexion. There has also been some concern that orthoses may be counterproductive by leading to trunk weakness; however, there is no evidence supporting this belief.

The Quebec Task Force has concluded that there is no evidence of efficacy for the use of orthoses in spinal disorders. Although they do not appear to weaken the trunk, they also do not appear to alter posture out of the brace, do not consistently diminish back muscle action during activities, and do not immobilize the spine. In fact, there is some evidence that spinal movement is paradoxically increased within the orthosis in selected cases. There have been no good studies demonstrating long-term gains or alterations of the natural history of back injury with the use of orthoses.

### Manipulation

Manipulation appears to be a potentially useful tool in the hands of a skilled clinician for the management of lumbar dysfunction. It appears to shorten the course of subacute back pain in certain individuals. Manipulation does not alter the natural history of back pain and alone is not efficacious in the management of chronic back pain.

## SURGICAL MANAGEMENT

### The Lumbar Spine

#### Back Pain

The validity of a facet joint syndrome is debated because facet joint injections as a diagnostic and therapeutic measure remain questionable. In a double-blind, randomized, placebo-controlled study, injection of methylprednisolone into facet joints had little effect in alleviating chronic low back pain. Another author noted that injection of saline was as effective as injection of local anesthetic and steroids in relieving pain. The response to injection did not correlate with the clinical result of posterior lumbar fusion. Therefore, the role of fusion for this entity appears limited, as does treatment with facet injections.

There appear to be enough basic scientific data to lend support to a possible discogenic etiology of low back pain. The rationale for spinal fusion and disk excision for discogenic pain is based on the premise that mechanical forces may elicit painful responses within nerve fibers and stimulate disk-derived nociceptive chemical mediators.

Surgical treatment for degenerative disk disease without a compressive etiology and in the absence of radicular symptoms can be recommended if certain criteria are observed. The following are considered surgical indications for the diagnosis of discogenic back pain: unremitting pain for more than 6 months; failed aggressive physical conditioning for more than 4 months; inability to partake in any gainful employment; inconclusive imaging studies and a negative work-up for other causes of low back pain; MRI results consistent with advanced degenerative disk disease, preferably at an isolated level; a positive diskogram; and a negative psychiatric evaluation.

### Radiculopathy

Intervertebral disk herniation is the most common indication for lumbar spine surgery, accounting for three quarters of all lumbar spine operations. In general, there are two indications for lumbar diskectomy. The first and absolute indication for lumbar decompression is cauda equina syndrome, reported to occur in 0.24% to 2% of patients who undergo surgery. The second and far more common indication is failure of nonoperative management in patients with sciatica, with or without a neurologic deficit.

A relative indication is functionally significant lower extremity weakness, which affects 5% to 20% of patients with lumbar disk herniation. Operative delays of up to 3 months have been shown to have a minimal effect on the ultimate recovery of strength, although many surgeons recommend earlier intervention. The most common indication is severe pain, and patients who have an unequivocal history of sciatica accompanied by one or more neuromuscular complaints, such as weakness or sensory loss, are the best candidates. Conversely, a dominant complaint of low back pain or atypical sciatica indicates that the results are likely to be less favorable.

The clinical signs should be unequivocal, and a positive nerve root tension sign is most predictive. The straight-leg raising test is highly predictive when it is less than 30 degrees, whereas its diagnostic significance is reduced when it is more than 50 degrees. A positive contralateral straight-leg raise test is highly specific for herniation.

The imaging studies should confirm the suspected pathology. The presence of pathology, however, in the absence of clear symptoms should induce substantial wariness. The decision about operative intervention should then be based first on the history and physical examination, with imaging studies used primarily for confirmation.

### Lumbar Spine Fusions

Although conditions such as traumatic injuries, spinal infections, and tumorous lesions remain indications for reconstructive spine fusion surgery, the vast majority of lumbar spinal fusion procedures are still focused on degenerative conditions affecting the spine's mechanical integrity. The following are diagnoses in which fusion should be strongly considered if operative management is employed:

1. Isthmic spondylolisthesis
2. Unstable spinal stenosis (degenerative spondylolisthesis or scoliosis)
3. Segmental instability (degenerative or iatrogenic)
4. Failed back surgery with instability or a destabilizing decompression

## NATURAL HISTORY, OUTCOME, AND PROGNOSIS

### The Lumbar Spine

#### Back Pain

As previously noted, back pain is a significant problem in our society. The lifetime prevalence in adults for an episode of low back pain alone has been reported to be as high as 80%. Approximately 90% of patients with idiopathic back pain have resolution within 6 weeks of symptom onset, and 4% to 5% of patients have persistent pain. In patients diagnosed with low back pain, a pathologic anatomic etiology is not found in 80%.

Intervention within the first 6 weeks may play a role in shortening the pain episode, but the literature is inadequate to define which patients and what types of interventions are effective. Perhaps the major intervention in the first 6 weeks should be a structured educational program.

#### Radiculopathy

In a randomized, prospective study by Weber, all patients presented with unequivocal clinical symptoms and signs of myelographically confirmed lumbar disk herniation. All 280 patients were hospitalized and treated with analgesics and bed rest. After exclusion of two groups of patients, the remaining 126 patients were randomized to receive conservative treatment, consisting of 6 weeks of physiotherapy and education, or conventional disk excision without fusion. The follow-up interval extended to 10 years.

Weber concluded that the major benefit of lumbar disk excision is early reduction of pain. After 4 years, the results, in terms of symptoms and function, were comparable for the operative and nonoperative groups.

Whether one performs surgery or chooses conservative management, the patient with a documented lumbar disk herniation appears to be at continuing risk for back disorders in the future. One study showed a 25% risk of significant recurrent low back pain occurring at work in those with a prior history of lumbar disk surgery, compared with 6% in the control group. An important point is that the patients who had surgery had fully recovered and returned to work, usually for long intervals.

## BIBLIOGRAPHY

Bell GR, Rothman RH: The conservative treatment of sciatica. Spine 9:54, 1984.

Belitsky RB, Odam SJ, Hubley-Kozey C: Evaluation of the effectiveness of wet ice, dry ice, and cryogen packs in reducing skin temperature. Phys Ther 67:1080, 1987.

Boden SD, Wiesel SW, Laws ER, et al: The Aging Lumbar Spine, Dignosis and Treatment, 1st ed. Philadelphia, WB Saunders, 1991, pp 1–51.

Bogduk N, Tynan W, Wilson AS: The nerve supply to the human lumbar intervertebral disc. J Anat 132:39, 1981.

Brumarski DJ: Clinical trials of spinal manipulation: A critical appraisal and review of the literature. J Manipulative Physiol Ther 7:243, 1984.

Crandall PH, Batzdorf U: Cervical spondylotic myelopathy. J Neurosurg 25:57, 1966.

Deyo RA: Conservative therapy for low back pain: Distinguishing useful from useless therapy. JAMA 250:1057, 1983.

Edeiken J, Pitt M: The radiologic diagnosis of disc disease. Orthop Clin North Am 2:405, 1971.

Gersh MR, Wolfe SI: Applications of transcutaneous electrical nerve stimulation in the management of patients with pain. Phys Ther 65:314, 1985.

Hurme M, Alaranta H: Factors predicting the results of surgery of lumbar intervertebral disc herniation. Spine 12:933, 1987.

Johnsson KE, Rosen I, Uden A: The natural course of lumbar spinal stenosis. Clin Orthop 279:82, 1992.

Jonsson B, Stromqvist B: Symptoms and signs in degeneration of the lumbar spine. A prospective, consecutive study of 300 operated patients. J Bone Joint Surg Br 75:381, 1993.

Kellgren JH: The anatomic sources of back pain. Rheumatol Rehabil 16:3, 1977.

Malmivaara A, Pohjola R: Cauda equina syndrome caused by chiropraxis on a patient previously free of lumbar spine symptoms. Lancet 2:986, 1982.

Melzack R, Jean ME, Strafford JG, et al: Ice massage and transcutaneous electrical stimulation: Comparison of treatment for low back pain. Pain 9:209, 1980.

Michlovitz S: Biophysical principles of heating and superficial heat agents. In Michlovitz S (ed): Thermal Agents in Rehabilitation, 2nd ed. Philadelphia, FA Davis, 1990, pp 88–108.

Nachemson AL: Newest knowledge of low back pain. A critical look. Clin Orthop Relat Res 279:8, 1992.

Simmons ED Jr, Simmons EH: Spinal stenosis with scoliosis. Spine 17:S117, 1992.

Waddell G, McCulloch JA, Kummel E, Venner RM: Nonorganic physical signs in low back pain. Spine 5:117, 1980.

Weber H: Lumbar disk herniation. A controlled, prospective study with ten years of observation. Spine 8:131, 1983.

# Special Orthopedic Problems

# 27

*Edward L. Chairman and David J. Secord*

There are multiple nontraumatic causes of neurologically induced deformity affecting the lower extremity. They fit into categories of genetic and hereditary etiology, metabolic dyscrasias, and tumor or tumor-like induced problems. The effects on the lower extremity can vary widely. Some of the diseases have a quick and definable influence on the biomechanics of the limb, and some are progressive in nature and need to be addressed in stages. This review is meant not to be totally exhaustive but to look at hoofprints and identify horses primarily and one or two zebras. With the identification of the malady, a short identification of possible treatment modalities is explored.

The prevalence of genetic deformities in our society lends itself to careful examination. These deformities are of two types: somatic chromosomal and sex chromosomal. Of the somatic chromosomal type, the one seen to affect the biomechanics of the lower extremity is Down syndrome (trisomy 21). The other forms of genetically induced mental retardation are grouped with Down syndrome, as they present with similar pedal deformity, and many of the other forms of mental retardation that are not induced by trauma (e.g., cri du chat) tend to cause high mortality rates in those afflicted before walking commences.[1]

Down syndrome presents in the lower extremity as a flat foot and an apropulsive gait, caused by a combination of germ defect and neurologic deficit.[2] It is important to correct this as the gait in these patients does not go through the normal propulsive cycle of heel strike to toeoff; instead, both heel and forefoot strike the ground and lift off again almost simultaneously. The long-term effects of this gait pattern are arthritic changes in the forefoot, rearfoot, and ankle and translational effects at the knees, hips, and axial spine that also cause arthritis (Table 27–1).

The use of a custom orthotic device in these patients' shoes helps to establish a more normalized and isolated gait pattern of heel strike to push off and is recommended for all Down syndrome patients.[3] Especially important to consider in the or-

thotic is a moderate arch and neutral to 5 degrees of posting in the medical rearfoot to address the hyperpronatory foot motion. Although the studies of the Down syndrome cohort did not include patients with other types of mental retardation, it is common to see a flat foot in this group as well, with a similar apropulsive gait. It is possible that a custom orthotic would be of benefit to this group as well.

Sex chromosome–linked deformities can affect both males and females and have different presentations. In males, the prevalent conditions are the muscular dystrophies. Duchenne's muscular dystrophy is most commonly seen and presents with an equinovarus rearfoot deformity and inability of the patient to bring the heel to the ground easily.[4] Although the effect of the disease is progressive and eventually leads to non–weight-bearing status of the patient, the treatment of choice for the ambulatory child is molded ankle-foot orthosis (MAFO), which gives support to the foot and ankle and allows a more steady gait. As the deformity progresses, a spring-loaded brace system that is attached to the shoe allows mechanically induced dorsiflexion of the foot on the ankle to clear the ground when the leg swings forward after push off.

Becker's muscular dystrophy, which is less prevalent, has a similar presentation, although the progression of deformity is slower and the morbidity and mortality are not as severe. The treatment is approximately the same, although the use of braces is delayed along with the onset of the muscle weakness.[4–6]

The sex chromosome–based dysfunctions as they present in the lower extremity in females include Turner's syndrome and Klinefelter's syndrome. Affected individuals develop a flatfoot deformity secondary to an equinus limitation in the Achilles tendon and resultant midfoot breakdown and flexible pes planovalgus.[1] These individuals have increased joint motion in places where it normally does not occur and have resultant degenerative joint disease and chronic pain. If recognized early, the problem may be addressed (if not completely corrected) by the use of orthotic control of

Table 27–1   **Representative Pathologies, Etiologies, and Treatment**

| Effect | Etiology | Treatment |
| --- | --- | --- |
| Flatfoot | Some forms of the myelodysplastic deformities such as spina bifida<br>Late-stage destructive neuropathies such as diabetes with Charcot's joint changes | Support of arch with custom-made orthotic if responsive to over-the-counter device or taping procedure<br>Surgical correction a salvage concept in cases of intractable pain |
| High-arched foot | Some forms of the myelodysplastic deformities such as spina bifida<br>Seen in the hereditary sensory and motor neuropathies, exacerbated by intrinsic muscle wasting<br>Uncorrected clubfoot deformity<br>Muscular dystrophies | Responds poorly to custom orthotic control in many cases. Elevation of the heel may decrease some problems, but increase weight bearing forces at metatarsal heads and encourage hammertoe deformities.<br>Accommodative orthotic will give relief in most cases. |
| Footdrop | Any sensory neuropathy, but especially in a toxin-induced, vitamin deficiency, dysproteinemia or glycogen-glucose dyscrasia<br>Trauma to peroneal nerve | Molded ankle-foot orthosis (MAFO) helpful in many cases<br>If patient is able to execute even minor abilities to dorsiflex foot, a spring-loaded Roberts plate with a leg brace assists dorsiflexion. |
| Breakdown and lesions | Sensory neuropathies with loss of protective sensation, with diabetes the primary concern, but also in syphilis and Hansen's disease<br>Vitamin deficiencies, with neuropathies and attendant tissue changes | Use of Plastisote insole material molded to the patient's foot type, leaving depressions for high-pressure areas or prelesional change areas.<br>Custom-molded extra-depth shoes with Plastisote insoles are better for long-term treatment. |

motion in conjunction with lengthening of the Achilles tendon to increase the dorsiflexion of the foot on the ankle. If unaddressed, the degenerative changes occurring in the foot will eventually have to be addressed by a fusion of the joints with the abnormal motion, primarily the talonavicular and calcaneocuboid joints and the subtalar joint.[7] This is an end-stage procedure that is designed for no other purpose but to end pain with range of motion.

Intrauterine position can cause problems with nerves that may be loosely considered traumatic but fit into this chapter by not being acute problems and also not being resolved without intervention, that is, are not ameliorated by palliative care. The most common of these is a position-induced damage to the peroneal nerve in the neonate that causes a clubfoot deformity.[8] Because of the usual position of the fetus in the womb, it is normally the right foot that is in the clubbed position; infrequently, the condition is bilateral in presentation.[9] The normal positional clubfoot is addressed by cast correction of the deformity after birth. If the deformity is not cast correctable, the Turco procedure with an Achilles tendon lengthening is performed.[9] The purely positional deformity is correctable because nerves are not damaged. Where there is damage to nerves, an imbalance of the eversional and inversional forces results and any correction achieved by casting or surgery fails due because of the muscle imbalance.[6] Where nerves are damaged and correction is expected to fail, a tendon transfer is considered to balance forces, including splitting the tibialis posterior tendon and passing part of the split to the area of the base of the fifth metatarsal after going through

the tibiofibular syndesmosis.[9] Rerouting of the tibialis anterior to a more lateral position can be added to the procedure, as well as consideration of fusion of the first metatarsal and medical cuneiform joint to correct elevation caused by the lack of action of the peroneus longus tendon.[9] Such a patient would also need a MAFO to maintain position of the ankle joint for the foot to clear the ground in the swing phase of gait.

Outside the womb, a large number of entities can cause neurologic loss of function that presents in the lower extremity. In the realm of infectious disease, a once prevalent cause of lower extremity deformity was polio.[10] This affected the anterior horn of the central nervous system and so is categorized as a lower motor neuron disease. The primary effect of the disease was motor loss, with muscle wasting and footdrop. The common treatment for this irreversible malady is the leg brace with an attached foot plate and dorsiflexory spring or, more likely at present, an MAFO and assistance with crutches or walker if the condition is bilateral.[11]

Other diseases that are less often seen also present in the lower extremity after a neurologic effect. These include Hansen's disease (leprosy) and syphilis. Because of the similarity of Hansen's disease to diabetic peripheral neuropathy, the two are discussed in the section on diabetes.

Syphilis in the tertiary stage causes tabes dorsalis and footdrop.[12] The footdrop is addressed with either an MAFO or tendon balancing-redirecting procedures, using the split posterior tibialis tendon or rerouting the peroneus brevis tendon. The latter procedure is preferred becuase it involves a phasic group that can undergo change in phasic activity more easily and through physical therapy can be retrained to act as a dorsiflexor of the foot on the ankle on intention by the patient during swing phase and early heel strike and discontinue to act as an evertor of the foot in midstance to push off.[9]

Lyme disease is more commonly encountered in the northern and northeastern areas of the country and has many effects on those afflicted. Although rare in presentation, a palsy induced by Lyme disease causes loss of the peroneal innervated muscle groups and a temporary (or rarely permanent) footdrop.[13] As with any other form of footdrop, the patient benefits most from an MAFO.

Also rare in appearance is Guillain-Barré syndrome induced by herpes. This is a viral disease that presents in the dorsal root ganglion and can flare up with stress and other causes. Guillain-Barré syndrome has a waxing and waning presentation and resolves as the herpes attack resolves.[14] This proximal muscle weakness is best treated by use of knee braces and a supportive walker and/or crutches until resolved. The effect on the lower extremity is related only to proximal muscle weakness, as Guillain-Barré syndrome affects only proximal muscles, but the instability of the patient during ambulation can cause ankle sprains and possible fractures when the lower extremity muscles attempt to compensate for the proximal deficiencies.

Cerebral palsy may be iatrogenically induced or caused by a cerebral or spinal cord lesion.[15] The effect in the patient is the same in either case: spastic paralysis of the lower limb, causing a toe-to-toe gait, inability to bring the heel to the ground except when standing, and instability in gait.[16] The long-term effects of this are pathologically high pressures on the forefoot and especially under the first metatarsal head, digital contractures that cause higher pressure at the metatarsal head(s) because of a retrograde force of tendon pull on the digit translated to the connecting metatarsal head, and pulling of the fat pad from under the metatarsal head to lie within the sulcus of the digit. The corrective approach to the pathognomonic "scissors" gait is less certain, but the equinus deformity is not corrected by lengthening the Achilles tendon. To do so would only cause the spastic contracture to reestablish the previous muscle position and reestablish the equinus deformity. The procedure commonly used for this group of patients is the Murphy advancement.[12, 17] This entails anterior placement of the insertion of the Achilles tendon off the normal posterior calcaneal position. It weakens but does not obliterate the ability of the tendon. To prevent the migration of the tendon to a more posterior position and resultant increase in the pull of the Achilles tendon and return of the deformity, rerouting of the flexor hallucis

longus tendon behind the reattached Achilles tendon is also done.

Toxin-induced neuropathies can involve the lower extremity as well. One of the neuropathies more commonly encountered in inner-city settings with usually older homes with older paint is that of lead poisoning. Lead is sequestered in the bones and has effects other than those on the neurologic system,[18] and the effects of lead poisoning largely mimic those of amyotrophic lateral sclerosis.[19] This is largely the effect of motor weakness and debilitation. Because of the footdrop induced, the MAFO is an important aspect of care, although the cavovarus foot type that is sometimes induced in the patient may require Achilles tendon release and subtalar joint fusion to provide a functional limb.[20]

Abnormalities in the lower extremities caused by tumors, mass-occupying lesions, and pseudotumorous lesions are frequently encountered. These may be broken down into upper motor neuron, lower motor neuron, and both upper and lower motor neuron lesions or tumors.[2]

In the upper motor neuron category are primary lateral sclerosis and lymphoma. Both of these cause a spastic paralysis in the lower extremity. The treatment options for these patients include conservative treatment with an MAFO if the deformity is controllable or possibly surgical transection of the Achilles tendon to reduce the spastic contracture in the crural muscle group, causing an equinus and toe-walking and apropulsive gait. Murphy's Achilles tendon advancement procedure may also help if the spasticity can be controlled.[9]

Lower motor neuron lesions tend to cause flaccid paralysis and include maladies such as tumor of the conus medullaris, tumor of the cauda equina and multifocal motor neuropathy with cord block, the motor-predominant peripheral neuropathies, and lower motor form amyotrophic lateral sclerosis.[2] Because of the flaccid nature of the deformity, surgery is not normally needed. Depending on the degree of deformity, a custom-formed orthotic device may give the needed support to the foot, using soft accommodative materials to support the arch and control the forefoot and rearfoot motion. If footdrop is encountered, it may necessitate the use of an MAFO.

When both an upper and lower motor neuron lesion is encountered, as in Charcot's disease (amyotrophic lateral sclerosis), gradually increasing spastic and flaccid paralyses cause problems in walking and controlled movements. In the lower extremities, the early manifestations can be controlled by custom orthotics to control hyperpronation (excessive rolling in of the foot) caused by the weakness in the dorsiflexors of the foot. As the weakness progresses and footdrop ensues, an MAFO is needed, as well as possible reattachment of the Achilles tendon or release of this tendon altogether with the use of the MAFO or ankle fusion to allow a foot stable enough to walk with and support weight bearing.[21]

A myriad of hereditary neuropathies affect the lower extremity.[2] The first category includes the hereditary motor and sensory neuropathies (HMSNs). The many diseases in this category include the following. HMSN I, or the hypertrophic form of Charcot-Marie-Tooth disease, is autosomal dominant in distribution and therefore severe in penetration.[22] HMSN II, the neuronal form of Charcot-Marie-Tooth disease, is also autosomal dominant in distribution and therefore severe in presentation and penetration of the affected individuals. HMSN III, or Dejerine-Sottas disease, is the third type of motor and sensory neuropathy. The fourth is HMSN IV, or Refsum's disease. The last is Friedreich's ataxia, which is also autosomal dominant. All of these motor and sensory neuropathies cause muscle wasting and weakness in the lower extremity, as well as the upper extremity in the more extreme forms and stages of these diseases.[23] The sensory losses must be considered as well, because the lack of sensory feedback to the individual leads (with the muscle loss changes) to apropulsive gait changes, abnormal pressures under weight-bearing areas of the foot, contractures of the digits with increased pressures under the metatarsal heads, and eventual ulceration and possible infection and limb loss. It is important in treating these patients to inspect the feet for callus or ulcerative changes, punctures, or abrasions and use the correct footwear with a supportive MAFO.[24] These patients, like those in the diabetic population, buy shoes that they feel "fit" the foot. As sensation decreases, the patient buys tighter shoes that can be felt on the foot. This leads to further abnormal pressures in the digits and weight-bearing areas of the foot, causing ulcerative changes and frank necrosis in some cases.

There are purely muscular neuropathies as well. The spinal muscular atrophies are of three types: infantile, childhood, and adolescent (called Wohlfart-Kugelberg-Welander disease).[2] Atrophy of the muscles in these patients affects the lower extremity in the typical footdrop pattern and, depending on the degree of deformity, is largely helped by the use of a custom orthotic to an MAFO device.

Arthrogryposis multiplex congenita causes a flaccid paralysis with muscle weakness resulting from a lower motor neuron dyscrasia. Also seen are joint immobility and talipes equinovarus (clubfoot) deformity.[25] This causes abnormal weight bearing on the lateral side of the foot, which may be balanced by orthotic control if the deformity is mild. If it is more severe, surgical release of the deforming forces involving subtalar joint fusion with Achilles tendon lengthening is needed to maintain the cor-

rection of the deformity and provide a firm foot to walk on. Later progression of the muscle weakness may necessitate the use of an MAFO to counter footdrop.

Multiple sclerosis presents as muscle weakness and loss of normal gait. Treatment is with bracing and crutches. In the regressive stages, residual deformity may need correction by custom orthotic control to balance forces and restore propulsive gait.

The hereditary sensory neuropathies affect individuals much as the other neuropathic diseases do, causing lack of balance and lack of ability to feel the ground under the foot.[2] The gait changes may be controlled by orthotics or MAFOs. The sensory losses need to be addressed like those in any other sensory neuropathy: inspection of the feet and use of custom-molded extra-depth shoes with an accommodative insole to distribute pressures and prevent breakdown of tissues under weight-bearing forces.

Myelodysplasias, including spina bifida, may be encountered in the lower extremity in two forms: a flat foot or high-arched foot.[17] The presentaton of the pes plano valgus foot is encountered when a vertical talus develops in the neonate. If no surgical correction is accomplished before full ossification of pedal bones, a rocker-bottom foot results and conservative care may help ameliorate pressure areas but does not correct the instability in the foot. A triple arthrodesis is the common surgical correction undertaken if an extra-depth molded shoe with a Plastisote insole does not alleviate the pain caused by the deformity. In patients with more commonly encountered pes cavus deformity, an elevated or "cock-up" hallux may be seen with the high arch.[24] Spinal cord–induced spasticity of the foot with attendant deformities may make using shoegear difficult. Pes cavus deformities respond less well to orthotic management than flatfoot deformities, but there may be some relief to the prominent metatarsal heads.[26] A soft, accommodative material should be used. Treatment of the hallux deformity is surgical if it is severe and involves a Jones tenosuspension of the flexor hallucis longus to the head of the first metatarsal.[27]

Metabolic disorders are widely varied and affect a large number of patients. The most prevalent is diabetes, and although the sequelae are numerous, only the aspect of neuropathy is addressed here. Along with peripheral neuropathy we discuss Hansen's disease, as the two tend to have parallel courses. Diabetes causes a neuropathy that is progressive and deforming. Advancing from distal to proximal and affected by the degree of disease, the neuropathy affects all components of the mixed nerves (autonomic, sensory, and motor) and influences the lower extremity in that order: loss of autonomic enervation, sensory loss, and muscle wasting with motor neuropathy.[28] The changes in patients with diabetes and Hansen's disease involve prominent metatarsal heads, contracted digits, and atrophied fat pad protection (to mention a few) with dysesthesia and loss of sensorium. This leads to ulceration, possible infection, and possible limb loss.[29] The problematic weight-bearing topology of the diabetic foot (assuming healed ulceration or surgical incision) is treated with extra-depth molded shoes with Plastisote insoles.[30] The muscle wasting may progress to a footdrop deformity, necessitating an MAFO, but this is not usually needed.[31]

Glycogen storage diseases and purine-pyrimidine dyscrasias cause problems with the formation of long-chain fatty acids and the maintenance of the myelin covering of nerves.[2] This also affects the central nervous system in most cases, but if the patient is ambulatory, the effect is like that of diabetes—a progressive distal polyneuropathy that causes deformity and muscle wasting as well as skin and vascular changes. The treatment also ranges from the soft accommodative orthotic device to the extra-depth custom shoe with Plastisote insole and possibly to an MAFO.

Alcoholism is another major cause (with diabetes and syphilis) of polyneuropathy and attendant deformity with possible formation of Charcot's neurotrophic osteoarthropathy (Charcot's joint).[2] The treatment for the distal sensory neuropathy is like that of diabetes and Hansen's disease. The sensory neuropathy seen in alcohol abuse (Wernicke's disease) can be complicated by the onset of Korsakoff's psychosis with cerebellar degeneration. This causes an ataxic gait and complicates attempts to normalize pressures under the foot.

Any of the lipid metabolism disorders can cause a problem with maintenance of the myelin sheath of the nerve and a peripheral neuropathy.[2] These include diseases such as Gaucher's disease, hypobetalipoproteinemias, Refsum's disease, and Niemann-Pick disease, to name a few. The approach to these patients, while they are ambulatory, ranges from a soft orthotic in the mild case to cushion prominences and use of an MAFO as the disease progresses to a footdrop deformity.

Dysproteinemias such as multiple myeloma and macroglobulinemia also cause peripheral neuropathy, among other things.[2] Treatment is also palliative and includes accommodative insoles or custom-made soft orthoses. Footdrop may or may not be encountered in these patients but is not common.

Vitamin deficiencies are rare in the United States unless caused by a resistance. Whether vitamin C (scurvy), vitamin D (ricketts), or vitamin $B_{12}$, $B_6$, or E deficiencies are seen, the effects are generally on the maintenance of the myelin sheath of the nerve with resultant peripheral neuropathy. These

conditions are treated as any other peripheral neuropathy would be. When more involved disease progression is seen (causing an ataxic gait, seen in vitamin E deficiency)[2] or more complicated gait patterns are encountered (seen in $B_{12}$ deficiency), the use of braces and crutches may be needed. Folate deficiency has the same effect on the peripheral nerves but has central nervous system effects as well and causes confused mentation, which further complicates the gait pattern.

Vitamin toxicity is not common, although it is a concern in oncology when retinoids are employed. The body's ability to excrete an overabundance of vitamins usually allows problems to be averted. Vitamin A toxicity has been described and can cause not only headache and coma but also nerve hyperesthesia.[1] This has been described only in the ulnar nerve and without lower extremity implication. Vitamin $B_6$ toxicity can cause a sensory polyneuropathy similar to that seen with a $B_6$ deficit.

Protein deficiency and fat deficiency secondary to malabsorption also cause problems leading to peripheral neuropathy.[2] These also tend to affect both the peripheral and the central nervous system and cause complex problems in gait and pressure distribution. A need for supportive braces and crutches while the patient is ambulatory is common.

Endocrine-induced neuropathy is uncommon but may be encountered in patients with either a thyroid or a renal crisis. In thyroid patients, thyrotoxicosis can present as amyotrophic lateral sclerosis. As amyotrophic lateral sclerosis involves both upper and lower motor neurons, the complex mixed spastic-flaccid paralysis results in a gait with a combination of a footdrop and apropulsion.[2] The condition is treated with an accommodative orthotic device in the early stages and an MAFO or spring-assist dorsiflexory leg-foot brace in patients with progressive disease. Patients with end-stage renal disease have both deficiencies in calcium metabolism (which affect nerve conduction) and $B_{12}$ absorption and transformation problems. These affect one-carbon chemistry and the maintenance of the myelin of the nerve.[32] Both problems with nerve conduction and the onset of a peripheral and central nervous system neuropathy can have a devastating impact on the patient and cause change in mentation as well as sensory and motor neuropathic complications. The use of an early-stage accommodative orthotic and a late-stage MAFO or leg braces is indicated.[17]

## REFERENCES

1. Kumar V, Cotran RS, Robbins SL: Basic Pathology. Philadelphia, WB Saunders, 1992.

2. Asbury AK: Diseases of the Peripheral Nervous System. *In* Harrison's Principles of Internal Medicine, 12th ed. New York, McGraw-Hill, 1991, pp 2096–2107.

3. Silby-Silverstein L: Use of custom orthotic control in the correction of congenital pes plano valgus in the Down's syndrome patient. Ph.D. dissertation, Thomas Jefferson University, Philadelphia, 1994.

4. Mendell JR, Griggs RC: Muscular dystrophy. *In* Harrison's Principles of Internal Medicine, 12th ed. New York, McGraw-Hill, 1991, pp 2112–2118.

5. Cohen-Sobel E, Darmocheval V, Coselli M, et al: Atypical case of Becker's muscular dystrophy. Early identification and management. J Am Podiatr Med Assoc 84(4):181–188, 1994.

6. Ando N, Fujimoto Y, Ando M, et al: A new method of gait analysis in Duchenne muscular dystrophy. Rinsho Shinkeigaku 32:962–968, 1992.

7. Schuberth JM: Fusions in the arthritic patient. *In* Oloff LM (ed): Musculoskeletal Disorders of the Lower Extremities, Philadelphia, WB Saunders, 1994, pp 560–562.

8. Feldbrin Z, Gilai AN, Ezra E, et al: Muscle imbalance in the aetiology of idiopathic club foot. An electromyographic study. J Bone Joint Surg Br 77:596–601, 1995.

9. DeValentine SJ, Blakeslee TJ: Congenital talipes equinovarus. *In* DeValentine SJ (ed): Foot and Ankle Disorders in Children. New York, Churchill Livingstone, 1992, pp 94–98.

10. Schuberth JM: Tendon transfers. *In* Oloff LM (ed): Musculosketetal Disorders of the Lower Extremities. Philadelphia, WB Saunders, 1994, pp 588–611.

11. Harter DH, Petersdorf RG: Viral diseases of the central nervous system: Aseptic meningitis and encephalitis. *In* Harrison's Principles of Internal Medicine, 12th ed. New York, McGraw-Hill, 1991, pp 2032–2034.

12. Wargon C, Risser J, Goldman FD: Afflictions of nerves and muscles. *In* Oloff LM (ed): Musculoskeletal Disorders of the Lower Extremities, Philadelphia, WB Saunders, 1994, 284–299.

13. Steere AC: Lyme borreliosis. *In* Harrison's Principles of Internal Medicine, 12th ed. New York, McGraw-Hill, 1991, pp 667–669.

14. Corey L: Herpes simplex viruses. *In* Harrison's Principles of Internal Medicine, 12th ed. New York, McGraw-Hill, 1991, pp 681–686.

15. Caviness VS: Neurocutaneous syndromes and other developmental disorders of the central nervous system. *In* Harrison's Principles of Internal Medicine, 12th ed. New York, McGraw-Hill, 1991, p 2058.

16. Koch TK: Neuromuscular disorders. *In* DeValentine SJ (ed): Foot and Ankle Disorders in Children. New York, Churchill Livingstone, 1992, pp 461–464.

17. Fenton CF: Neurological disorders. *In* McGlamry ED (ed): Comprehensive Textbook of Foot Surgery, 2nd ed. Baltimore, Williams & Wilkins, 1992, pp 970–971.

18. Graef JW, Lovejoy FH: Heavy metal poisoning. *In* Harrison's Principles of Internal Medicine, 12th ed. New York, McGraw-Hill, 1991, pp 2182–2185.

19. Lipscomb MF: Environmental diseases. *In* Kumar V, Cotran RS, Robbins SL, Basic Pathology, 5th ed. Philadelphia, WB Saunders, 1992, pp 229–231.

20. Akiyama H, Tamura K: Microsurgical treatment for duplicated hallux. J Bone Joint Surg Br 76:500, 1994.

21. Banks AS, McGlamry ED: Charcot foot. J Am Podiatr Med Assoc 79(5):213–235, 1989.

22. Duvrier RA, McLeod JG, Conchin TE: Hypertrophic forms of hereditary motor and sensory neuropathy. Brain 110:121–148, 1987.

23. Dyck PJ, Lambert EH: Lower motor and primary sensory neuron diseases with peroneal muscle atrophy. Part II. Arch Neurol 18:625, 1968.

24. Koch TK: Neuromuscular disorders. *In* DeValentine SJ (ed): Foot and Ankle Disorders in Children. New York, Churchill Livingstone, 1992, pp 461–464.

25. Bamshod M, Walkins WS, Zenger RK, et al: A gene for distal arthrogryposis type I maps to the pericentromeric region of chromosome 9. Am J Hum Genet 55:1153–1158, 1994.

26. Wickstrom J, Williams RA: Shoe corrections and orthopaedic foot supports. Clin Orthop Relat Res 70:30–42, 1970.

27. Cowell HR: Shoes and shoe corrections. Pediatric Clin North Am 24:791–797, 1977.

28. Cavanagh PR, Ulbrecht JS: Biomechanics of the diabetic foot: A quantitative approach to the assessment of neuropathy, deformity, and plantar pressure. *In* Jahss MH (ed): Disorders of the Foot and Ankle: Medical and Surgical Management, 2nd ed. Philadelphia, WB Saunders, 1991, pp 1864–1870.

29. Delbridge L, Ctercteko G, Fowler C, et al: The aetiology of diabetic neuropathic ulceration of the foot. Br J Surg 72:1–6, 1985.

30. Figge J, Figge HL: Recent advances in diabetic care and management. Clin Orthop Relat Res 296:31–36, 1993.

31. Horowitz SH: Diabetic neuropathy. Clin Orthop Relat Res 296:78–85, 1993.

32. Ganong WF: Review of Medical Physiology, 15th ed. Norwalk, CT, Appleton & Lange, 1991.

# Impact of the Americans with Disabilities Act on Neurologic Impairments of the Lower Extremities

# 28

*Alan S. Gold and Marie Sambor Reilly*

In 1990, the U.S. Congress enacted the Americans with Disabilities Act (ADA). The ADA can be found at 42 USC §12101 *et seq.* The ADA has the potential to revolutionize the way society treats individuals with disabilities. It affects almost every aspect of our lives. It potentially changes the way schools treat handicapped children, the way hospitals treat patients, and even the way doctors interact with patients. Failure to understand how this act limits one's ability to deal with people considered disabled, as defined therein, could lead to substantial legal liability as well as exclusion from federal and state programs. The ADA provides onerous penalties, including punitive damages and compensatory damages. It was also one of the first discrimination laws to provide a trial by jury.

To understand the scope of the ADA and the impact on decision-making processes, you must explore, in depth, the provisions of the act and how the courts have interpreted them. First, we analyze what is provided for by the ADA.

The act expressly prohibits discrimination in employment. It states:

No covered entity shall discriminate against a qualified individual with a disability because of the disability of such individual in regard to job application procedures, the hiring, the advancement, or discharge of employees, employee compensation, job training or other means, conditions and privileges of employment.

*See* 42 USC §12112. The act defines discrimination, which includes limiting, segregating, or classifying a job applicant or employee in a way that adversely affects the opportunities or status of such applicant or employee because of the disability of such applicant or employee. It also forbids participation in a contractual or other arrangement or relationship that has the effect of subjecting a covered entity's qualified applicant or employee, with a disability, to discrimination prohibited by the ADA. It forbids the utilization of standards, criteria, and methods of administration that have the effect of discrimination on the basis of disability even if there is no intent. It also prohibits denial of a job or benefit to a qualified employee because of a known disability of an individual with whom the qualified employee has a relationship or association. This means that one cannot refuse to hire an employee because the employee has a handicapped child or a terminally ill wife or husband. This is a provision of the law that is often ignored.

The ADA also forbids medical examination for purposes of determining the nature or severity of a disability. *See* 42 USC §12112(d). An employer may make preemployment inquiries into the ability of an applicant to perform job-related functions but cannot make general inquiries, not specifically related to the job, designed only to find out whether a disability exists. A medical examination cannot be utilized for this purpose either. An employer may require a medical examination after an offer of employment has been made to a job applicant, before the commencement of employment, and may condition an offer of employment on the results of such examination if all new employees are subject to such an examination. It is required that any determination of disability and all information obtained regarding the medical condition or history of the applicant be maintained in separate medical files

233

and be treated as confidential medical records. Any medical examination has to be limited to determining the existence of disabilities that are job related and consistent with business necessity. Although this issue has not yet been decided, a doctor could incur liability by conducting unlawful medical examinations for employers. The act also severely limits the ability of doctors to decline to treat patients because of disabilities, including acquired immunodeficiency syndrome (AIDS).

The courts interpreting the act have imposed liability against doctors who fail to treat patients because of the patients' disabilities. The courts have taken an expansive view of the definition of disability. Many medical professionals, in the past, have refused to treat patients who are human immunodeficiency virus (HIV) positive or who actually have AIDS. The courts have uniformly concluded that unless the physician can establish a specific danger of contamination, the physician must treat the patient. The U.S. Justice Department has taken a particularly hard stand against health care professionals who refuse to treat potential patients who are HIV positive. The Justice Department has initiated many actions against doctors all over the country and been successful in collecting substantial attorneys' fees from those individuals. Various state human relations commissions, employing state law, have also concluded that doctors have no right to refuse to treat a patient who suffers from AIDS.

The Justice Department sued a dentist pursuant to the ADA on the basis of that dentist's practice of referring HIV patients to another dentist. The court concluded that the dentist had no right to refuse HIV-positive patients even though another dentist was willing to provide treatment. The mere referral violated the ADA. The dentist defended his action on the basis of the following:

> [N]othing in this title shall require an entity to permit an individual to participate in or benefit from the goods, services, facilities, privileges, advantages and accommodations of such entity where such individual poses a direct threat to the health or safety of others. The term "direct threat" means a significant risk to the health and safety of others that cannot be eliminated by a modification of policies, practices or procedures or by the provision of auxiliary aids or services.

The court concluded that an HIV-positive patient failed to present, as a matter of law, a direct threat to the health or safety of others.

The ADA also affects the provision of hospital services. In one case[1] a hospital attempted to withhold medical treatment from an anencephalic infant girl. The girl was found to be permanently unconscious, could not hear or see, and had only brain stem function. The mother insisted that the girl be kept alive with ventilator treatment. The family had no ability to pay for the treatment but insisted that the hospital provide free treatment. It was possible that the girl could live for years. The U.S. Court of Appeals for the Fourth Circuit held that, pursuant to the ADA, the hospital had to continue to provide treatment to the girl and had to keep her alive. This decision greatly limits a hospital's discretion to withhold treatment. If a court would not allow withholding of treatment in this case,[1] it is difficult to imagine a situation in which a court would conclude that a hospital or doctor acted properly in withholding treatment.

Courts have also utilized the ADA to ensure that doctors treat patients equally in their offices. A doctor must ensure that patients who suffer from neurologic diseases of the lower extremity, who are unable to walk or who have difficulty walking, have access to the office facilities equal to that of patients who do not have these problems. Courts even conclude that it is inappropriate to have special waiting rooms that are closer to the entrance than other waiting rooms because this may be viewed as discriminatory and as isolation of a patient.

In another case,[2] a deaf patient contended that she had been refused full and equal medical treatment in the physician's office. She argued that the physician had previously paid for an interpreter to assist the patient in communicating with him. The physician, however, indicated that he might not pay for an interpreter in the future. The court concluded that such a decision established a case of discrimination.

A physician has the duty to make reasonable modifications of policies, practices, or procedures when such modifications are necessary to accommodate a patient's disability. Obvious modifications consist of ensuring that someone who cannot walk or who has difficulty in walking has access to restroom facilities and to all portions of the office necessary for treatment. This would include the waiting room. As stated previously, the use of a special waiting room, however, may be discriminatory. It also includes accommodations that would not be readily apparent, such as an interpreter for people who are deaf and special assistance for the blind.

The ADA, as it applies to physicians and others providing services to the public, contains a broad definition of discrimination. It is discriminatory to fail to make reasonable modifications of policies, practices, or procedures when such modifications are necessary to afford goods, services, facilities, privileges, and advantages or accommodations to individuals with disability unless it can be demonstrated that making such modifications would fundamentally alter the nature of such goods, services, facilities, privileges, advantages, or accommodations. It is also discriminatory to fail to remove architectural barriers and communication barriers that are structural in nature in existing facilities. Thus, when treating individuals with neurologic diseases of the lower body, physicians have a duty to ensure that they have complete and total access to every relevant part of the physician's office. The physician cannot decide to meet them at the hospital instead of the office unless medical necessity requires it. You must treat them like every other patient.

The extent to which courts require accommodation can be shown by the decision of the court in a case[3] in which the court concluded that the plaintiff, the Attorney General of New York, had stated a cause of action against a medical group that had refused to provide sign language interpreters and medical examinations for the hearing impaired. The court concluded that, depending on the financial viability of the medical group, it may have a responsibility to provide such services at no extra charge.

In order to determine the applicability of the ADA, we must first discuss the definition of "disability" as contained in the ADA. The ADA contains a three-pronged definition of disability. If any one prong exists, the ADA applies. The ADA defines a person with a disability as someone who (1) has a physical or mental impairment that substantially limits that person in one or more major life activities or (2) has a record of such a physical or mental impairment or (3) is regarded as having such a physical or mental impairment. The various committee reports of the ADA describe a physical or mental impairment as any physiologic disorder or condition, cosmetic disfigurement, or anatomic loss affecting one or more of the neurologic, musculoskeletal, special sense organs, respiratory including speech organs, cardiovascular, reproductive, digestive, genito-urinary, hemic and lymphatic, skin, or endocrine body systems or any mental or psychologic disorder. It does not include simple physical characteristics. Thus, many neurologic diseases of the lower body, depending on their effect on the patient, could constitute a disability within the definition of the act.

The second prong of the definition of disability applies to individuals who had a physical or mental impairment but have since recovered in whole or in part. Congress included this provision in the ADA to prevent those individuals from being discriminated against on the basis of prior medical history. Congress also intended to protect those inappropriately classified as handicapped such as the mentally ill or the mentally retarded. *See* 120 Cong Rec 3531, 3534. Consequently, a person who had a serious heart disease or cancer that prevented them from engaging in a major life function for a substantial period of time but has since recovered could invoke the act if that person could establish discrimination on the basis of his or her prior impairment.

The third prong of the definition of disability covers a person who is "regarded" as having a physical or mental impairment. This applies to persons who have a physical or mental impairment that does not substantially limit a major life activity but are treated by others as suffering from such a limitation or who have a physical or mental impairment that substantially limits a major life activity only as a result of the attitude of others toward that impairment. It also applies to a person who does not have a physical or mental impairment but is treated by someone covered by the ADA as having a physical or mental impairment that substantially limits a major life activity. This third prong applies in many instances to those who suffer from neurologic diseases of the lower body. Difficulty in walking and problems with coordination may be viewed by employers as limiting the individual's ability to perform a job when in fact they do not.

What about a person with a temporary impairment that substantially limits the person in a major life activity? The definition of disability does not require that the impairment be of any particular duration. The statute covers a person with a physical or mental impairment that substantially limits one or more life activities. The fact that an impairment is temporary may mean that the impairment is of a kind that does not substantially limit the person in any major life activity. The focus of the ADA however, is on limitation of a life activity. If an impairment substantially limits a life activity, such an impairment would meet the statutory requirements regardless of the duration of the impairment. By contrast, an impairment that does not substantially limit a major life activity would not be covered under the ADA even if it were a chronic or permanent impairment.

A welder suffers an injury to her arm. She contends that it adversely affects her in that she is unable to perform jobs that require her to do substantial climbing. The court concluded that she is not disabled because she retains the ability to perform work in general and is limited only with regard to a narrow range of jobs.

A person with one arm missing was able to work. Notwithstanding that such a person could meet the requirements for disability under the ADA. According to the court, such a person might be able to claim substantial limitation in any number of major life activities not related to work. In another case,[4] a plaintiff contended that he was disabled because he had bone spurs, ligament damage, and gout in his right leg. The court concluded that all of these conditions were temporary. Thus, he did not meet the disability requirements of the ADA. To the extent that any neurologic diseases of the lower body may be temporary or that its most egregious effects are temporary, there would be no disability under the ADA.

As previously indicated, the ADA defines discrimination as including failure to make reasonable accommodation for the known physical and mental limitations of an otherwise qualified person with a disability. This is true unless it can be demonstrated that the accommodation would impose an undue hardship on the operation of the business involved. The ADA defines "reasonable accommodation" as making an existing facility used by employees readily accessible to and usable by individuals with disabilities. It also includes job restructuring; part-time or modified work schedules; reassignment to a vacant position; acquisition or modification of equipment or devices; appropriate adjustment or modifications of examinations, training materials, or policies; the provision of qualified readers or interpreters; and other similar accommodations for individuals with disabilities. *See* USC §12119. The ADA defines "undue hardship," which limits the necessity of making a reasonable accommodation, as including an action requiring significant difficulty or expense when considered in light of various factors set forth in the ADA. Those factors include (1) the nature and cost of the accommodation; (2) the overall financial resources of the facility or facilities involved in the provision of the reasonable accommodation; (3) the overall financial resources of the covered entity, the overall size of its business with respect to the number of its employees, and the number, type, and location of its facilities; and (4) the type of operation or operations of the covered entity, including the composition, structure and function of the work force of such an entity, the geographic separateness, and the administrative or physical relationship with other facilities. *See* 42 USC §12111(10).

Some courts have tried to define what employers need to do and have tried to interpret the reasonable accommodation requirement as defined in the ADA. Most courts have concluded that an employee unable to meet attendance requirements fails to be a qualified individual within the meaning of the ADA. Those courts require the employer to make some accommodation for the employee's attendance schedule, but they view continuing inability to appear at work on a regular or continuous basis as lack of ability to perform the job. For example,[5] a telephone company employee had excessive absences because of migraine headaches. The court concluded that the essential functions of her job included regular and predictable attendance. The employee's suggested accommodation that she be allowed to work whenever she felt able was deemed unreasonable by the court.

In another case,[6] the court concluded that reasonable accommodation under the ADA did not require an employer to allow a disabled worker to work at home without supervision. It did not require the employer to install a computer in the disabled worker's home so that she could stay home and work without giving up sick leave.

A majority of courts have also concluded that reasonable accommodation under the ADA does not include reallocating job duties and changing the essential function of jobs. This is true especially when the changes would result in other employees having to work harder or longer hours or would alter the nature of the employer's business.[7] Some courts have concluded that requiring an employer to hire a helper to assist a disabled employee in performing the essential functions of a position is not a reasonable accommodation. The employer, furthermore, is not required to offer a promotion or advancement to a disabled employee as a reasonable accommodation.[8] But some courts have required granting a leave of absence to seek medical treatment where some evidence existed that it would alleviate the problem. In one case,[9] the court concluded that the employer should have granted a leave of absence to a salesman to allow him to enter into a 28-day alcohol treatment program. The court held that the failure to do so violated the act. An insurance claims adjuster asked to work at home as an accommodation for his disability. The court concluded that this request was not per se unreasonable and depended on the specific nature of the job and the disability.[10]

As a physician, you may be called upon to support a patient's claim of discrimination pursuant to the ADA either in the context of access to public facilities or in a claim involving discrimination. Your function is extremely important. It does not end when you determine what the patient can or cannot do. In the employment context, you need to understand the plaintiff's job and determine what the plaintiff has the physical and mental ability to do and what accommodation, if any, could be required. You must be extremely specific in determining the nature of the accommodation that could work. Medically, you must be able to state how any accommodation will increase, and to what extent, the ability of the employee to perform a job. General statements and reports such as "the patient has the ability to perform the essential requirements of the job" are simply not helpful.

## SUMMARY

The ADA has already revolutionized our society. It has enabled disabled individuals or those perceived to have disabilities to participate in a whole range of activities that were previously closed to them. We are all only an automobile accident away from joining the minority group known as "the disabled." The benefits given to the disabled by the ADA benefit society as a whole, but every revolution has a price. We all have to change the way in which we approach our professions and our employees to guarantee compliance. It is hard, at first, but we will all benefit in the end.

## REFERENCES

1. *Baby K*, US App Lexis 2215 (4th Cir 1994).
2. *Mayberry v Van Baltier*, 4 ADD 1 (ED Mich 1994).
3. *New York by Vacco v Mid-Hudson Medical Group*, PC, 877 F Supp. 143 (SD NY 1995).
4. *Rogers v International Marine Terminals*, 8 ADD 81 (ED Ala 1995).
5. *Barfield v Bell S. Tele Communications*, 886 F Supp 1321 (SD Miss 1995).
6. *Vande Zande v Wisconsin Dept of Admin*, 44 F3d 538 (7th Cir 1995).
7. *Milton v Scribner, Inc*, 53 F3d 1118 (10th Cir 1995).
8. *Ricks v Xerox Corp*, 877 F Supp 1468 (Dist Kan 1995).
9. *Corbett v National Products Co*, 9 ADD 23 (ED Pa 1995).
10. *Anzalone v Allstate Insurance Co*, 8 ADD 29 (ED La 1995).
11. *Garcia-Baz v Swift Textiles*, 873 F Supp 547 (D Kan 1995).

# Clinical Neurogenetics

# 29

*Brian K. Kelly*

An in-depth discussion of clinical neurogenetics is beyond the scope of this chapter. An attempt is made to outline briefly our understanding of the various mechanisms of genetic disease as it pertains to neurologic disorders, with a concentration on the clinical effects involving podiatric medicine. The influences of genetics on neurologic disease is varied and complex, and certain basic principles of inheritance patterns should first be understood.

In the classic mendelian approach to inherited disorders, certain physical traits are genetically expressed by particular areas on a chromosome, which we designate as a gene. There are 46 chromosomes in the nucleus of a human cell, of which 22 pairs are autosomal, and one pair contains the sex chromosomes X and Y. A mutation in any gene may produce physical signs and symptoms, and the location of that mutation gives rise to a variety of recognizable neurologic disorders.[1] Of the 22 pairs of chromosomes, one half of each pair is inherited maternally and the other half derives from the paternal parent. There are two copies of each gene, one appearing on the maternally derived chromosome and the other appearing at the same site on the paternal chromosome. These homologous sites are designated alleles and, if identical on the paternal and maternal chromosomes, are designated homozygous. If the genetic information on the two chromosomes differs at an allelic site, they are designated heterozygous.

In classical mendelian genetics, autosomal alleles may be dominant or recessive. An understanding of dominant versus recessive is aided by the concept of genotype versus phenotype. The genotype of an organism is the genetic content of the chromosomes. The phenotype refers to the physical expression of the genetic content. With a dominantly inherited trait, the genotype may be either heterozygous or homozygous at a particular allele. The phenotype, or physical expression of this trait, is that of the dominant gene. With a recessive allele, the genotype must be homozygous for the recessive trait for it to be expressed in the phenotype. For offspring to receive a homozygous pair, this allele would have to be carried by both parents. If a mating pair were heterozygous carriers of a particular allelic trait, the offspring of that pair would have a

25% chance of inheriting the homozygous allele. In X-linked disorders, the offspring of a carrier female has a 50% chance of receiving the affected gene. The male offspring who inherit the affected gene exhibit the disease phenotype. The female offspring who inherit the affected gene from the mother but receive a nonaffected gene from the father are carriers of the trait and may not express the phenotype. The female offspring of an affected male are at 100% risk of receiving the affected X chromosome. Male offspring are not at risk of receiving X-linked disorders from the paternal parent, as the paternal contribution consists of the Y chromosome. In these disorders, only males are at risk for expressing the mutation, and there is never male-to-male transmission. With X-linked dominant inheritance, female offspring may express the disease, but the condition is usually more severe in the affected males. In X-linked recessive disorders, occasionally female carriers may express the disease through a phenomenon known as random X inactivation.[2] There are no identified neurologic disorders related to the Y chromosome.

The proportion of gene carriers who express a trait clinically determines the penetrance of a gene. Penetrance may be age related, with increasing clinical expression coinciding with increasing age.[3]

Chromosomal aberrations may give rise to structural defects in the gene. Large defects may result in severe abnormalities not compatible with life. In surviving offspring, neurologic deficits may be severe. Examples of structural abnormalities include trisomies, insertions or inversions, duplications or deletions, and translocations of genetic material. Most chromosomal abnormalities are sporadic, with small risk of recurrence. However, certain common neurologic disorders such as myotonic dystrophy and Down syndrome are examples of inheritable chromosomal aberrations.[4]

Research has revealed that several disorders are related to mitochondrial DNA mutations.[5] Inheritance of mitochondria is dependent on cytoplasmic inheritance and thus is limited to maternal transmission, as no mitochondria are inherited from the paternal sperm. Although all children of an affected mother are at risk for receiving the affected mitochondria, the degree to which each offspring re-

**239**

ceives the mitochondria is variable. For this reason, there is extreme variability among families in the expression of a given disorder.

Several inherited disorders are caused by inheritance of an abnormal number of chromosomes. Normally, a chromosomal pair consists of a single maternally derived chromosome paired with a single paternally derived chromosome. The possession of an abnormal number of chromosomes is known as aneuploidy. When an organism contains an extra chromosome, yielding three matched chromosomes, the condition is referred to as trisomy. This condition has been most commonly associated with chromosome 21. Trisomy 21 gives rise to Down syndrome. Absence of a chromosome, yielding an unmatched chromosome, is referred to as monosomy. The most frequently observed monosomy involves the sex chromosomes, yielding the 45,XO karyotype, which is seen in Turner's syndrome. Other aneuploidies involving sex chromosomes include Kleinfelter's syndrome, yielding a 47,XXY karyotype; the 47,XYY syndrome; and the 47,XXX syndrome.

## MUTATIONS

In order to understand the mechanisms of mutation, a basic understanding of the structure of the chromosome is necessary. The reader is referred to basic texts in genetics for a more in-depth review of the structure and function of chromosomes.

In brief, genetic information is stored and transmitted using a library of coded instructions contained in deoxyribonucleic acid (DNA) and ribonucleic acid (RNA). DNA is a double-stranded helix, containing complementary strands composed of deoxyribose sugar molecules bound together by phosphodiesterase links, with each sugar attached to a nucleic acid base. These nucleic acids consist of the purines (adenine and guanine) and the pyrimidines (cytosine and thymine). Adenine base pairs with thymine, and cytosine base pairs with guanine. This base pairing ensures that each strand bears a complementary representation of the nucleic acid information contained on its partner's strand. The double helix unwinds during replication and during the process of transcription. In transcription, RNA is formed from the DNA template. The RNA template is then used to construct proteins in the process of translation. Each of these processes relies on accurate reproduction of the parent template for consistent transmission of genetic information. RNA formed from the DNA template is dubbed messenger (mRNA) and encodes the blueprint for protein synthesis. The mRNA contains codons, or triplets of nucleic acids, that code for particular amino acids.

As each amino acid is added in sequence, a protein is formed.

Mutations may occur at a single point or by insertion, or deletion, or substitution of nucleic acids. Depending on the size, location, or type of mutation, the protein product may be normal or altered to varying degrees of severity. Mutations may also occur by way of structural alterations, resulting in rearrangement or deletion of large segments of the DNA. Genetic research has shown that several neurologic disorders are created by trinucleotide repeat expansions. These are unstable mutations, consisting of a repetitive sequence of trinucleotides, which may change in size in succeeding generations, often resulting in a more severe form of the disorder.

## PHYSICAL FINDINGS

The inherited neurologic disorders pertinent to podiatry are those that affect the peripheral nerves, muscles, motor neurons, and neuromuscular junction. Aberrations in the form or function of these systems may directly or indirectly affect the structural appearance or performance of the lower extremity and the patient's gait.

In disorders leading to chronic peripheral polyneuropathies, deformities may be observed in the spine, foot, or hands. These deformities are often most severe in long-standing neuropathies, beginning early in life. Austin's paper on the syndrome of hypertrophic neuritis described foot deformity findings in 30% of patients with inherited polyneuropathies.[6] The deformity of talipes equinus has been observed with weakening of the peroneal and pretibial musculature, with subsequent unopposed action of the calf muscles. The phenomenon of clawfoot can be observed with disorders causing paralysis and atropy of the intrinsic muscles of the foot. This is due to the unopposed pull of the long extensors of the toes causing dorsiflexion of the proximal phalanges, with flexion of the distal phalanges caused by unopposed pull of the long flexors of the toes. Shortening of the foot and elevation of the arch may also be noted.[7]

Chronic denervation of a muscle leads to its atrophy. Significant sensory loss can lead to loss of pain perception, leaving the foot susceptible to repetitive trauma with serious consequences for the skin and joints. Pressure sores may erode into deep ulcerations and set up reactions in the subcutanoous tissue and underlying bone. Osteomyelitis may develop, and the affected region may be threatened with amputation. The skin may lose its flexibility, taking on a tight and shiny appearance, and thickening of the subcutaneous tissue may be noted.

Curving and ridging of the toenails may be seen. The inability to perceive deep pain also results in chronic traumatic injury to the joints, which accumulates to produce joint deformity and disintegration, such as may be seen in Charcot's arthropathy.

In most chronic polyneuropathies there is a glove-and-stocking distribution of sensory loss, with decreased sensation first appearing in the toes and ascending proximally. By the time hand sensory loss is noted, lower extremity loss should be prominent. In mild forms of a disease, only lower extremity loss may be noted. Atrophy of affected muscles tends to proceed subacutely over weeks to months. The severity of atrophy is proportional to the degree of nerve damage. In long-standing atrophy, the denervated muscle fibers degenerate and die. If reinnervation does not occur within a 3- to 4-year period, complete degeneration of the muscle fibers occurs. For reinnervation to restore muscle volume and function, it must occur within a year of denervation.

In general, neuropathies tend to diminish tendon reflexes, with the degree of decrease proportional to the severity of the disorder. Paresthesias, often described as tingling or burning sensations involving the feet and hands, may be a prominent complaint in sensory neuropathies. Sensory complaints range from stabbing pain, electric-like sensations, and prickling to an anesthetic-like effect. In some patients, otherwise innocuous stimuli, such as a light touch, may produce extremely unpleasant or painful sensations. Pain may radiate beyond the local area of stimulation or may persist long after removal of the stimulus. Proprioceptive loss, with retention of motor function, may result in an ataxia of gait by virtue of the sensory loss alone.

## INHERITED DISORDERS

The reader is referred to specific sections for in-depth discussions of these disorders.

### Peripheral Neuropathies

Genetically transmitted disorders of the peripheral nervous system have significant overlap of symptoms. These disorders may involve primarily the motor, sensory, or autonomic nervous system, or any combination of the three. In addition, the disorders may exhibit primarily demyelinating or axonal features.

One of the most common forms of neurogenetic disease is Charcot-Marie-Tooth disease, also known as hereditary motor and sensory neuropathy type I. This disorder was first recognized in 1886 in independent reports from Jean Martin Charcot and Pierre Marie in France and Howard Tooth in England.[8, 9] Patients with the disorder typically have symmetric involvement of motor and sensory function, with clinical findings of decreased sensation, diminished to absent reflexes, and distal muscle weakness with atrophy. Weakness and atrophy of the intrinsic muscles of the foot may result in clawfoot and pes cavus. Eventually, all muscles of the calf and the distal third of the thigh may become weak and atrophic, with the presentation of the classic "inverted champagne bottle" appearance of the lower extremities. With progressive loss of nerve function in the calves, the ability to plantarflex the foot is lost. Varying degrees of cramps and paresthesias have been described, with some degree of sensory loss in the hands and feet. The patient may present to the podiatrist with complaints of gait dysfunction, and examination discloses evidence of a sensory ataxia and weakness of the distal extremities, often accompanied by footdrop.

Hereditary motor and sensory neuropathy type I is an autosomal dominantly inherited disorder. Clinical symptoms usually first become evident at the time of adolescence, although milder forms may have a later onset. Charcot-Marie-Tooth (CMT) disease has been subdivided into a variety of disorders with either primarily demyelinating or primarily axonal features.[10] The most common of these is a demyelinating disorder referred to as CMT1a, which has been mapped to chromosome 17. Other forms have been mapped to chromosome 1 (CMT1b) and to the X chromosome (CMTX). Approximately three fourths of the patients with CMT1 have been found by use of positional cloning to exhibit DNA duplication in chromosome 17 site p11.2-12.

A neuronal form of CMT was described by Dyck and Lambert.[10] This form of the disease, called CMT2, usually has a later onset of symptoms and slow progression. The disorder has been mapped to chromosome 1.[11] Hereditary motor and sensory neuropathy type III, also known as Dejerine-Sottas disease, is a severe demyelinating polyneuropathy with early onset. It is inherited as an autosomal recessive trait and progresses slowly, with the appearance of pain and paresthesias in the feet followed by symmetric weakness and wasting of the distal extremities. Patients are confined to a wheelchair at an early age. In 1993 Roa and colleagues[12] described Dejerine-Sottas syndrome associated with a point mutation in the peripheral myelin protein 22 gene.

Hereditary neuropathy with pressure palsy (HNPP), formerly known as tomaculous neuropathy, has an autosomal dominant inheritance and, like CMT1a, has been mapped to a locus on chromosome 17.[13] The specific regions on the chromosome associated with CMT1a have also been associated with

HNPP. It is theorized that duplication of the chromosome at site 17p11.2-12 in CMT1a and deletion of the chromosome at the same site in HNPP may be the reciprocal products of DNA crossing over.

Hereditary sensory neuropathies represent a diverse group of inheritance patterns, with a variety of clinical syndromes. Hereditary sensory neuropathy type 1 is an autosomal dominantly inherited disorder with clinical signs of slow loss of pain and temperature sensation, predominantly in the feet, with progression to the legs and hands. Lancinating pain may be present, and other neurologic systems are often involved. Hereditary sensory neuropathy types 2, 3, and 4 are autosomal recessively inherited, and sensory abnormalities may be present from birth.[14]

Friedreich's ataxia is an autosomal recessive disorder that has been mapped to the long arm of chromosome 9.[15] Although it is primarily known as the most commonly inherited cerebellar disorder, leading to ataxia, there is also notable loss of large-fiber sensory neurons. Thus, in addition to the cerebellar ataxia, a sensory ataxia with areflexia and proprioceptive loss can be seen.

Familial amyloidotic polyneuropathy is dominantly inherited and has clinical features of motor, sensory, and autonomic neuropathy. A variety of clinical presentations have led to the identification of different inherited types. Several of these types involve mutations affecting transthyretin, an amyloid fibril protein.[16]

## Inherited Disorders of Muscle

Muscular dystrophies and congenital myopathies are a diverse group of disorders characterized by their clinical presentations and pathologic findings. Abnormalities of muscular development may produce postural fixations of limbs with fibrosis of the musculature and ligamental shortening. A common effect of fibrous contracture related to podiatry is the development of clubfoot. This deformity takes several forms: plantarflexion of the foot and ankle (talipes equinus), inversion of the foot (talipes varus), eversion of the foot (talipes valgus), or dorsiflexion of the foot (talipes calcaneus). These disorders may arise from an embryonic abnormality of the tarsal and metatarsal bones, congenital dystrophy of the musculature, or a primary neurologic disorder. In arthrogryposis multiplex congenita, there is a failure of development of the anterior horn cells, which results in asymmetric lack of development and weakness of limb musculature, unopposed contraction of the unaffected muscles, and fixed deformities.

In the congenital polymyopathies, there may be retardation of motor development, with early onset of hypotonia and weakness. Central core disease is considered a prototype of congenital myopathies.[17] This is a dominantly inherited disorder in which normal motor milestones are delayed. Walking may not be achieved until the age of 5. Proximal weakness is characteristic of muscular disorders, and difficulty may be observed with attempted stair climbing or rising from a seated position.

Denborough and colleagues[18] demonstrated a possible genetic link between the malignant hyperthermia syndrome and central core disease. The chromosomal locus of both of these disorders has been identified as a region on chromosome 19 that codes for the ryanodine receptor.[19]

Nemaline myopathy is associated with genetic heterogeneity, including both autosomal dominant and recessive inheritance types. Affected children present with hypotonia and impaired motility in infancy. However, unlike the findings in central core disease, marked thinning and hypoplasia of the musculature are seen. The dominantly inherited form has been localized by linkage analysis to chromosome 1.[20]

Centronuclear (myotubular) myopathy has been described with autosomal dominant and recessive forms and a sex-linked form. Linkage analysis of the sex-linked form has identified a deletion on the X chromosome that is also identified with Hunter's syndrome and the fragile X syndrome.[21]

Duchenne's muscular dystrophy is one of the most common lethal inherited disorders. It has been estimated that 1 in every 10,000 germ cells (sperm and ova) demonstrate spontaneous mutations of the gene involved. As males produce millions of sperm in a lifetime, the mutation is present in every male. Difficulty in ambulation and proximal weakness progress to confinement in a wheelchair by adolescence. Pseudohypertrophy of the weakened calves is notable. Contractures of tendons may produce toe walking and instability. Duchenne's muscular dystrophy was the first inherited disorder to be genetically identified. Mutations were localized by positional cloning to the p21 region of the X chromosome.[22] The specific protein product of this region was named dystrophin.[23] Becker's muscular dystrophy is also caused by abnormalities of dystrophin but to a lesser degree than in Duchenne's muscular dystrophy.

Myotonic dystrophy is a highly prevalent dystrophy that may affect adults and children. This disorder has been found to be caused by a trinucleotide repeat of sequence CTG on chromosome 19.[24] The phenomenon of anticipation refers to the expansion of this trinucleotide repeat sequence in successive generations, often leading to a more severe form of the disease. Variability in the size of the abnormal trinucleotide repeat sequence and variability in the penetrance of the gene have led to a wide range of phenotypic expression of the disorder. The site of mutation has been mapped to the 3′ region of the myotonin protein kinase gene.[25] It has been postulated that the myotonia seen in affected patients may be due to altered membrane excitability caused by abnormalities in the phosphorylation of the skeletal muscle sodium channel.[26] It is now possible to diagnose affected fetuses in utero.

Inherited disorders of mitochondrial metabolism affect multiple systems and may come to the podiatrist's attention because of the dystonia or weakness associated with many of these disorders. These disorders are caused by enzymatic defects in the transport of fatty acids into the mitochondria or in the biochemical pathway of beta oxidation of long-chain fatty acids.

## Metabolic Disorders

Of the large variety of inherited disorders whose presentations are due to metabolic malfunctions, only brief mention is made here. Ceramidase deficiency is an autosomal recessive disorder with deficient activity of the lysosomal enzyme ceramidase leading to accumulation of ceramide. Affected patients have painful, deformed joints, hypotonia, ataxia, and muscular atrophy. This disorder was first described by Farber and coworkers in 1957.[27] Onset of symptoms occurs shortly after birth. Psychomotor deterioration and seizures are often present. The triad of subcutaneous nodules, vocal hoarseness, and arthropathy is classically found.

Metachromatic leukodystrophy comprises a group of disorders related to a deficiency of the lysosomal enzyme sulfatidase leading to abnormal accumulation of cerebroside sulfate. Disorders with infantile onset are characterized by developmental delay with late onset of walking. Flaccid paralysis and peripheral neuropathy progress to inability to walk or stand. Ataxia, upper extremity hypotonia, and lower extremity spasticity develop. Death occurs in childhood. Juvenile-onset forms involve intellectual decline, loss of ambulation, hypertonicity with leg scissoring, and talipes equinovarus. Blindness, neuropathy, and seizures may appear, with death usually before adulthood. Adult-onset forms present in adolescence to early adulthood, with intellectual decline, ataxia of gait, hypertonicity, pes cavus, and hyperactivity of tendon reflexes. The classical form involves deficiency of the enzyme arylsulfatase A, whose gene has been localized to chromosome 22. A large number of point mutations have been identified that affect the production of the enzyme.[28]

Fabry's disease is an X-linked recessive disorder resulting from deficiency of α-galactosidase A. Affected males experience episodes of severe burning pain in the fingers and toes, beginning in childhood, with progression into adolescence.[29]

A variety of inherited disorders may produce ataxia, including adrenoleukodystrophy, Refsum disease, mitochondrial encephalomyopathies, Hartnup disease, Friedreich's ataxia, olivopontocerebellar atrophy, ataxia telangiectasia, Machado-Joseph disease, Bassen-Kornzweig disease, hexosaminidase deficiencies, and Krabbe's disease. A description of these disorders is beyond the scope of this chapter.

## GENETIC RESEARCH

Genetic research has been greatly assisted by the use of restriction endonucleases. They are bacterial enzymes that cleave foreign DNA into fragments at specific restricted sites within the DNA molecule. Each restriction endonuclease recognizes a specific DNA sequence, at which the foreign DNA may be cut, yielding fragments of DNA that may then combine with the host DNA by complementary base pairing. The fragments produced can be used to construct a map showing the cutting sites of the various enzymes used in relation to each other.

Prokaryotic organisms such as plasmids, phage, and cosmids are known as vectors, and foreign DNA may be grafted onto them for cloning. Plasmids are small, circular DNA molecules found in bacteria and yeasts. The genes they carry may convey certain desirable traits on which the host cell is dependent (e.g., resistance to specific antibiotics). Plasmid, phage, and cosmid DNA used in genetic research contains regions in which fragments of cloned DNA may be inserted using cleavage sites for one or more restriction enzymes.

The cloning of sets of DNA fragments in various vectors may be used to construct a genetic library. A human genetic library can be assembled using DNA fragments from human tissue in combination with DNA of a vector. The human DNA is cleaved by specific restriction enzymes and then incorporated into the vector DNA. These segments of DNA combined with the vector's DNA are placed in bacterial hosts, where they replicate. The DNA sequences are retrieved by use of radiolabeled DNA or RNA probes that are specific for the sequences of interest and hybridize with the designated sequences. A genetic library is a collection of different clones containing the organism's entire genome. When a library is constructed, a variety of probes are available for the identification of specific clones that carry traits of interest.

Gel electrophoresis allows recognition of a particular DNA fragment by separation of complex molecules into smaller fragments on the basis of their molecular weight or size. A specific DNA fragment in a size-fractionated gel is identified through the technique of Southern blotting.[30] Separation and labeling of mRNA size fractionated on a gel matrix with subsequent hybridization to a DNA probe are employed in Northern blotting. Proteins are detected using Western blotting.

DNA fragments can then be sequenced using the Sanger dideoxy chain termination method.[31] Analysis of DNA has been greatly enhanced by use of the polymerase chain reaction. This method allows amplification of tiny DNA fragments for analysis. The study of human genetic mutations, such as trinucleotide repeat expansions, has been made possible by this method. Mapping of the human genome has been significantly enhanced by the use of linkage analysis. Linkage analysis is based on the simple concept that certain genes are physically close to one another on the DNA molecule. The closer two genes are to one another, the less likely a recombination event (such as crossing over in meiosis) is to occur between the two. The frequency of recombination events between two genes is a function of the distance between them. Linkage analysis is useful for families affected with a particular disease in which a polymorphic marker is present on the genome. A familial pedigree yields useful information on the location of the disease gene relative to the genetic marker.

The objective of positional cloning is to isolate a gene for a particular disease trait. Once isolated, the gene can be studied to understand the pathophysiology of the disease. When the genetic origins of a disease trait are understood, a rational approach to therapy can be undertaken. Detection of mutations within the gene can be used as a diagnostic tool.[32]

## CLINICAL APPLICATIONS

Specific genetic markers that have been closely linked to the genomic locus of a disease may be used in the presymptomatic identification of gene carriers.[33] The closer the disease gene is to the genetic marker, the more likely the two gene loci are to be transmitted together.

This information may allow the identification of at-risk individuals for genetic counseling. In order to perform genetic counseling, the disease must be accurately diagnosed on the basis of the history and physical examination, laboratory data, and family pedigree. When an accurate diagnosis has been made, the patient may be educated regarding the risk of both the patient and other family members inheriting the disease trait. Patients should be provided with an accurate description of the disease, expected signs and symptoms, the natural course of the disorder, and the long-term prognosis. Patients should understand the variability in age of onset and severity of expression among carriers of the gene.

The development of genetic engineering techniques has opened the door to potential use of gene therapy to transfer replacement genetic material into defective cells. This concept is best demonstrated in the inherited metabolic disorders, wherein a gene encoding an enzymatic product is defective. Attempts have been made to encode a functioning gene within a vector and then transfer the vector into intact organisms.[34] Unfortunately, to date, success in maintaining a stable vector population and transmitting the vector to intact cells has been limited. Despite these difficulties, the gene therapy approach to treatment of inherited disorders is promising, and a large number of clinical trials are under way.

## REFERENCES

1. Martin JB: Molecular genetics in neurology. Ann Neurol 34:757, 1993.
2. Lyon MF: Some milestones in the history of X-chromosome inactivation. Annu Rev Genet 26:16, 1992.
3. Lupski JR, Zoghbi HY: Molecular genetics and neurologic disease: An introduction. In Rosenberg RN, Prusiner SB, DiMauro S, Barchi RL (eds): The Molecular and Genetic Basis of Neurologic Disease. Boston, Butterworth-Heineman, 1997, p 3.
4. Zoghbi HY, Caskey CT: Inherited disorders caused by trinucleotide repeat expansions. In Harris H, Hirschorn KH (eds): Advances in Human Genetics. New York, Plenum (in press).
5. DiMauro S, Moraes T: Mitochondrial encephalomyopathies. Arch Neurol 50:1197, 1993.
6. Austin JH: Observations on the syndrome of hypertrophic neuritis. Medicine (Baltimore) 35:187, 1956.
7. Adams RD, Victor M: Diseases of the peripheral nerves. In Principles of Neurology, 4th ed. New York, McGraw-Hill, 1989, 46, p 1028.
8. Charcot J-M, Marie P: Sur une forme particuliere d'atrophie musculaire, souvent familiale, debutant pars les pieds et jambes et atteignant plus tards les mains. Rev Med 6:97, 1886.
9. Tooth HH: The Peroneal Type of Progressive Muscular Atrophy. London, HK Lewis, 1886.
10. Dyck PJ, Lambert EH: Lower motor and primary sensory neuron diseases with peroneal muscular atrophy. I. Neurologic, genetic, and electrophysiologic findings in hereditary polyneuropathies. Arch Neurol 18:603, 1968.
11. Ben Othmane K, Middleton LT, Loprest LJ, et al: Localization of a gene (CMT2A) for autosomal dominant Charcot-Marie-Tooth disease type 2 to chromosome 1p and evidence of genetic heterogeneity. Genomics 17:370, 1993.
12. Roa BB, Dyck PJ, Marks HG, et al: Dejerine-Sottas syndrome associated with point mutation in the peripheral myelin protein 22 (PMP22) gene. Nat Genet 5:269, 1993.
13. Marimann ECM, Gabreels-Festen AAVM, van Beersum SEC, et al: The gene for hereditary neuropathy with liability to

pressure palsies (HNPP) maps to chromosome 17 at or close to the locus for HMSN type 1. Hum Genet 93:87, 1993.

14. Dyck PJ, Chance P, Lebo R, et al: Hereditary motor and sensory neuropathies. *In* Dyck PJ, Thomas PK, Griffen JW, et al (eds): Peripheral Neuropathy, 3rd ed. Philadelphia, WB Saunders, 1993, p 1094.

15. Chamberlain S, Shaw J, Rowland A, et al: The mutation of Friedreich's ataxia maps to human chromosome 9p22-cen. Nature 334:248, 1988.

16. Benson MD, Uemichi T: Transthyretin amyloidosis. Amyloid 3:44, 1996.

17. Fardeau M, Tome FMS, Samson F, et al: Congenital myopathies. *In* Rosenberg RN, Prusiner SB, DiMauro S, et al (eds): The Molecular and Genetic Basis of Neurological Disease, 2nd ed. Boston, Butterworth-Heinemann. 49:867, 1997.

18. Denborough MA, Dennett X, Anderson R: Central-core disease and malignant hyperpyrexia. BMJ 1:272, 1973.

19. MacKenzie AE, Korneluk RG, Zorzato F, et al: The human ryanodine receptor gene: Its mapping to 19q13-1. Placement in a chromosome 19 linkage group, and exclusion as the gene causing myotonic dystrophy. Am J Hum Genet 46:1082, 1990.

20. Laing NG, Majda BT, Akkari PA, et al: Assignment of a gene (*NEM1*) for autosomal dominant nemaline myopathy to chromosome 1. Am J Hum Genet 50:576, 1992.

21. Dahl N, Samsom F, Thomas NST, et al: X-linked myotubular myopathy MTM1 mapped between DXS304 and DXS305, closely linked to the DXS455 VNTR and a new, highly informative microsatellite marker (DXS1684). J Med Genet 31:922, 1994.

22. Greenstein RM, Reardon MP, Chan TS: An X/autosome translocation in a girl with Duchenne muscular dystrophy (DMD): Evidence for DMD gene localization. Pediatr Res 11:475A, 1977.

23. Hofffman EP, Brown RH, Kunkel LM: Dystrophin: The pro-

tein product of the Duchenne muscular dystrophy locus. Cell 51:919, 1987.

24. Mahadevan M, Tsilfidis C, Sabourin L, et al: Myotonic dystrophy mutation: An unstable CTG repeat in the 3' untranslated region of the gene. Science 255:1253, 1992.

25. Brook ID, McCurrach ME, Harley HG, et al: Molecular basis of myotonic dystrophy: Expansion of a trinucleotide (CTG) repeat at the 3' end of a transcript encoding a protein kinase family member. Cell 68:799, 1992.

26. Mounsey JP, Xu P, John JE Jr, et al: Modulation of skeletal muscle sodium channels by human myotonin protein kinase. J Clin Invest 95:2379, 1995.

27. Farber S, Cohen J, Uzman LL: Lipogranulomatosis: A new lipoglycoprotein storage disease. J Mt Sinai Hosp 24:816, 1957.

28. Polten A, Fluharty AL, Fluharty CB, et al: Molecular basis of different forms of metachromatic leukodystrophy. N Engl J Med 324:18, 1991.

29. Ohnishi A, Dyck PJ: Loss of small peripheral sensory neurons in Fabry disease. Arch Neurol 31:120, 1974.

30. Southern EM: Detection of specific sequences among DNA fragments separated by gel electrophoresis. J Mol Biol 98:503, 1975.

31. Sanger F, Nicklen S, Coulsen AR: DNA sequencing with chain terminating inhibitors. Proc Natl Acad Sci U S A 74:5463, 1977.

32. Cotton RGH: Current methods of mutation detection. Mutat Res 285:125, 1993.

33. Kan YW, Dozy AM: Polymorphism of DNA sequence adjacent to human beta-globin structural gene: Relationship to sickle mutation. Proc Natl Acad Sci U S A 75:5631, 1978.

34. Rogers S, Lowenthal A, Terheggen HG, et al: Induction of arginase activity with the Shope papilloma virus in tissue culture cells from an argininemic patient. J Exp Med 137:1091, 1973.

# 30

# Cutaneous Manifestations of Neurologic Diseases in the Lower Extremity

*Paul Shneidman and Steffi Hamarman*

This chapter discusses diseases and pathologic processes that involve both the nervous system and the feet and lower extremities. It does not cover peripheral and central neurologic processes that primarily cause weakness, atrophy, and muscle imbalance that can result in foot, ankle, and leg deformity. Such illnesses are discussed elsewhere in this text. Neurologic conditions can be manifest directly in visible cutaneous findings (e.g., hereditary neurocutaneous disorders) or as painless sores on the feet (e.g., peripheral neuropathies associated with diabetes or amyloidosis). Alternatively, infections, neoplasms, and some other disease processes may affect the skin and the peripheral nervous system (PNS), or the skin and the central nervous system (CNS). These diseases are commonly manifest in the lower extremity. Their recognition alerts the podiatric clinician to focus on historical information, physical findings, and diagnostic tests that take into account the predilection for involvement of these sites.

## HISTOLOGY OF THE SKIN

Microscopically, the skin is composed of two layers, the outer epidermis and the underlying dermis, which are separated by a basement membrane. Cells in the basal layer of the epidermis are bounded by the underlying basement membrane and are the mitotically competent precursor cells for the successive layers of the epidermis, which include spinous (prickle) cells, granular cells, and anucleate horny cells (corneocytes or keratinized cells). In each of these successive layers the cells become flatter and express more keratin. The life span of an epidermal cell from birth after division of a basal cell to exposure at the skin surface and sloughing off of an anucleated keratinized cell is about 40 to 56 days.[1] The underlying dermis contains fibroblasts, histiocytes, mast cells, blood and lymphatic vessels, and nerves, as well as abundant extracellular fibers (collagen, elastin, and others) and ground substance. Below the dermis is the subcutis (or deep subcutaneous connective tissue), which contains cellular elements, fat lobules, connective tissue, and underlying fascia. In looking at skin, one is looking at epidermis and dermis, with coloration resulting from melanocytes and blood vessels in the dermis and upper subcutis.

Embryologically, the epidermis is derived from ectoderm, the dermis from mesoderm. Skin melanocytes, dorsal root ganglion cells, and sympathetic ganglion cells arise from neural crest, a distinct population of migrating cells derived from developing spinal cord.

Eccrine sweat glands, a tubular system traversing the dermal and epidermal layers, open directly on the skin and are responsible for the bulk of sweating. They are innervated by postganglionic sympathetic fibers containing acetylcholine and neuropeptides as transmitters.[2] In addition, sympathetic fibers innervate blood vessels in dermis and deeper connective tissue and are responsible for vasoconstriction of these vessels. Hair follicles consist of a complex of multiple tissues: the shaft, sheath, and protruding hair; two separate glands (sebaceous and apocrine sweat glands), which open into the space around the follicle shaft; and an arrector muscle near the hair shaft.[1]

Abundant sensory and efferent sympathetic nerves are found in the dermis, and fine nerve fibers penetrate into the epidermis.[3] There are specialized structures surrounding large-fiber sensory nerve endings in the upper dermis (Meissner's corpuscles and Merkel's disks, which include sensory cells in the epidermis) and in the lower dermis and deeper subcutaneous connective tissue (pacinian corpuscles and Ruffini's endings). These endings represent the terminations of individual sensory nerves and detect the tactile modalities of touch pressure, flutter, tickle, texture, vibration, and direction of skin movement.[4] Naked or free nerve endings that are present in dermis and penetrate into epidermis detect sharp and dull pain, itch, warmth, and cold.[4] Receptor and terminal nerve fiber damage and loss[5] occur in a number of "dying back" axonal neuropathies, in which the longest axons of sensory nerve cells located in the dorsal root ganglia are most vulnerable to damage and are preferentially lost.[6] Loss of nerve fibers also occurs with aging, skin trauma, and disease. The ensuing sensory symptoms can be both positive (paresthesias, pain) and negative (sensory loss, hypesthesia, anesthesia) and are an important part of syndromes that affect both the skin and nervous system. Both neuropathies and primary skin disease can damage or otherwise perturb the tissue organization of the skin and lead to visible alterations. The skin acts as a protective barrier, an immune recognition and effector organ,[7] a surface in which the receptive endings for the somatosensory system are embedded, the primary site for evaporative thermoregulation, and a site where disease processes can occur. The skin develops and is maintained by a complex set of cellular lineage decisions and inductive interactions.

On a macroscopic level, the skin of the dorsum of the foot is thin and loosely attached to subcutaneous tissue. The skin of the sole is thick and glabrous and is firmly attached to the subcutaneous tissue and to the deeper plantar aponeurosis through a set of septa alternating with fat, which acts as a cushion against the force generated during weight bearing. The epidermis is thickest over the heel and ball of the foot in the areas involved with weight bearing. Plantar skin lacks hair follicles but has an abundance of eccrine sweat glands.[8] In the leg above the foot, the skin is attached to a layer of fat and connective tissue that concentrically surrounds the crural fascia, inside the boundary of which are located muscles, bones, and major vessels and nerves.[9]

## SMALL-DIAMETER AXONOPATHIES AND FOOT ULCERS

Many abnormal metabolic toxic or deficiency states cause a subacute injury that damages the integrity of the longest axons and leads to loss of nerve fibers, first in the tips of the toes and then in adjoining areas of the feet. Long-standing diabetes causes such a dying back or axonopathic type of neuropathy that can affect primarily either small-diameter or large-diameter axons.[6] Pathologically, there is microangiopathy with thickening of the basement membrane of capillaries and perineureum, loss of nerve fibers, and spotty areas of demyelination.[11] It may be difficult to demonstrate the selective loss of small-diameter fibers by nerve biopsy because of partial regeneration by the small fibers.[12] These patients usually have a history of insulin-dependent diabetes for a significant period of time. Clinically, pain and temperature perception and autonomic functions such as sweating are lost in small-fiber neuropathy. The neuropathy affects toes and feet in a symmetric "stocking" distribution, is worst distally at the tips of the toes, and shows a proximal to distal gradient. Lack of sweating is due to loss of sympathetic efferents and is manifest as dryness of the skin (xerosis). The "trophic" status of the skin and underlying tissue is abnormal—the skin is scaly, hyperkeratotic, shiny, and darkened; may feel cool when touched; and has poor capillary refill after release of focal pressure.

Diabetic foot ulceration is a serious and common complication of diabetic neuropathy. It is strongly correlated with sensory loss.[10] It may be associated with neuropathy alone or seen in association with neuropathy and vascular disease but is seldom seen with diabetic vascular disease alone.[10] Thus, the affected foot can be warm and have intact pulses or can lack pulses and show evidence of superimposed ischemia. Ulcers are thought to be caused by repeated mechanical trauma to the foot, inapparent to the patient because of the profound small-fiber sensory neuropathy. Autonomic neuropathy, leading to dryness and cracking of skin, edema or hyperemia,[10] and defects in wound healing, may also contribute. Studied radiographically, 22% of diabetic patients with foot ulcers has unrecognized fractures, usually of the shafts of the metatarsal bones, a finding absent in diabetic patients with neuropathy but without ulcers and in nondiabetic control subjects.[13] Diabetic neuroarthropathy (Charcot's joints) is a form of traumatic arthritis seen in distal joints of the foot and is strongly associated with coexisting ulcers and sensory neuropathy.

In addition to diabetes, foot ulcers are seen in several uncommon hereditary neuropathies affecting small-diameter sensory and autonomic axonal fibers. Hereditary sensory and autonomic neuropathy (type I) is a rare autosomal dominant neuropathy that presents in the second decade and is associated with a small-fiber neuropathy affecting pain and temperature sensation and sweating. It is associated with mutilation of the feet.[6] Hereditary sensory and autonomic neuropathy types II and IV are rare autosomal recessive conditions with onset at birth or early childhood. They present with profound sensory loss and hand and foot mutilation and fractures.[6] Autosomal dominantly inherited amyloid neuropathies are due to mutations affecting the transthyretin protein that cause aggregation and deposition of the abnormal product in nerve and elsewhere. This gives rise to small-fiber axonal loss and clinically causes loss of pain and temperature sensation, loss of sweating, and commonly trophic changes and foot ulcers.[6] Staining of skin, lip, or fat pad biopsy specimens for amyloid is a useful diagnostic test. Commercially available laboratory tests assay the mutant gene sequence directly and can be used to confirm the diagnosis in the commonest forms of hereditary amyloid neuropathy. Some acquired forms of amyloidosis give rise to small-fiber axonal neuropathies but do not commonly cause foot ulcers or mutilation.

## NEUROGENETIC SYNDROMES: THE PHAKOMATOSES

Neurofibromatosis type 1 (NF1) or von Recklinghausen's disease, is an autosomal dominant condition with a frequency of 1 in 3000 births. Up to 50% of cases lack a family history, because there is a high spontaneous mutation rate at the genetic locus and disease can arise de novo. The mutation is completely penetrant (all adult patients have Lisch's nodules, small hamartomas involving the iris of the eye), but the expressivity is widely variable. The mutation results in loss of function (and apparently dominant negative mutation) of a guanosinetriphosphatase (GTPase)-activating protein that acts to turn ras-GTP into ras-GDP,[14] normally inactivating a cellular signaling pathway that is involved in cell proliferation. The NF1 gene is widely expressed embryonically but is restricted to neurons and glia of the CNS and PNS, as well as cells of the adrenal medulla.[15] Abnormally proliferating or functioning melanocytes and Schwann cells, both neural crest derivatives, give rise to café au lait spots and neurofibromas. Histologically, the peripheral tumors are both schwannomas and neurofibromas. The neurofibromas have abundant collagen and fibroblasts, Schwann cells, and fewer mast cells. Café au lait macules show an increase in melanin in melanocytes and keratinocytes. Giant melanin particles may be present in these cells.[16]

Clinical diagnosis is based on a presentation with at least two of seven criteria: (1) six or more café au lait spots; (2) two or more neurofibromas or one plexiform neuroma; (3) freckling in axillary, inguinal, or other intertriginous areas; (4) two or more Lisch nodules (hamartomas of the iris); (5) optic nerve glioma; (6) distinctive bone lesions; and (7) a first-degree relative with NF1.[17] These manifestations develop as the individual ages, are mostly absent at birth, but are usually present by late adolescence.[16]

Café au lait spots are brown, uniformly colored macules, mostly less than 10 cm in diameter but with a range of 0.5 to 50 cm. They occur anywhere on the skin, including the feet and ankles. The diagnosis is based on finding multiple spots larger than 0.5 cm in children and larger than 1.5 cm in adults. Up to three café au lait spots are commonly found in normal persons. Neurofibromas are flesh-colored or pink, raised or pedunculated growths, soft and deformable to palpation. They enlarge as the individual ages and may become pruritic during puberty or pregnancy. Markedly increased growth can indicate malignant change, and biopsies of such lesions should be performed. Deep neurofibromas, termed plexiform neuromas, encase a peripheral nerve, often at its termination, and are associated with overgrowth of overlying skin and subcutaneous tissue, which can hang in folds. This may involve just one leg, giving a picture of elephantiasis-like overgrowth. Neurofibromas of the spinal roots and spinal meningiomas occur and can affect the lower extremities. Skeletal abnormalities include dysplasia of the sphenoid bone and the internal auditory canal, scalloped vertebrae leading to severe scoliosis, absence of the radius or fibula,[18] and pseudoarthrosis of the tibia.[19] There is an increased risk of malignant tumors.[15]

No treatment of the underlying defect is available. Neurofibromas and other tumors can be excised. Diagnosis can lead to appropriate evaluation, monitoring for complications, and genetic counseling.

Tuberous sclerosis (TS) is inherited as an autosomal dominant condition with variable penetrance and expressivity. The gene frequency may be 1 in 5800, and up to 60% may be new mutations.[20] The triad of mental retardation, epilepsy, and adenoma sebaceum on the face are the classical criteria for diagnosis, but hamartomas can also exist in the eyes, kidneys, lungs, and skeleton in this multisystem disease. Two unlinked genes are associated with TS; the defective gene on chromosome 16 has been identified, and the protein has a region of homology to GTPase-activating protein.[20]

The cutaneous pathology includes depigmented areas, which are areas of skin that lack melanocytes; angiofibromas; and subungual fibromas, which are mixtures of fibroblasts and angiomatous tissue. The brain lesions consist of discrete, whitish, firm lesions, or tubers, which microscopically consist of abnormal, hamartomatous neuronal and astrocytic cells. They occur in a subependymal or cortical location. Optic nerve or retinal hamartomas occur in 50% of patients. Rhabdomyomas occur in the heart; angiomyolipomas and multiple cysts occur in the kidneys. Abnormalities can also be found in bones and lung.[21]

The clinical diagnosis depends on cutaneous findings, some of which may be revealed by inspection of the lower extremities. The cutaneous findings include hypopigmented macules, angiofibromas, periungual fibromas, forehead plaques, and shagreen patches.[21] The underpigmented skin lesions are dull white and have three shapes. The "ash leaf" macule is 1 to 12 cm in size, oval with pointed ends, and is characteristic of TS. Polygonal areas of depigmentation measuring 0.5 to 2 cm and 1- to 3-mm macules occurring in clusters are also seen. Hypopigmentation of scalp hair and eyelashes occurs. Hypopigmented skin lesions are present in 70% of TS patients at birth. Illumination with Wood's light, which is a filtered long-wavelength ultraviolet light source, makes the skin macules more visible. Wood's light is needed to visualize the lesions, which may be inapparent.[21] Café au lait patches occur in about 10% of cases.[19]

Angiofibromas are smooth, dome-shaped papules, pink to brown in color, that appear on cheeks, nasolabial folds, and chin, with sparing of the upper lip. These lesions are known as adenoma sebaceum and often occur in a "butterfly" distribution on the face. Angiofibromas often do not appear until puberty and are present in 80% to 90% of adult patients with TS. Periungal fibromas often appear at puberty and arise next to or underneath fingernails or toenails. They can cause grooving of the nail. Shagreen patches are yellow, raised plaques that are found on the trunk or back.[21]

Seizures occur in 80% of patients. Infantile spasms are the most common seizure type in TS, but generalized, partial, and atypical absence seizures also occur. Laboratory tests that can be useful include the Wood's lamp test, computed tomographic and magnetic resonance imaging studies of the brain, electroencephalography, echocardiography, and imaging studies of the internal viscera and bones. Treatment is symptomatic and is directed at seizures, which can be difficult to control, and at cardiac and renal lesions.[21]

Incontinentia pigmenti is a rare X-linked condition appearing in female infants. Hemizygosity may be embryonic lethal to males.[21] It affects the skin with vesicles and verrucae which evolve into brown or gray macules in whorls and linear bands, seen at age 4 months to 2 years. Patients then develop hypopigmented and atrophic linear streaks, which they may carry into adulthood.[21] Patients have mental retardation, seizures, ataxia, and upper and lower motor neuron weakness.[19, 21] The skin lesions are characteristic, and magnetic resonance imaging shows focal atrophy in patients with neurologic symptoms and signs.[22]

Hypomelanosis of Ito is a rare disorder characterized by hypopigmented macular streaks and whorls on the skin and neurologic and eye abnormalities. It may be related to incontinentia pigmenti.[21] In both conditions, the characteristic skin bands can be seen in the legs. Another condition,

basal cell nevus, can present with pigmented nevi on the neck, trunk, and limbs. It is associated with macrocrania and mild mental retardation.[19]

## INFECTIONS AND INVOLVEMENT OF PERIPHERAL NERVOUS SYSTEM, CENTRAL NERVOUS SYSTEM, AND LOWER EXTREMITIES

Infectious disease often affects both skin and nervous system. Abnormalities visible on inspection of the lower extremities are important clinical data. For example leprosy affects 5.5 million people worldwide,[23] and is a frequent cause of painless foot ulcers and peripheral neuropathy.[23, 24]

Secondary syphilis[25, 26] can present with skin rash that involves the lower extremities. Tertiary syphilis can present with several syndromes that involve the nervous system and the feet and lower extremities. Syphilitic infection may be more rapidly progressive or take a more virulent form in patients coinfected with human immunodeficiency virus (HIV). Syphilis is caused by *Treponema pallidum*, which can be visualized microscopically in material derived from the primary chancre or from lesions of secondary syphilis. The spirochetal organism is transmitted from one person to another during intimate contact, most commonly during unprotected sex. A chancre develops at the site of primary infection, usually the genitals, with an incubation period averaging 3 weeks, and then heals over weeks. Secondary syphilis is marked by systemic symptoms: fever, lymphadenopathy, malaise, weight loss, sore throat, arthralgias, splenomegaly, headache, photophobia, and stiff neck.[25] A papulosquamous rash affects the face, palms, soles, and other areas. Initially, the rash consists of red or pink macules, 0.5 to 1 cm in size, that may resemble the rash of measles or other viral exanthems. These lesions then evolve into papules. Lesions on the palms and soles become hyperkeratotic and scaly.[26] A meningitis occurs at this time, with cells present in the spinal fluid.[25, 26] This stage resolves after weeks and is followed by a latency stage that can last for years. The patient may remain asymptomatic. Alternatively, tertiary syphilis can develop with cardiovascular, mucocutaneous, or neurologic syndromes, or destructive lesions involving other tissues. Cutaneous lesions of tertiary syphilis appear as plaques, nodules, and ulcerations. Gummas, or localized collections of granulomatous tissue, can appear in the calf or long bones of the legs. The tertiary neurosyphilitic syndromes tabes dorsalis and general paresis are now rare, but meningovascular syphilis, cranial neuropathies, and CNS gummas[27] are seen. Meningovascular syphilis causes chronic meningitis, obliterative endarteritis, lymphocytic vasculitis of larger vessels (Heubner's arteritis), perivasculitis, gummas, and adhesive arachnoiditis around the brain. Patients develop a chronic meningitis, cranial neuropathies, hydrocephalus, and syndromes of dementia, headache, confusion, optic atrophy, and stroke.[25] General paresis involves many of the pathologic elements of meningovascular syphilis but includes parenchymal infection of the brain causing atrophy and gliosis. Dementias, psychosis, and motor symptoms are seen. Congenital syphilis can be transmitted to the fetus, even during latency.[26] Diagnosis of any of the preceding syndromes is based on clinical presentation, blood serology, and cerebrospinal fluid serologic analysis. The serum rapid plasma reagin and Venereal Disease Research Laboratory tests (reaginic tests) are used for screening, but 20% to 40% of positives are false positives. The more specific fluorescent treponemal antibody absorption test can be used for confirmation. Neurosyphilis is treated with high-dose intravenous penicillin for 10 to 14 days. Patients require follow-up reaginic serologic tests and clinical evaluation.

Lyme disease is caused by a spirochete, *Borrelia burgdorferi*, and is common in endemic areas of the northeastern United States. A bite by an infected tick commonly occurs on the leg. The initial red macule spreads over adjacent skin over days to weeks as a large red ring with a central clearing. This skin lesion is termed erythema migrans but is absent in 20% to 40% of cases.[28] Without treatment, it resolves spontaneously, but it is followed in 15% to 20% of patients by a neurologic syndrome of painful radiculitis, meningitis, and facial palsies, which are often bilateral.[23] Late in the infection patients also develop carditis, joint arthritis, polyneuropathy, or a specific skin lesion, acrodermatitis chronica atrophicans. Acrodermatitis chronica atrophicans presents as a bluish-red skin lesion on the lower extremities that evolves into an atrophic area.[28] Diagnosis is based on testing for antibodies by enzyme-linked immunosorbent assay or, more definitely, by Western blot. Treatment is with ceftriaxone, tetracycline, or ampicillin.

Cutaneous pathology of the lower extremities, with concomitant involvement of the PNS and CNS, is frequently seen during the latter stages of infection with HIV. Patients with CD4+ lymphocyte counts of less than 100 are at risk for a variety of opportunistic infections. Reactivation of a latent pulmonary infection with the fungus *Cryptococcus neoformans* occurs in about 5% of patients with acquired immunodeficiency syndrome (AIDS). The fungus disseminates hematogenously. Ten percent of these patients have skin involvement, which most frequently takes the form of painless, erythematous macules that progress to nodules or ulcers, oc-

curring mainly on the face.[29] The lesions may also resemble those of molluscum contagiosum, a poxvirus infection, but lack the central umbilication or keratin plug seen in the viral lesions. Of 30 consecutive patients with AIDS and cryptococcal meningitis, 10% had papulonodular lesions, 10% had molluscum contagiosum–like lesions, and 7% had pustular-ulcerative lesions.[30] Cutaneous cryptococcosis can also take the form of erythematous macules, plaques, folliculitis, acneiform lesions, and herpes-like vesiculations.[31] Cryptococcal meningitis is common in this group of patients and presents with headache, fever, stiff neck, vomiting, malaise, or obtundation. Blood, cerebrospinal fluid, and urine cultures often yield the organism, and cryptococcal antigen titers are diagnostic in these body fluids.[31] Treatment is with intravenous amphotericin B and oral flucytosine, fluconazole, or itraconazole.[32] Other deep fungal infections with *Histoplasma capsulatum* or *Coccidioides immitis* can simultaneously involve the skin and nervous system. These can occur in immunosuppressed patients who have been previously exposed to aerosolized spores in the endemic geographic areas. Both can manifest as papules, plaques, pustules, and nodules on the skin; granulomas or meningitis in the CNS; and granulomas elsewhere in the body.[31] Superficial fungal infections, such as tinea pedis caused by infection with *Trichophyton rubrum*, are common on the feet and nails of AIDS patients and can be difficult to eradicate.

Varicella-zoster virus, the causative agent of chickenpox, latently infects dorsal root ganglion nerve cells and can be reactivated as herpes zoster (HZ). HZ presents with localized symptoms of pain, pruritus, and paresthesias, followed rapidly by the appearance of skin lesions in the distribution of a single or several adjacent dermatomes. The discrete, raised lesions are initially erythematous papules, which progress over 1 day to vesicles and over the next 2 days to pustules. By 7 days the pustules dry, followed by scabbing and crust formation at 10 to 12 days. The scabs fall off by 2 to 3 weeks. There may be a transient viremia and constitutional symptoms.[33] The dermatomes of the lower extremities are commonly involved, and associated complications include motoric weakness in the legs, bladder and anal sphincter dysfunction, and myelitis. Segmental motor weakness occurs in 5% of cases of HZ.[34] In 90%, weakness occurs in the same dermatome as the rash, and recovery occurs in most cases.[33] Bladder or anal sphincter dysfunction can occur after HZ involving the sacral dermatomes,[35] with an excellent prognosis for recovery. Postherpetic neuralgia commonly develops in elderly patients. HZ in any location can be followed by a postinfectious leukoencephalitis or Guillain-Barré syndrome.[33]

Immunosuppressed patients, such as those with AIDS, can develop disseminated varicella-zoster virus infection with pneumonia, visceral involvement, and encephalomyelitis. Treatment with acyclovir is indicated for HZ involvement of the eye, distribution in multiple dermatomes, or HZ in immunosuppressed patients.

## CANCER INVOLVING BOTH NERVOUS SYSTEM AND LOWER EXTREMITIES

Neoplasms can affect the skin of the lower extremities and nervous system simultaneously. Kaposi's sarcoma (KS) is a tumor of endothelial cells of blood and lymphatic vessels. KS is seen in homosexual men infected with HIV and in elderly patients from the Mediterranean area. It presents as purplish raised lesions. Of AIDS patients with KS, 45% have involvement of the lower extremities and 70% have tumor affecting the oral cavity and hard palate.[29] KS can invade peripheral nerve, plexus, or rarely brain.[36] It has been linked to human herpesvirus 8, also called Kaposi's sarcoma–associated herpesvirus. Evidence of infection is found in 95% of cases of KS of all types, and seroconversion to this virus antedates the appearance of KS in HIV-infected homosexual men.[37] Treatment is by local radiation therapy, chemotherapy, and interferon alfa. Human chorionic gonadotropin has been shown to induce regression.[38]

Malignant melanoma (MM) is a common cancer and is the third most common cancer to metastasize to the brain, after lung and breast carcinoma.[39] Congenital melanocytic nevi, moles larger than 10 cm, have a 6% lifetime risk of developing into MM and should be removed. Congenital melanocytic nevi smaller than 1.5 cm have a much lower chance of malignant transformation, and careful observation may be appropriate. MM lesions are irregular in shape and coloration. They display the ABCD characteristics: asymmetry of shape, border irregularity, color variegation, and diameter greater than 6 mm. Four subtypes of MM are superficial spreading MM, nodular MM, lentigo maligna MM, and acral-lentiginous MM.[40] Acral-lentiginous MM can present as a dark brown, blue-black, or black lesion on the foot or sole or as melanonychia striata, which is an enlarging fingernail bed. The overwhelming majority of acquired melanocytic nevi (moles) are benign and have a regular, round border and uniform coloration. Those that are not should be examined by biopsy or excised. Lymphomas and metastatic lesions can also be seen on the skin of the lower extremities.

## SUMMARY

A large number of processes affect both the skin and the nervous system. The nervous system is not available for direct inspection (except for the optic fundus), but the clinician can readily inspect the skin. Frequently, relevant skin findings are visible on the feet and lower extremities. The histology of the skin gives clues to the cells that can be involved, for example, in disorders of pigmentation or in neoplasia. The enormous surface area of the skin ensures that a systemic vasculitis or a recurrent embolic process has a high chance of being visible. Trophic influences and the importance of pain perception are highlighted in neuropathies that involve foot ulcers.

## REFERENCES

1. Mehregan A: Pincus' Guide to Dermatohistopathology, 6th ed. Norwalk, CT, Appleton & Lange, 1995.
2. Ogawa T, Low PA: Autonomic regulation of temperature and sweating. *In* Low PA (ed): Clinical Autonomic Disorders. Boston, Little, Brown, 1993.
3. Arthur RP, Shelley WB: The innervation of human epidermis. J Invest Dermatol 32:397–410, 1959.
4. Lindblom U, Ochoa J: Somatosensory function and dysfunction. *In* Asbury AK, McKhann GM, McDonald WI: Diseases of the Nervous System—Clinical Neurobiology. Philadelphia, WB Saunders, 1992.
5. McCarthy BG, Hsieh S-T, Stocks A, et al: Cutaneous innervation in sensory neuropathies: Evaluation by skin biopsy. Neurology 45:1848–1855, 1995.
6. Schaumburg HH, Berger AR, Thomas PK: Disorders of Peripheral Nerve. Philadelphia, FA Davis, 1992.
7. Baer RL: Allergic contact dermatitis and Langerhans cells: Comments on recent developments. Cutis 52:270–272, 1993.
8. Sammarco GJ: *In* Sammarco GJ (ed): Foot and Ankle Manual. Philadelphia, Lea & Febiger, 1991.
9. Clemente CD: Anatomy—A Regional Atlas of the Human Body. Baltimore, Urban & Schwarzenberg, 1981.
10. Thomas PK, Griffin JW: Neuropathies predominantly affecting sensory or motor fuction. *In* Asbury AK, Thomas PK (eds): Peripheral Nerve Disorders—2. Oxford, Butterworth Heinemann, England, 1995.
11. Vital C, Vital A: Peripheral neuropathy. *In* Ducket S (ed): The Pathology of the Aging Human Nervous System. Philadelphia, Lea & Febiger, 1991.
12. Llewelyn JG, Gilbey SG, Thomas PK, et al: Sural nerve morphometry in diabetic autonomic and painful sensory neuropathy: A clinicopathological study. Brain 114:867–892, 1991.
13. Cavanaugh PR, Young MJ, Adams JE, Boulton AJM: Radiographic abnormalities in diabetic feet. *In* Boulton AJM, Conner H, Cavanaugh PR (eds): The Foot in Diabetes. Chichester, England, Wiley, 1994.
14. Ballester R, Marchuk D, Boguski M, et al: The NF1 locus encodes a protein functionally related to mammalian GAP and yeast IRA proteins. Cell 63:851–859, 1990.
15. Pleasure JR, Chance PF, Pleasure DE: Neurofibromatosis types 1 and 2. *In* Asbury AK, Thomas PK (eds): Peripheral Nerve Disorders—2. Oxford, Butterworth Heinemann, 1995.
16. Mackool BT, Fitzpatrick TB: Diagnosis of neurofibromatosis by cutaneous examination. Semin Neurol 12:358–363, 1992.
17. Mulvihill JJ, Parry DM, Sherman JL, et al: Neurofibromatosis 1 (Recklinghausen disease) and neurofibromatosis 2 (bilateral acoustic neurofibromatosis). An update. Ann Intern Med 113:39–52, 1990.
18. Ausman JI, French LA, Baker AB: Intracranial neoplasms. *In*

Joynt RJ (ed): Clinical Neurology. Philadelphia, JB Lippincott, 1992.

19. Baraitser M: Neurocutaneous disorders. *In* Asbury AK, McKhann GM, McDonald WI. Diseases of the Nervous System—Clinical Neurobiology. Philadelphia, WB Saunders, 1994.

20. European Chromosome 16 Tuberous Sclerosis Consortium: Identification and characterization of the tuberous sclerosis gene on chromosome 16. Cell 75:1305–1315, 1993.

21. Wiss K: Neurocutaneous disorders: Tuberous sclerosis, incontinentia pigmenti, and hypomelanosis of Ito. Semin Neurol 12:364–372, 1992.

22. Pascual-Castroviejo I, Roche MC, Martinez Fernandez V, et al: Incontinentia pigmenti: MR demonstration of the brain changes. AJNR 15:1521–1527, 1994.

23. Said G: Neuropathies due to Lyme disease, leprosy and Chagas disease. *In* Asbury AK, Thomas PK (eds): Peripheral Nerve Disorders—2. Oxford, Butterworth Heinemann, 1995.

24. Parson M: A Colour Atlas of Clinical Neurology. Weert, Netherlands, Wolfe, 1983.

25. Reik L: Spirochaetal infections of the nervous system. *In* Kennedy PGE, Johnson RT (eds): Infections of the Nervous System. London, Butterworth, 1987.

26. Johnson RA, White M: Syphilis in the 1990s: Cutaneous and neurologic manifestations. Semin Neurol 12:287–298, 1992.

27. Roeske LC, Kennedy PR: Syphilitic gummas in a patient with human immunodeficiency virus infection. N Engl J Med 335:1123, 1996.

28. Coyle PK: Lyme disease. *In* Feldman E (ed): Current Diagnosis in Neurology. St. Louis, Mosby–Year Book, 1994.

29. Stratigos AJ, Johnson RA, Dover JS: Cutaneous manifestations of human immunodeficiency virus infection. Semin Neurol 12:299–311, 1992.

30. Manfredi R, Mazzoni A, Manetti A, et al: Morphological features and clinical significance of skin involvement in patients with AIDS-related Cryptococcosis. Acta Derm Venereol 76:72–74, 1996.

31. Stratigos AJ, Laskaris G, Stratigos MD: Behçet's disease. Semin Neurol 12:346–357, 1992.

32. Sanford JP, Gilbert DN, Gerberding JL, Sande MA: Guide to Antimicrobial Therapy 1994. Dallas, Antimicrobial Therapy, 1994.

33. Kennedy PGE: Neurologic complications of varicella-zoster virus. *In* Kennedy PGE, Johnson RT (eds): Infections of the Nervous System. London, Butterworth, 1987.

34. Thomas JE, Howard FM: Segmental zoster paresis—A disease profile. Neurology 22:459–466, 1972.

35. Jellinek EH, Tulloch WS: Herpes zoster with dysfunction of bladder and anus. Lancet 2:1219–1222, 1976.

36. Gorin FA, Bale JF, Halks-Miller M, Schwartz RA: Kaposi's sarcoma metastatic to the brain. Arch Neurol 42:162–165, 1985.

37. Goa SJ, Kingsley L, Hoover DR, et al: Seroconversion to antibodies against Kaposi's sarcoma–associated herpesvirus-related latent nuclear antigens before the development of Kaposi's sarcoma. N Engl J Med 335:233–241, 1996.

38. Gill PS, Lunardi-Iskandar Y, Louis D, et al: The effects of preparations of human chorionic gonadotropin on AIDS-related Kaposi's sarcoma. N Engl J Med 335:1261–1269, 1996.

39. Amer MH, Al-Sarraf M, Baker LH, Vaitkevicius VK: Malignant melanoma and central nervous system metastases: Incidence, diagnosis, treatment, and survival. Cancer 42:660–668, 1978.

40. Rivers JK, Rossi SF: Malignant melanoma. Semin Neurol 12:338–345, 1992.

# Physical Therapy in the Treatment of Lower Extremity Pain and Impairment

# 31

*John M. Barbis*

Chronic lower extremity pain and impairment related to neuromusculoskeletal dysfunction pose significant management problems to both the physician and the physical therapist. It is often difficult to ascribe the pain and impairment to a single pathoanatomic source and, as a result, it is difficult to establish and complete an adequate intervention plan. Lower extremity impairments caused by acute orthopedic and/or neurologic conditions (sprains or strains, fractures, joint disorders, neurologic compromise, and postsurgical conditions) usually have more definitive pathoanatomic loci and, as a result, are easier to diagnose and treat. Numerous textbooks on physical medicine and physical therapy deal with the management of acute lower extremity pain and impairment.[1-3] This chapter discusses the use of physical therapy in the management of chronic lower extremity pain and movement impairment. It describes the evaluation and diagnostic processes that therapists use to come to treatment conclusions, which are not familiar to most physicians. It also describes treatment approaches and modalities that therapists may use in the management of chronic lower extremity pain and impairment.

## OVERVIEW

As with all of health care, research and changes in reimbursement patterns have changed the practice of physical therapy. Before these changes, the emphasis of care during the treatment was on therapist-applied procedures. Modalities (e.g. heat, cold, ultrasound, electrical stimulation, diathermies), massage, joint mobilizations, and therapeutic exercise performed either manually by the therapist or using equipment in the clinic were the major components of the care plan. The patient was dependent on the therapist for the direct application of the treatment procedures. Now, the emphasis in physical therapy is on the development of treatment plans in which

the patient is the primary provider of the care. Although the traditional therapist-applied procedures are still components of the treatment, their role is now adjunctive and their use is limited. Education of patients and the development of independent care approaches that allow patients to assume the responsibility for their care as soon as possible are emphasized. This changes the role of the therapist and requires the therapist to be a better communicator, coach, and teacher. It also requires the therapist to be more skilled in examining the patient and prioritizing key problems (diagnoses) and selective in the use of adjunctive therapeutic procedures.

The changes in the health care environment have also affected the relationship between the physician and the therapist. Therapists can no longer rely on the physician's prescription as evidence of the necessity and appropriateness for the treatment. Therapists are responsible for the care they provide. Differences often arise between a physician's referral and the therapist's assessment of the most appropriate treatment plan. When such differences arise, clear and effective communication between the physician and the therapist is essential to resolve them.

## PHYSICAL THERAPY EXAMINATION

The physician's examination and the physical therapist's examination of a patient with chronic lower extremity pain and impairment are different.[4] The physician's examination is most concerned with identifying the pathoanatomic or pathophysiologic source of the symptoms. The therapist's examination is more limited in focus and more concerned with identifying the pathokinesiologic source of the pain and impairments.[5, 6] Pathoanatomic or pathophysiologic diagnoses are important to the therapist because they establish parameters within which the therapist must work. They are particularly important for their exclusionary effect. Although a specific pathoanatomic or pathophysiologic diagnosis may not specifically indicate the physical treatment to be performed (the pathokinesiologic diagnosis does), it indicates what procedures are inappropriate or are to be performed with caution. The pathoanatomic or pathophysiologic diagnostic categories that would be either a contraindication to the use of physical therapy or indicate its use with caution are listed in Table 31–1.

Although there are some similarities between the physician's and the physical therapist's examinations, there are several differences that emphasize the focus that physical therapy places on the management of factors that prevent normal pain-free movement and function. In the subjective component of the examination, the therapist is concerned about the history and onset of the problem and the health history of the patient, but the examination focuses more on the effect of the symptoms on function and the effect of function on the symptoms. Assessing the patient's limitations and the irritability of the condition are major components of the subjective assessment because that information helps not only in leading to the development of a diagnosis and treatment plan but also in guiding the direction of the objective examination.

The objective examination includes few of the standard physical examination procedures normally performed by the physician. Unless there are profound reasons for doing otherwise, only a brief systems evaluation occurs. The majority of the examination is designed to assess the degree of impairment of movement and the effect of movement on the symptoms. The major areas of the objective examination are as follows.

## Movement Assessment

The examination of movement is concerned less with the absolute degree of limitation of movement than with how the symptoms and movement limitations change with repeated movements or sustained positions and what factors (disruptions in the quality of the movement, loss of joint accessory motion, and disruptions in normal movement pathways or tracking) produce the limitations of movement or

**Table 31–1  Contraindications to the Use of Physical Therapy**

| |
|---|
| Unstable fractures |
| Acute infection |
| Acute inflammatory disease |
| Nonorganic syndromes |
| Pain of visceral origin |
| Malignancy |

function (gait deviations, joint mechanics during transfers, work activities, activities of daily living). In addition, the physical therapy examination assesses whether the symptoms are produced upon end-range motion or during motion. Often, upon testing repeated joint motions, rapid changes in joint motion and symptom intensity and location can be seen. These changes are not seen when a movement is tested only once or twice. Passive movement testing of joint accessory motions, observation of the quality of active movement in the peripheral joints, and observation of posture and joint-body mechanics during movement are essential components of the examination.

## Neuromuscular Assessment

Although the quantification of the force generated by the muscle when it is required to contract can be an important component of this assessment, whether it is a technologic assessment (e.g., dynamometers, force plate evaluation) or a manual assessment (manual muscle test or isometric strength testing), its use is limited. More important in the development of a physical therapy diagnosis and treatment plan are the relationships of weakness and pain during a muscular contraction, the quality of the contraction, fatigue produced by repeated contractions, and functional limitations caused by the weakness.

## Neurologic Status

Sensory, muscle strength, and reflex tests are part of the physical therapy examination. Neural mobility testing is an important component of the physical therapy examination of the status of the neurologic system in patients with chronic lower extremity pain. In neural mobility testing, combination movements at multiple joints are used to place stress on specific components of the central or peripheral nervous system.[7] By proper positioning and movement, the mobility of individual peripheral nerves can be assessed. Neural entrapments, intraneural adherences, and extraneural adherences can be demonstrated through careful manipulation of the spine and lower extremities. As Butler[7] indicated, many chronic pain problems in the lower extremity that have not responded to normal care or have been aggravated by normal care are caused by these restrictions in the normal movement of the nervous system.

## Postural Examination

Observation of the patient's posture and joint positioning, especially during standing, is valuable in assessing for anomalies that might be the primary cause of the pain or hinder normal recovery. In assessing posture, it is not enough to notice an anomaly. Most patients have at least one postural or positional anomaly that is benign and does not affect the recovery from the primary problem. For the anomaly to be considered relevant to the patient's management, the postural examination must demonstrate a positive correlation between the anomaly and the production or reduction of the symptoms.

## Functional Status

Observation of body mechanics and joint movements during activities of daily living, work or recreational activities, and ambulation is important for assessing the extent of the impairment. This observation is also important for understanding how the joint, muscle, or nerve problems affect function and how function may affect the primary problems at the joint, muscle, or nerve. Functional capacity evaluations can give a quantitative measure of the patient's impairment. They do not, however, provide sufficient pathokinesiologic information about the problem to be helpful in the direct development of the treatment plan. They are not performed during a normal examination. Functional capacity evaluations are special examinations that are normally performed when the patient is considered for return to work or has attained maximum medical improvement.

## PHYSICAL THERAPY DIAGNOSES

The diagnostic categories that are most important in the development of physical therapy treatment programs for chronic pain and impairments of the neuromusculoskeletal system in the lower extremities are listed in Table 31–2. In addition to the diagnostic categories in Table 31–2 is a descriptor, irritability, that can apply to each of these diagnoses and is important for directing the resultant management plans. Irritability is based on an assessment of the ease with which a symptom complex can be aggravated by movement or positioning. It is an important component of the physical therapy diagnostic process that must be assessed before determining the vigor of the examination and treatment. As stated by Maitland,[8] irritability "is determined by relating the vigour of an activity

**Table 31–2  Physical Therapy Diagnoses for Lower Extremity Pain and Impairment**

Nonmechanical diagnoses
    Complex regional pain syndrome
    Reflex sympathetic dystrophy
Mechanical diagnoses
    Peripheral joint and musculotendinous syndromes
        Hypermobility
        Hypomobility
        Joint derangement
        Abnormal joint tracking
        Musculotendinous syndromes
    Regional pain and impairment syndromes
        Postural and positional anomalies
        Neural dynamic syndromes
        Axial referral syndromes

which causes the pain, first to the degree of the pain that ensues, and then to the length of time taken for the increased pain to subside to its usual level." Practitioners often confuse irritability with inflammation. Although stimulation of an inflammatory process through movement or sustained positioning can be a cause of irritability, it is not the only cause. Irritability can also be a measure of the ease with which pain can be produced and remain elevated on mechanical deformation of musculoskeletal structures or by structures in the peripheral or central nervous system. The latter can be an important component in the production and maintenance of neurogenic or neuropathic pain. Often, anti-inflammatory medication has no effect in controlling pain when the irritability of the tissue is due to these noninflammatory causes. The determination of irritability is important in developing a prognosis for the patient and in setting the length of care. As the irritability becomes greater, the prognosis becomes poorer and the projected period of care longer. The irritability should change as treatment progresses. Failure to change the irritability in a reasonable period of time is one of the first indicators of a need to reevaluate the treatment plan and prognosis.

## Nonmechanical Diagnoses

Nonmechanical diagnoses are those in which movement and position have no or an inconsistent effect on symptoms. Nonorganic problems, pain of visceral origin, inflammatory processes, and malignancies are examples of diagnoses in this category. Patients whose symptoms fall in this category are not candidates for physical therapy and should be referred to other health care practitioners for management.

### Complex Regional Pain Syndromes and Reflex Sympathetic Dystrophy

For physical therapy management, complex regional pain syndromes and reflex sympathetic dystrophy are placed within the same category of diagnoses. Because these syndromes are characterized by severe, unremitting pain and impairment that can be aggravated by movement and activity but not abolished or relieved by movement, positioning, and rest, physical therapy often has little or no effect on the primary symptoms. Physical therapy, however, can have a positive effect on the patient's level of function. Training the patient in more efficient patterns of movement, desensitization procedures, and behavioral interventions can often improve the quality of function and life. If secondary mechanical problems exist, physical therapy can decrease the patient's level of discomfort by assisting in the management of the secondary mechanical problems.

## Mechanical Diagnoses

Mechanical diagnoses encompass syndromes in which movement or position has a direct influence on the production and reduction of the symptoms. There are two broad categories of mechanical diagnoses related to the lower extremity that are important in the management of chronic lower extremity pain and/or impairment: peripheral joint–musculotendinous syndromes and regional syndromes.

### Peripheral Joint–Musculotendinous Syndromes

#### Hypermobility

Pain and impairment produced by syndromes in this diagnostic category are caused by excessive joint motions that often produce instabilities. Hypermobility can have many causes. Ligamentous or capsular laxity or compromise is the most important cause of hypermobility. Irregularities in the structure and shape of the lower extremity joints can also be sources of hypermobiltiy. Hypermobility is best managed through exercise, neuromuscular reeducation, and functional training. The purpose of these procedures is to stabilize the joint through strengthening of the musculature and consistent use of appropriate postures. Assistive devices such as braces or orthotics are often needed to stabilize the joint.

#### Hypomobility

Pain and impairments produced by syndromes in this diagnostic category are caused by loss of joint motion. Hypomobility is produced as a result of scarring or adhesions of the soft tissues around a joint after injury or trauma, adaptive shortening of the soft tissue around a joint (the natural tendency for tissue to adapt to the stresses placed on it—in this case, loss of the soft tissue's normal length because of failure to move the soft tissue consistently through its normal range of motion), and osseous changes within or around a joint. Hypomobility caused by soft tissue shortening responds well to physical therapy, particularly therapeutic exercise and manual therapy techniques. The most important clinical sign confirming this diagnosis is production of symptoms when the affected tissue is placed at end-range stretch and the reduction or loss of symptoms as the tension is removed from the tissue. Hypomobility caused by abnormal osseous formation in or around the joint does not respond well to active physical therapy interventions but may respond to interventions that involve splinting, bracing, and joint conservation training.

### Joint Derangement Syndromes

Pain and impairments produced by syndromes in this diagnostic category are caused by disruptions in joint motions that can be rapidly affected by repeated or sustained joint loading activities. Derangements are often caused by disruptions of the menisci or loose bodies within a joint. With joint derangements, an obstruction in the movement of the joint is seen in at least one direction and one or more of the following behaviors may be demonstrated with repeated motions or sustained loading:

- Joint obstruction and/or symptoms increase and remain worse after the application of repeated or sustained loading procedures.
- Joint obstruction and symptoms decrease and remain decreased after the application of repeated or sustained loading procedures.
- Joint obstruction persists and symptoms may decrease or remain unchanged with repeated or sustained loading procedures but never remain improved.[9]

Joint derangements are often reducible and one or more directions can be found in which the symptoms decrease and function improves; however, at times derangements can be irreducible and no movement or position improves the signs and symptoms. Reducible derangements can respond rapidly to physical therapy through the use of neuromuscular reeducation, exercise, and manual techniques. Management of the reducible derangement often takes longer because of the inability of the patient to maintain the reduction during the periods between treatments. Education and training of patients are crucial in the successful management of reducible derangements. Irreducible derangements respond poorly to physical therapy. It often takes several visits to determine that a derangement is irreducible.

### Abnormal Joint Tracking Syndromes

Pain and impairments produced by syndromes in this diagnostic category are caused by disruptions in the normal pathways of movement in the joint. Abnormal tracking is seen during active motion at the joint. It is often present even when passive motions are full and pain free. Joint tracking problems can occur as a result of trauma (either sudden or overuse), muscle imbalances, anatomic anomalies, or disease. Once the abnormal motion has developed, it is often maintained by muscle imbalance, tissue tightness, and poor neuromuscoloskeletal movement patterns (particularly gait patterns and compensatory movements). The knee, particularly the patellofemoral joint, often develops tracking problems that can lead to significant pain and impairments of lower extremity function. Subtle joint tracking problems can develop at other joints, leading to pain and movement impairments whose causes are difficult to diagnose. Pain and impairments brought on by joint tracking problems are usually managed well with physical therapy. Neuromuscular reeducation, exercise, manual therapy techniques, education and training of patients, and, at times, the use of orthotics or braces are probable components of an appropriate treatment plan.

### Musculotendinous Syndromes

Pain and impairments produced by syndromes in this diagnostic category are caused by pain and/or weakness within the musculotendinous complex. These syndromes can occur as a result of trauma, surgery, and/or neural injury. In evaluating musculotendinous problems, it is important to recognize the influence of pain on the perception of muscular weakness. If pain is present, muscles appear to be weak because of the inhibitory effects of pain on voluntary muscle contraction. When pain is abolished, strength returns to normal almost immediately. True muscle weakness caused by rupture of the muscle or tendon, neurologic compromise, or atrophy of the muscle fibers usually does not produce pain when the muscle contracts maximally. The patient just cannot develop the required tension. The presence of pain along with weakness usually indicates some damage to the musculotendinous structure. If pain accompanies weakness, the pathology producing the pain needs to be addressed before weakness is addressed. Musculotendinous

syndromes usually respond well to physical therapy. These problems can be treated by the procedures included later in this chapter. The specific procedures used to treat a specific syndrome are determined by the irritability, severity, and location of the damaged tissue.

### Regional Pain and Impairment Syndromes of the Lower Extremity

Pain in the lower extremity is often referred from or caused by other structures. The spine, sacroiliac joints, and central and peripheral neural structures can all refer pain or produce impairment in the lower extremities. Recognition of the importance of pathologies that can have a regional effect on the symptoms is critical in the successful management of lower extremity pain and impairment. These syndromes can also be secondary diagnoses that complicate and confuse the management of the primary diagnoses.

### Postural and Positional Anomalies

Specific anomalies in postures and position that can produce impairments in the lower extremities can be acquired through poor posture, poor mechanics of movement, injury, or disease. Anomalies of posture and position can also have congenital sources. Because of the compressive, shearing, and torsional forces placed on all of the structures from the lumbar spine to the foot during normal weight-bearing activities, anomalies in the position of one joint can have profound effects on other joints in the kinetic chain. A positional or postural anomaly can directly cause a disruption in the function of that joint or another joint in the weight-bearing chain.[2] However, an anomaly at a specific joint is often benign until an injury or unusual stresses occur at that or another joint. The forces placed on the injured joint by the abnormal position or posture prevent the injured joint from healing normally. This phenomenon is often seen with knee pain as anomalies in foot position can maintain abnormal tracking patterns of the patella. Before injury of the knee, the abnormal tracking may have been benign, but after the injury the stresses caused by the abnormal tracking prevent normal healing. It is important to evaluate the posture and position of all of the joints from the lumbar spine to the foot in both lower extremities when impairments in one lower extremity fail to resolve.

The fact that a positional anomaly exists does not mean that it will have a deleterious effect on the treatment process. Most abnormal postures or positions are benign. The therapist should be able to demonstrate a rather rapid change in the impairment through correction of the deformity if it is implicated in the problem. When the deformity is relevant to the patient's problem and is correctable, physical therapy can be successful in producing a positive change in the deformity and the patient's symptoms. Procedures that emphasize training of the patient and strengthening and lengthening of specific soft tissue structures are needed to correct and maintain the correction of the deformity. If the patient cannot maintain the corrected postures independently, braces or orthotics may be needed.

### Neural Dynamic Syndromes

Pain and movement impairments produced by syndromes in this diagnostic category are caused by limitations in the mobility or compression of the neural elements in the spine or lower extremity. Pain, weakness, sensory change, loss of normal motion, and at times signs of sympathetic activity can be produced by entrapments or restrictions of normal nerve mobility. These symptoms often present in patterns that are well recognized. Tarsal tunnel syndrome, peroneal entrapments, pyriformis syndrome, and adherences of the sciatic nerve are well recognized and can present with objective evidence of motor or sensory loss. Entrapments of these and other peripheral nerves or nerve branches can occur after trauma or surgery. The pain produced by these problems may not appear in classical referral patterns and results of electrodiagnostic testing are often negative. As a result, acceptance of these diagnoses is controversial, especially when pain is the only complaint.[7] Studies of the upper extremity have demonstrated that damage to the small unmyelinated fibers of the peripheral nerves can occur without objective neurodiagnostic evidence of nerve damage.[10] Butler[7] goes into great depth in discussing the pathology involved in the development of these minor (no direct evidence of neural compromise) but troublesome neural lesions, and his book is essential reading for those involved in managing these problems. Selective tension movements that stress particular nerves or parts of the nerves are at this time the best tests to indicate the presence of these problems. Butler demonstrates how to perform these tests. Neural mobilization, education and training of patients, exercise, and postural supports can be used to treat these syndromes when the irritability is low. When the irritability is high, rest, postural support, and education and training are most commonly used to control the symptoms. Active exercise and manual techniques often exacerbate the symptoms when the syndrome is irritable.

### Axial Referral Syndromes

Pain and impairments produced by syndromes in this diagnostic category are caused by mechanical problems in the lumbar spine or sacroiliac joint. Disk lesions, facet degeneration, stenosis, and other problems in the lumbosacral area can cause significant symptoms in the lower extremities. In most cases, the lower extremity symptoms are accompanied by back or buttock pain, which make the discovery of the spinal source of the symptoms easier. Lower extremity symptoms can be produced by problems in the lumbar spine without back pain or with minimal back pain. In these cases, the presence of spinal pathology is often overlooked as the cause of the symptoms. The system of spinal examination developed by McKenzie[11] is commonly used for lumbar spine problems in physical therapy.[12] A positive correlation was found between the predictive capabilities of the McKenzie examination of the lumbar spine and the confirmation of disk pathology through the use of diskogram or magnetic resonance imaging examination.[20] The McKenzie examination system uses repetitive movements, sustained positions, and changes in the patient's signs and symptoms to discern the presence and type of mechanical problem in the lumbar spine.[11] The diagnoses used in the McKenzie system are based on symptom response to movement and position rather than pathology. The diagnoses and their definitions are listed in Table 31–3.[11] The sacroiliac joint can also cause pain to be referred into the lower extremity. Like the lumbar spine, the sacroiliac joint can at times refer pain to the lower extremity (especially the hip and thigh areas) without producing back pain. The work of Laslett and Williams[13] is particularly valuable in determining the relevance of sacroiliac pathology to the production of lower extremity symptoms.

---

**Table 31–3 McKenzie Classification of the Mechanical Disorders of the Lumbar Spine**

Postural syndrome
  Pain is intermittent.
  Pain is not referred.
  No loss of motion or provocation of symptoms occurs with repeated movements.
  Pain is produced by prolonged maintenance of specific postures.
Dysfunction syndromes
  Pain is intermittent.
  Pain is not referred (except in a nerve root adherence).
  Pain is felt at end range and not during movement.
  No centralization or peripheralization of symptoms is seen on repeated movements.
Derangement syndromes
  Symptoms may change in intensity, character, and location with repeated motions and changes in posture.
  Spinal motions can show a rapid gain or loss of motion on repeated movements.
  Symptoms can be referred.
  Pain can be constant or intermittent.
  Centralization or peripheralization is seen with repeated motions.

The treatment program developed by McKenzie is the best studied and best supported one for the lumbar spine and sacroiliac joint in physical therapy.[14] McKenzie's program uses repeated motions, sustained positions, postural correction, education of the patient, and postural supports to treat axial syndrome symptoms.

## PHYSICAL THERAPY TREATMENT

In the management of any patient with lower extremity impairment, it is important not only to match appropriate treatment procedures to the patient but also to match the patient to the procedures.[9] Treatment procedures, no matter how appropriate or well performed, cannot be effective if the patient, because of cognitive, emotional or behavioral, financial, physical, employment, or other resource limitations, cannot be compliant. In designing an intervention program for a patient with a specific impairment, therapists must not lose sight of the fact that they are treating a patient with a particular syndrome, not just the syndrome. This orientation to treatment is particularly important in the management of chronic pain and impairment, because the pain and impairment have usually affected many aspects of the patient's life.

## Teaching

Effective teaching of patients provides information about the cause and treatment of the condition. Patients who are knowledgeable about their condition are more likely to change their behavior. Behavioral changes and compliance are the cornerstones of the treatment plan. Teaching must be an integral part of each treatment with the ultimate goal of helping patients realize their maximal potential through self-management. To be effective, the education program must

- Use easily understandable, simple explanations to describe the cause and the potential solution for the symptoms.

- Describe and demonstrate the cause and the effect of positions, activities, and exercise on the reproduction or reduction of the symptoms.

- Be integrated with the other treatment options.

- Reinforce appropriate behaviors, static and dynamic postures, and proactive interventions.

- Adapt the teaching to the specific needs of the patient.

- Emphasize function and activity over temporary pain reduction.

- Repeat the information within the same or similar contexts.

One-on-one instruction appears to be more effective in development of the patient's knowledge and behaviors than the use of printed materials and audiovisual presentations. Although printed materials and audiovisual presentations are valuable in augmenting and clarifying the desired concepts, they cannot serve as a substitute for the continual reinforcement that must occur during each individual treatment. Telephone conversations can also be used to monitor and reinforce specific behaviors and results of the treatment plan. Patients seldom grasp all of the information that they need to manage their problem in one or two sessions. The information must be repeated in formats that do not bore or belittle the patient with repetition but challenge the patient to adapt the information to new problems and circumstances.

## Training of Patients

Training involves the performance of activities during the patient's education and includes neuromuscular reeducation (postural training, ergonomic and joint conservation training, and gait training) and self-management training (correct use of modalities, independent exercise, and other self-treatment techniques).

### Neuromuscular Reeducation

Neuromuscular reeducation trains patients to use their joints and muscles more efficiently, produce less strain and stress on joint neural and muscular structures during activity, and perform work and recreational activities more efficiently and effectively. Neuromuscular reeducation is more than just exercise. It is designed to use the increased strength, flexibility, and endurance produced by therapeutic exercise to produce better functional movement through training in the coordinated control of all of the structures in the trunk and lower extremity during activity. Neuromuscular reeducation requires supervised repetition of movements and activities under increasing stresses (load, speed, positioning) while still maintaining the the quality of the movements. Training usually proceeds from the joint and muscle level (using guided movements and specific exercises to produce normal joint tracking, sequence of muscular contraction, and coordinated movements) to higher order levels leading to training in the proper performance of specific activities. During this training, the patient is taught how to perform the movements correctly, given activities (exercises and performance tasks) to enhance performance and compliance, and taught to recognize warning signs of poor technique.

For neuromuscular reeducation to be successful, the therapist must impress upon patients the importance of practicing the activities or exercises frequently during the day and incorporating the correct movement patterns into their daily activities. The success of this treatment technique relies on frequent and correct completion of the home activities so that they become patterned into patients' normal movements. Patients are often instructed to perform 1 to 2 minutes of neuromuscular reeducation exercises or activities every 1 to 2 hours between treatments. Included in this group of treatments are closed-chain kinetic exercises. These exercises involve movements and activities in positions in which the joints in the lower extremity are weight bearing and the foot is usually fixed on the floor. There is evidence that exercises and training using these joint loading positions are more effective than non–weight-bearing exercises in producing good functional outcomes, because the patient is trained in positions that best mimic the normal functional positions and movements of the lower limb.[15]

### Self-Management Training

Because of the changes in the health care environment, patients need to be trained in providing much of their own care. This is particularly true when long-term use of specific procedures may be required. The use of cryotherapy, moist heat, transacutaneous electrical nerve stimulation and intermittent compression may be needed by patients with chronic lower extremity pain and impairment for pain relief or edema management. When such long-term use of a procedure is necessary, the patient should be instructed in the use of the procedure and should receive the necessary equipment. Patients also need to be trained in the proper use and care of braces and orthotics. Of particular importance in relation to chronic pain and impairment is training of the patient or the patient's family in the performance of specific exercises or other procedures that can be used to decrease the pain or improve function. The patient or the patient's family can be taught to perform specific manual techniques to relieve the symptoms or observe for and correct specific postures, movement patterns, or behaviors that may cause the symptoms to recur or be exacerbated. Developing the patient's and the family's con-

fidence in their ability to manage the patients pain and impairment must be a critical component of the long-term management.

## Therapeutic Exercise

Therapeutic exercise includes resistive exercise (isometric, isotonic, or isokinetic exercise), passive exercise (range-of-motion exercises, stretching, and self-mobilization), and aerobic exercise. Its purpose is to increase strength, range of motion, and endurance. Therapeutic exercises are based on the principle that tissue must be stressed or loaded to produce beneficial effects. In therapeutic exercise the effects on specific structures or systems are isolated. Therapeutic exercises must be combined with neuromuscular reeducation to be effective.

Therapeutic exercise performed in a water environment (pool or exercise tank) can be an important element in the rehabilitation of patients with lower extremity impairment. When resistive or endurance exercise cannot be performed because of pain or instability produced during weight bearing, the buoyancy and gentle, variable resistance of the water can be used to exercise the lower extremity. Pool therapy or aquatherapy is often successful in helping severely debilitated patients to initiate a rehabilitation program and allowing them to progress to a standard therapeutic exercise program.

### Resistive Exercise

Although the type of exercise is important for safety and effectiveness, any therapeutic exercise program designed to improve strength requires the specific muscle group or groups to be loaded to an appropriate level. The specific load placed on the muscle or muscle group during treatment is determined by the condition of the patient. General guidelines for strengthening usually suggest that three sets of 10 to 15 repetitions at a resistance level that maximizes effort on the 15th repetition be performed each day or at least three times a week.[2] Lower intensities are often required because of the patient's condition, and exercise intensities less than this can be effective in producing improvements in strength. Greater gains, however, are produced by more intense work. Isometric exercise can also be performed to increase strength when joint motion is limited or stability is a concern, but resistive exercise that requires resistive movements throughout the functional length of the muscle is more effective.[2]

Resistive exercise can be performed with high-technology equipment, free weights, and rubber bands. Muscle strength does not appear to be produced more effectively by any single piece of equipment when the loads placed on the musculature remain constant. Eccentric resistive exercise is often thought to produce more rapid increases in strength, but this appears to be a function more of the increased loads that can be placed on the muscle during eccentric exercise than of any other factor.[16]

### Endurance Exercise

Depending on whether the endurance that needs to be improved is muscular or cardiovascular, the type and amount of exercise vary. Muscular endurance depends primarily on muscle strength. Generally, as muscle strength improves, muscle endurance improves because the additional strength allows the muscle to function at lower percentages of its maximal strength. As a muscle functions closer to its maximal level of contraction, the time during which it can maintain that function decreases. Resistive exercise is the primary procedure used to increase muscular endurance.

Aerobic exercise to improve cardiovascular endurance is generally low-intensity exercise that involves the use of large muscle groups (e.g., walking, jogging, swimming, biking) to stress or load the cardiovascular system.[2] If cardiovascular pathology is suspected or significant risk factors are noted in the examination, a stress test should be performed before an aerobic exercise program is started. If there is no indication of potential cardiovascular pathology, most patients can be instructed to start their aerobic program by working at levels that make them slightly winded but not so much that they cannot maintain a normal conversation while exercising. To produce a cardiovascular training effect it is normally necessary to perform the exercise at the desired intensity for at least 20 minutes three times a week. If the patient's condition allows longer periods of exercise, higher intensities, and more frequent participation, the patient should be encouraged to exercise at the higher level.[2]

### Stretching

In developing a stretching program, it is important to design each exercise for a specific structure. Different tissues respond to stretching differently. Musculotendinous structures respond best to slow, sustained stretches usually lasting for 1 to 2 minutes and performed several times per day. The use of modalities or muscle inhibitory activities (maximal contraction of the specific muscle followed by relaxation or inhibitory responses upon contraction of the muscle's antagonist) can increase the effectiveness of the stretching. The stretching should also be followed by active exercises that assist in maintaining the added length of the structures.

Noncontractile structures (joint structures and neural tissue) appear to be more effectively stretched or mobilized by repetitive movements with moderate stresses (at or just below the onset of pain or strain) placed on the tissue for short durations (1 to 5 seconds) but repeated for periods of 30 seconds to 2 minutes. Neural tissue responds particularly poorly to sustained stretch and can be injured by it. These exercises should also be performed many times per day, usually every 1 to 2 hours for greatest effectiveness.

## Manual Therapy Procedures

Manual therapy procedures differ from stretching procedures in that the therapist usually performs these techniques rather than having the patient perform the techniques as self-treatment. In addition, manual therapy techniques are usually targeted to producing or effecting a specific change in a specific tissue rather than a global effect in a specific direction of movement.

### Joint Mobilization and Manipulation

Joint mobilization and manipulation techniques can be used for pain reduction, restoration of the normal joint accessory motions that accompany all gross motions, stretching of specific joint and periarticular structures, and reduction of joint derangements. There are several philosophies and schools of thought in the chiropractic, osteopathic, and physical therapy communities on the correct performance of specific techniques and the rationale for the use of specific techniques. There is no scientific evidence to support one philosophy or school of thought over another. Scientific evidence, however, does support the use of these procedures for limited periods of time.[17] Joint mobilization techniques are usually performed passively with the joint at rest in either midrange or end-range joint positions. A group of mobilizations called mobilizations with movement use therapist-generated forces to change the pattern of joint movement passively while the patient actively moves the lower limb.[18] Mobilization with movement can be particularly valuable in managing joint tracking problems at the knee or ankle. Mobilization or manipulative procedures must be accompanied by education of the patient and a home program to ensure that the gains produced by the procedures are maintained.

### Soft Tissue Mobilization

Deep massage, myofascial release procedures, and spray and stretch procedures have as their basic purpose improvement of the mobility and status of the musculature and connective tissues. Adhesions, tight fascial bands, trigger points, and scar tissue in muscle or its surrounding connective tissues can all prevent normal motion and produce pain. These abnormalities often occur after injury, surgery, prolonged maintenance of poor postures, or prolonged periods of inactivity and insufficient movement. Although these soft tissue mobilizations can produce beneficial results in the management of soft tissue immobility and pain, their beneficial effects are short lived unless active home programs and training of the patient is started to maintain the improvements.

### Neural Mobilization

Restoration of neural mobility is often the forgotten element in the rehabilitation after lower extremity injury or surgery, and this can lead to significant impairment and pain if not addressed. As the lower limbs are moved, the neural elements in the lower extremities must change their positions relative to other tissues. The nerves need to move longitudinally (lengthening and shortening) and perpendicularly (bowstringing as tension is applied as the nerve traverses a joint).[7] Failure to allow either perpendicular or longitudinal movement can produce tension within the nerve or compress the nerve against other structures. Although the basic structure of the nerve protects it against injury by tension or compression, in specific situations neural tissue is more vulnerable to injury. Previous injury, swelling, inflammatory environments, and anatomic anomalies (soft tissue, osseous, or neural) are potential provocateurs of neural entrapment or injury. If repetitive motions that place compressive or tension forces on the nerve are performed over an extended period of time in the presence of the risk factors previously mentioned, the axonal and/or nonaxonal structures in the peripheral nerve can be injured. Axonal injury (especially of the large-diameter sensory and motor fibers) is well recognized and objectively determined through the use of neurodiagnostic studies. The production of pain through neural injury of nonaxonal or small unmyelinated fiber origin is controversial because there are no well recognized neurodiagnostic tests to confirm its presence.

Neural mobilization is of particular importance in the management of the later form of neural entrapment or injury. Mobilizing the nerve longitudinally through the use of repetitive extremity movements or mobilizing the nerve perpendicularly through the use of plucking or massage-like movements can assist in freeing the nerve from its entrapment, decreasing neural inflammation and swelling, and possibly improving the blood flow and nutrition to the nerve. Care must be taken when the mobilization is being performed. Before the mobilization the therapist must clearly define its purpose. If the purpose of the mobilization is to decrease inflammation and swelling, gentle mobilization must be performed and the patient must be taught how to protect the nerve from irritation that may occur with normal lower extremity function. If the irritability of the nerve is low and the purpose of the mobilization is to free the nerve and increase mobility, the mobilization can be vigorous and the patient must be taught exercises to maintain the mobility after the mobilization. As indicated previously, nerve tissue responds poorly to sustained pressures and the mobilizations are usually performed with a cycle of one repetition every 1 to 5 seconds.

## Physical and Electrical Procedures

Physical and electrical procedures can be used to decrease pain, decrease inflammation and swelling, increase strength, and assist in gait training. Although these procedures can have beneficial effects in the treatment of acute injury, their use in the treatment of chronic lower extremity pain and impairment is often limited because their beneficial effects are usually temporary. They have roles in the treatment of specific conditions, but those roles are limited in their application and duration. Use of these modalities can often have a negative effect in the management of the patient with chronic pain[19] because these passive procedures do not foster independence and encourage patient responsibility. Passive modalities should be used only as temporary adjuncts to interventions that encourage active movement and patient independence. When long-term use of the modality may be beneficial, as in the use of transcutaneous electrical nerve stimulation to control pain or intermittent compressive therapy to control swelling, the patient should be instructed in how to use the equipment at home.

Superficial heating modalities and electrical stimulation can have analgesic effects during and for short periods after their application. Cryotherapy can be used to provide temporary pain relief and decreased swelling and inflammation after injury or exercise. Deep heating modalities, such as ultrasound and diathermy, selectively heat subcutaneous tissues. Ultrasound is particularly valuable for heating tissues at the bone-muscle interface, and diathermy is more effective in heating larger volumes of tissue with high water contents such as muscle. Phonophoresis (sonophoresis) and electrophoresis use ultrasound waves and electrical currents, respectively, to deliver specific medications (usually anti-inflammatory or analgesic medications) to tissues that are located relatively close to the skin. They are often used to treat tendinitis or bursitis. All of these modalities have limited applications in the treatment of chronic pain or impairment.

Muscle can be strengthened by using electrical stimulation. Although electrical stimulation is not as effective as resistive exercise in increasing muscle strength, it can play a significant role in either maintaining or increasing muscle strength after injury or surgery when strong contractions cannot be performed. Functional electrical stimulation uses a heel switch that is activated as the patient's heel strikes the floor. Compressing the switch causes the anterior tibialis muscle to be electrically stimulated and contract. The dorsiflexion produced by the contraction is used to assist the patient in clearing the forefoot during the swing phase of gait. Functional electrical stimulation can be used both as a training device during gait training and as short-term assistance for clearing the foot during ambulation.

## Use of Braces, Taping, Orthotics, and Assistive Devices

Braces, taping, orthotics, and assistive devices can be valuable in the management of chronic lower extremity pain and impairment. They can be used to protect, support, and unload weight from painful, irritated, or injured tissue. The patient's ability to bear weight during ambulation, transfer, performance of activities of daily living, and work can be enhanced by the appropriate use of this type of equipment. The effect of the brace or orthotic can be apparent in areas other than the area being supported. Supportive devices that correct positional problems at the foot have been shown to have beneficial effects in the management of knee and back pain.[2] The patient with chronic lower extremity pain and impairment that is worsened or caused by weight-bearing activities should be evaluated by the therapist or physician to determine whether an assistive device is needed to improve the effectiveness of treatment being given or provide long-term assistance with weight-bearing activities.

## THE USE OF PHYSICAL THERAPY FOR LOWER EXTREMITY PAIN AND IMPAIRMENT

Physical therapy can be extremely valuable in the treatment of lower extremity pain and impairment. Physical therapy can be particularly valuable when the pain or impairment is produced by weakness and mechanical sources. Physical therapy also has its limitations. Conditions in which pain or impairment is produced by nonmechanical sources are more likely to respond poorly to physical therapy and require a more coordinated effort between the physician and the therapist. Physical therapy has limited ability to produce prolonged relief from inflammation, pain, or swelling, except when procedures can be used to decrease or eliminate the mechanical factors that produce the symptoms. Close coordination between the physician and the therapist is needed in managing these conditions to maximize the effectiveness of each participant. Medication, injection, or surgical procedures are often critical components of the treatment plan that can be delivered only by the physician and they are often needed to allow the procedures performed by the physical therapist to produce any beneficial outcomes. Changes in behavior and increases in strength, motion, and pain-free function are critical components of the treatment plan that can be produced by physical therapy and are often needed to allow the physician-directed modalities to produce a beneficial outcome.

Clear physician-therapist communication is essential. To foster that communication, the physician's referral to physical therapy should include a diagnosis, treatment goals, precautions if necessary, and a general treatment plan. If a specific treatment procedure is necessary, the physician should indicate it. Generally, the treatment process is best served if the therapist has the option to use the procedures that best match the problems and diagnoses found on examination. The physician should expect a report from the therapist. As treatment continues, the physician should expect periodic communications indicating the patient's progress and ultimate prognosis or lack of progress and factors preventing improvement.

## REFERENCES

1. Nicholas JA, Hershman EB: The Lower Extremity and Spine in Sports Medicine. St. Louis, CV Mosby, 1995.
2. Gould JA: Orthopaedic and Sports Physical Therapy. St. Louis, CV Mosby, 1990.
3. Kottke FJ, Lehman JF: Krusen's Handbook of Physical Medicine and Rehabilitation. Philadelphia, WB Saunders, 1990.
4. Wolf SL: Clinical Decision Making in Physical Therapy. Philadelphia, FA Davis, 1985.

5. Delitto A, Snyder-Mackler L: The diagnostic process: Examples in orthopaedic physical therapy. Phys Ther 75:203, 1995.
6. Fosnaught M: A critical look at diagnosis. P.T. 4:48, 1996.
7. Butler DS: Mobilisation of the Nervous System. New York, Churchill Livingstone, 1991.
8. Maitland GA: Peripheral Manipulation. Toronto, Butterworths, 1977.
9. Laslett M: Mechanical Diagnosis and Therapy: The Upper Limb. Auckland, NZ, 1996.
10. Lang E, Claus D, Neundorfer B, Handwerker HO: Parameters of thick and thin nerve-fiber function as predictors of pain in carpal tunnel syndrome. Pain 60:295, 1995.
11. McKenzie RA: The Lumbar Spine: Mechanical Diagnosis and Therapy. Upper Hutt, NZ, Spinal Publications, 1981.
12. Jette AM, Smith K, Haley SM, Davis KD: Physical therapy episodes of care for patients with low back pain. Phys Ther 74:101, 1994.
13. Laslett M, Williams W: The reliability of selected pain provocation tests for sacroiliac joint pathology. Spine 19: 1243, 1994.
14. Barbis JM, Rath W: McKenzie approach to intervention. Orthop Phys Ther Clin North Am 4:1059, 1995.
15. Mangine R: Physical Therapy of the Knee. New York, Churchill Livingstone, 1995.
16. Basmajian J: Therapeutic Exercise. Baltimore, Williams & Wilkins, 1990.
17. Agency for Health Care Policy and Research: Acute Low Back Problems in Adults: Clinical Practice Guideline 14. Rockville, MD, Department of Health and Human Services, 1994.
18. Mulligan, BR: Manual Therapy. Wellington, NZ, Plane View Services, 1995.
19. Fordyce WE, Brockway JA, Bergman JA, Spengler D: Acute low back pain: A control-group comparison of behavioral vs traditional management methods. Behav Med 9:127, 1986.
20. Donelson R, Aprill C, Medcalf R, Grant W: A prospective study of centralization of lumbar and referred pain. A predictor of symptomatic discs and annular competence. Spine 22:1115, 1997.

# Index

Note: Page numbers in *italics* refer to illustrations; page numbers followed by a t refer to tables.